Coming into the World:
A Dialogue between Medical and Human Sciences

Edited by
Giovanni Battista La Sala, Piergiuseppina Fagandini, Vanna Iori, Fiorella Monti, Isaac Blickstein

Coming into the World

A Dialogue between Medical and Human Sciences

International Congress "The 'normal' complexities of coming into the world", Modena Italy 28–30 September 2006

Editors
Giovanni Battista La Sala, Piergiuseppina Fagandini, Vanna Iori, Fiorella Monti

Production Editor
Isaac Blickstein

W DE G
Walter de Gruyter
Berlin · New York

Editors
Giovanni Battista La Sala
Department of Obstetrics and Gynaecology
S. Maria Nuova Hospital
Reggio Emilia, Italy

Piergiuseppina Fagandini
Department of Motherhood and Infancy
S. Maria Nuova Hospital
Reggio Emilia, Italy

Vanna Iori
Family Pedagogy
Catholic University of Milan
and Family Observation
Reggio Emilia, Italy

Fiorella Monti
Faculty of Psychology
University of Bologna, Italy

Production Editor
Isaac Blickstein
Department of Obstetrics and Gynecology
Kaplan Medical, Rehovot, Israel
Hadassah-Hebrew University School of Medicine
Jerusalem, Israel

This work contains 40 figures und 7 tables.

ISBN: 3-11-019018-4
ISBN-13: 978-3-11-019018-2

Bibliographic information published by the Deutsche Nationalbibliothek

The Deutsche Nationalbibliothek lists this publication in the Deutsche Nationalbibliografie; detailed bibliographic data are available in the Internet at http://dnb.d-nb.de.

Production: Druckhaus „Thomas Müntzer“ GmbH, Bad Langensalza, Germany

List of Contributers

Francesca Agostini
Department of Psychology
University of Bologna, Italy

Beth Alder
Napier University
Edinburgh, United Kingdom

François Ansermet
European School of Psychoanalysis
University of Lausanne, Switzerland

Paola Benvenuti
Department of Neurological
and Psychiatric Sciences
Faculty of Medicine
University of Florence, Italy

Natascia Bertoncelli
Mother and Chield Department
Neonatal Division
University Hospital
Modena, Italy

Isaac Blickstein
Department of Obstetrics and Gynecology
Kaplan Medical, Rehovot, Israel
Hadassah-Hebrew University School
of Medicine
Jerusalem, Israel

Johannes Bitzer
Department for Social Medicine
Clinic of Obstetrics
University of Basel, Switzerland

Jacky Boivin
Cardiff University, United Kingdom

Giulia Dante
Unit of Obstetrics
Mother-Infant Department
University of Modena and Reggio Emilia,
Italy

Angela Maria Di Vita
Faculty of Educational Sciences
University of Palermo, Italy

Paul Durning
Department of Educational Science
University of Paris X-Nanterre, France

Manuela Errante
Tourist Marketing
University of Palermo, Italy

Fabio Facchinetti
Unit of Obstetrics
Mother-Infant Department
University of Modena and Reggio Emilia,
Italy

Piergiuseppina Fagandini
Department of Motherhood and Infancy
S. Maria Nuova Hospital
Reggio Emilia, Italy

Ramona Fava
Modena, Italy

Tajeb Ferradji
Centre of Ethnopsychiatry
University Hospital of Avicenne
Bobigny, France

Fabrizio Ferrari
Department of Neonatology
University of Modena and Reggio Emilia,
Italy

Véronique Francis
University Teachers Training Centre of
Orleans-Tours
Bourges
University of Paris-X-Nanterre, France

Vittorio Gallese
Departments of Neuroscience
and Physiology
University of Parma, Italy

Alessandro Gennaro
Department of Pedagogical and Didactic
Psychological Sciences
University of Lecce, Italy

Vanna Iori
Family Pedagogy
Catholic University of Milan
and Family Observation
Reggio Emilia, Italy

Giovanni Battista La Sala
Department of Obstetrics and Gynaecology
S. Maria Nuova Hospital
Reggio Emilia, Italy

Giovanna Bestetti
Faculty of Medicine
University of Milan and Milan Bicocca, Italy

Adriana Lis
Department of Psychology of Development
and Socialisation
University of Padua, Italy

Mauro Mancia
Professor Emeritus of Neurophysiology
Training Analyst of the Italian
Psychoanalytical Society
University of Milan, Italy

Claudia Mazzeschi
Department of Human
and Educational Sciences
University of Perugia, Italy

Lynda Miller
The Tavistock and Portman NHS Trust
London, United Kingdom

Fiorella Monti
Faculty of Psychology
University of Bologna, Italy

Gina Ferrara Mori
Italian Society of Psychoanalysis
Florence, Italy

Graham Music
The Tavistock and Portman NHS Trust
London, United Kingdom

Romana Negri
Infantile Neuropsychiatry
University of Milan, Italy

Adolfo Pazzagli
Department of Neurological
and Psychiatric Sciences
Faculty of Medicine
University of Florence, Italy

Sandra Piccinini
Nursery and Pre-School Institution
Reggio Emilia, Italy

Marisa Pugliese
Department of Mother and Chield
Psychosocial Division
University Hospital
Modena, Italy

Anita Regalia
Gynaecology and Obstetrics Clinic
S. Gerardo Hospital
University of Milan-Bicocca, Italy

Alba Ricchi
Unit of Obstetrics
Mother-Infant Department
University of Modena and Reggio Emilia, Italy

Maria Federica Roversi
Mother and Child Department
Neonatal Division
University Hospital
Modena, Italy

Bernadette Tillard
Department of Educational Science
University of Paris X-Nanterre, France

Ed Tronick
Departments of Pediatrics and Psychology
Harvard Medical School
Cambridge, Massachusetts, USA
School of Psychology
Fielding Graduate University
Santa Barbara, California, USA

Vania Valoriani
Department of Neurological
and Psychiatric Sciences
Faculty of Medicine
University of Florence, Italy

Daria Vettori
Parma, Italy

Maria Vinciguerra
University of Palermo, Italy

Annibale Volpe
Unit of Obstetrics
Mother-Infant Department
University of Modena and Reggio Emilia,
Italy

Table of Contents

Foreword

In October 1998, I was invited to attend a meeting in Reggio Emilia. As a first-time visitor to this region of Italy, I was initially introduced to the world famous parmigiano, prosciutto di parma, and to the aceto balsamico di Modena. However, these palatal delights were only the seasoning to a conference with a highly intriguing theme: *"Special Children and Parents: From the desired to the real child"*. At this weekend in Reggio Emilia I learnt about the keen interest of the conference president – Dr. La Sala – in a holistic approach towards patients undergoing infertility treatment.

Since that meeting, my ways with Dr. La Sala crossed numerous times, in scientific meetings as well as in research collaborations. In addition, during this period, I became acquainted with La Sala's group and their close teamwork with humanistic disciplines in Reggio and Bologna.

It was thus only natural to learn about the Modena congress – *"Coming into the world: a dialogue between medical and human sciences"* – which is, to the best of my knowledge – the first scientific attempt to encompass the myriad humanistic aspects of the complexities of reproduction. I was honored to accept the invitation extended by the Editors – La Sala, Fagandini, Iori, and Monti – to be responsible for the English version of a book that will be cover the main topics of the Modena congress in September 2006.

The production of this book had several difficulties that had to be resolved. First, it was the duty of the Editors to select the topics for this book from the presentations of the congress – not a simple mission at all given the high quality of the speakers as well as importance of all subjects. I am indebted to the Editors for their outstanding work.

Second, we had to translate multilingual contributions into English. This mission was skillfully done, supervised, and coordinated by Gillian Mansfield (Associate Professor of English Language, University of Parma), and by the Parma team including Niamh Boland, M.A, Michela Canepari, Ph.D, Alex Gillan, B.A., Natasha Huff, B.A. and Joan Rundo. I am deeply thankful for their efforts to make my editorial work much easier. The reader should however note that differences in style were inevitable, owing to differences in citations used by medical as compared to humanistic disciplines.

Third, the Editors are happy to illustrate this book with drawings from Reggio Children (Diana Municipal Preschool of Reggio Emilia) compiled by Annamaria Mucchi. These paintings best illustrate the authentic voice of childhood, in line with the theme of this book.

Finally, special thanks should be given to the Publishing house – Walter de Gruyter GmbH & Co, Berlin, and especially to Dr. Stephanie Dawson – Editor of Medicine & Sciences, for the invaluable help in all production steps.

Isaac Blickstein, MD

1. Preface: The "normal" complexities of coming into the world

Giovanni Battista La Sala; Department of Obstetrics and Gynecology, S. Maria Nuova Hospital, Reggio Emilia, Italy

The sound of the first cry of a newborn is a joyful event, yet full of conscious and unconscious mysteries of the past and the future. It is the symbol of the "normal" and, one might add, "mysterious" complexity of coming into and being in the world.

During life, birth is an intermediate stage of a long journey which "is born" from a desire-project of the parents, it is made materially possible by means of pregnancy and childbirth, and it is given concrete realization in extra-uterine life. Birth is a link between the past and the future, it is an important and complex piece within an even more important and complex totality, such as is human life.

The author of this text is an example of a gynecologist-obstetrician who has been trained and exercises his profession in a contemporary western society. My institutional role is that of supervising as best as I can the biology and anatomy of pregnancy and childbirth. In that respect, society has not only taught me how to do so, it requires me to do so. On the other hand, as far as I know, my institutional role symbolizes the division of medicine, which, as a model exerts its power not only in Italy but in all Western civilization.

During my thirty years of professional career, I gradually became aware of the objective and subjective limitations, at times very frustrating, of my "technical" role in pregnancy and childbirth. Indeed, I began to feel the need to go beyond the institutional "ghetto" in order to seek "help" from other sciences, such as the humanistic ones, in order to perform better my role as a "technician" and to learn more about what occurs before and after pregnancy and childbirth. I attempted to discuss my frustrations and my desire to try and modify the present state of affairs and re-build the existing bridge between medical and human sciences with Pinuccia Fagandini and Fiorella Monti, psychologists, and with Vanna Iori, family pedagogist. I was truly and pleasantly surprised to realize that we share the same wavelength and that we would be able to work together.

This is how the idea of this International Congress in Modena was conceived. This was then followed by the idea of publishing the proceedings of the Congress in Modena not only in Italian but also in English, as if to leave a message in a bottle that makes its way round the world.

The Modena Congress and this publication have been made possible thanks to the work of so many people to whom I give my sincere thanks. Particular thanks go to Serono S.p.A., who following a generous tradition known to obstetricians and gynecologists has provided an important financial contribution for the realization of this Congress and the publication of this volume.

2. Let children speak

Sandra Piccinini; Nursery and Pre-School Institution,
Reggio Emilia, Italy

"What am I doing here? Tell me".

You may wonder why a quotation from Alice in Wonderland should be used at the opening of an International Congress such as this by the President of a Children's Institution.

It is correct to let children speak, as if we were borrowing from learning. In times such as these, children are great help to us in extending our knowledge, in times when – as Loris Malaguzzi claimed – "it is necessary to reunite disciplines, since each on its own is helpless, each one needs to find some sort of trans-cultural solidarity". This interaction between disciplines and between different forms of learning becomes necessary if our thoughts are to be more connected than up to now.

This, I think, is also the aim of this congress: to compare various points of view on *coming into this world.*

The collaboration between the pre-schools of Reggio Emilia (in particular Diana – recognized internationally as a high level pedagogical project that is both qualitative and innovative) and Prof. La Sala did not begin today: "Mamma Onda" was the first of a series of collaborations in which we were able to find a common research approach. Research and exchanging knowledge will be the common denominator of this Congress, which we hope will achieve further competence in the daily work of all of us.

With this, let children speak:

The sea is born from mother wave.
The weather is born from the storm.
The wind is born from the air and takes shape by flapping
Time is born from years.

3. Modern reproductive medicine and the definition of parenthood: Praeter Naturam

Isaac Blickstein, MD; Department of Obstetrics and Gynecology, Kaplan Medical Center, Rehovot, and the Hadassah-Hebrew University School of Medicine, Jerusalem, Israel

Introduction

God blessed them. God said to them, "Be fruitful, multiply, fill the earth, and subdue it ..." Genesis 1: 28.

Reproduction is an intrinsic component of life. Without reproduction, life does not seem to be complete and, therefore, reproduction is an existential drive. As the passage from Genesis clearly states, reproduction is also a divine command. From a biological perspective, reproduction is quite simple and entails the mixture of DNA from male and female gametes to form a zygote. This zygote is then protected by a specialized organ of the female to allow differentiation and growth of the embryo-fetus. Finally, the products of conception are expelled in a timely fashion to allow the delivery of an offspring that is capable to survive.

This pattern of reproduction is followed, as a rule, in the entire animal kingdom and reproduction is considered impaired if one of these components is defective. Species-specific differences in this pattern are believed to represent clever ways that nature selected to circumvent specific obstacles to a successful outcome. In the human, the formation of the zygote in the oviduct by the post-coital unification of a single spermatozoon and a single oocyte, is followed by implantation, pregnancy, and birth. However, as far as we know, there are no natural solutions to overcome reproductive obstacles, and hence, the inability to reproduce is essentially unresolved unless some form of man-made intervention is implemented.

The probably oldest intervention in reproduction is cesarean section, aimed to help women who are unable to conclude the reproductive sequence. At the same time, no other advances have been made for centuries to overcome other reproductive obstacles. A distinct change in this construct occurred when effective infertility therapy became available and about three decades ago when the first in vitro fertilization (IVF) baby was born. These novel methods created puzzling deviations in the classical definition of parenthood, and re-shuffled all that we consider as natural reproduction.

This chapter discusses several examples of current reproductive medicine that significantly depart from the natural course. As Aristotle (300 BC) described similar circumstances, the argument will be that such deviations are beyond the nature's common course – praeter naturam.

Fatherhood

Data from more than twenty years suggest that the male factor is at least partly responsible in about 50% of infertile couples (approximately 30% of man only, and in 20% both man and woman are abnormal). The deviation from the natural course of reproduction begins in these cases with artificial insemination, whereby sperm is injected rather then ejaculated into the lower female genital tract and circumvents the natural way of conception. In even a more sophisticated way, sperm is directly injected, in vitro, into the female gamete, in a method called intracytoplasmic sperm injection (ICSI). One step further was the observation that sperm is actually not needed for fertilization. This led to sampling primordial spermatic forms from the testicles or ejaculatory tract (epididimis) by methods like TESA (testicular sperm extraction) or MESA (microsurgical epididymal sperm aspiration) followed by ICSI.

Whatever autologous method is used, it is expected that in a monogamic relationship, the male partner is the father of the child born to a given woman. However, using donor sperm for artificial insemination or for ICSI, the offspring is obviously not a biological product of the couple. Fatherhood should therefore be considered according to other levels of parent-child relationship.

Motherhood

A popular adage implies that one cannot be sure who was his father, but can be certain who his mother is. This somewhat chauvinistic cliché is no longer valid in the era of modern treatment of infertile women. First and foremost was the acceptance that, in practice, women need their uterus but do not need their ovaries in order to conceive. Since the 1990s, pregnancies with donor oocytes have become commonplace in many countries. This finding, namely that fertility is dependent on ovarian-age but not on uterine age, was the basis for pushing maternal age to upper limits which were never encountered before. For example, the BBC announced on January 23, 2005, that a 66-year-old Romanian woman, Adriana Iliescu, become the world's oldest mother. Dr Bogdan Marinescu, who carried out the fertility treatment, justified the procedure by saying she was in an appropriate condition to give birth and needless to say that the mother encountered immense joy when her baby was born, five weeks early, after undergoing nine years of fertility treatment. The case has prompted criticism from health professionals concerned about the medical risks and the impact on the child, since it is not clear how long the child will enjoy his mother.

Having said this, one should realize that there are pros and cons for pregnancy beyond reproductive age. Oocyte donation to postmenopausal women can be defended by societal practices, gender equality, and reproductive freedom. For societal practice, one may argue that there is no reason to assume that society, at large, will be harmed by allowing older women to conceive and that the parents have no physical and psychological resources for raising children at older age. Moreover, older parents are likely to be economically stable, more responsible, and have a more mature family unit. Regarding gender equality, one may argue that since older men are qualified to have children, denying women from this privilege is prejudicial and discriminative, albeit the offspring is not genetically her own child (as is the case with older fathers). Finally, if our society respects the rights of patients with life-limiting disease to procreate, the life expectancy of older mothers should not be a factor in reproductive choices.

The main argument against oocyte donation to women beyond reproductive age is that they exceeded a "natural" limit of reproductive capability, and compared this situation to oocyte donation to prepubertal girls. Thus the fact that teenager can sometimes be successful mothers is not an argument favoring teenage pregnancies. Conversely, the fact that grandparents can sometimes successfully raise children does not imply that older parents have emotional and physical energy to raise children. Finally, the increased risk of many pregnancy complications at older maternal age, for both mother and child, is also a strong argument against pregnancy beyond reproductive age.

The main ethical issue, raised by the American Society of Reproductive Medicine (http://www.asrm.org/Media/Ethics/postmemo.html), is whether the ultimate bearing and rearing of a child contribute to mutual well being of both parties – the women as well as the children – are served by assisted reproductive technology (ART) using donor oocytes. It could well be that societal and cultural pressures might push women beyond reproductive age to become mothers and it could be that children would eventually resent having mothers as old as grandmothers of their peers, and thus be adversely affected psychologically and socially by having older parents. In any case, postmenopausal pregnancy should always be discussed with both maternal and child interests considered together.

Going back to the cliché cited above, with modern infertility treatment, one may also be unsure whether the pregnant woman is the biological mother of the fetus. Surrogacy means that the surrogate mother, who has no genetic contribution to the offspring, is hired to substitute the biological mother and carry a baby that is given to those who employed her to do that job. It goes without saying that surrogate motherhood, albeit performed worldwide, is still controversial. Those in favor assume that surrogacy is beneficial to all parties involved: the infertile couple will have a biological child and the surrogate mother will receive a fair financial compensation. This view does not consider commercial surrogacy (i.e., not performed by a family member, friend, or driven by altruism) as potentially unethical. Those who are against surrogacy maintain that the risks outweigh the potential benefits, and that motherly emotions and antepartum bonding with the fetus that arise during pregnancy do not permit a genuinely informed consent by the surrogate mother to relinquish the baby postpartum.

Surrogacy is not restricted just to the uterus using a biologically distinct embryo produced by ART. One form of surrogacy is, in fact, carrying a 'semi'-autologous embryo, namely one that was conceived using the sperm of the male partner for intrauterine insemination. In such circumstance, the reproductive sequence just circumvents the coital act and the surrogate mother is also the genetic mother. Irrespective of how much the biological relationship between the surrogate mother and the unborn child is altered by the type of surrogacy, no doubt exists that all combinations form, in one way or another, profound medical, ethical, legal, and undoubtedly – also psychological – consequences. Consider, for example, the case of a British woman pregnant with twins that sued a California couple, alleging that couple who hired her surrogacy service backed out of the contract after she refused to perform a two to one reduction of the twins. (CNN, August 14, 2001; http://archives.cnn.com/2001/LAW/08/13/surrogate.dispute/index.html) The surrogate mother wants to carry the twins to term and find adoptive parents for them because she holds that the biological parents – wanting to perform an unselected reduction – are unfit to become parents of these children. In simple terms, a circumstance involving intimacy, love, parenthood, joy, and pleasure became a rent-a-womb situation, whereby the surrogate mother was interested in carrying the pregnancy in exchange for a fee whereas the biological parents were looking to rent space for the pregnancy period. This situation is certainly a challenge to the definition of parenthood.

Parenthood

Infertility and the derived bizarre situations are not restricted to the question of the 'real' mother in surrogacy. Consider the "five-person pregnancy" or "Angela" case which is a curious and controversial example of the consequences of ART, and casts serious doubts on the definition of parenthood. In March 1997, Reuter Information Service reported that a 37-year-old Italian mother of two, identified only as "Angela," had been implanted with two embryos created from the sperm and eggs of two different couples, after she agreed to act as a surrogate mother simultaneously for two infertile couples. The surrogate mother, a Roman Catholic herself, disagreed with the Church's opposition to both IVF and surrogate motherhood, and considered her altruistic effort to help others as undeserving of condemnation. It was then reported (Lancet, 1997) that Angela gave birth to a healthy boy and girl at 36 weeks' gestation but parenthood (i.e., which baby belongs to which couple) was only established by postpartum DNA fingerprinting. This is probably the first example of twins who share no parents, share no genetic relationship with the surrogate mother, and share no genetic relationship with each other.

Another example was reported in May 2003 (http://www.smh.com.au) whereby the Supreme Court of New South Wales had to decide if frozen embryos implanted and born after their grandmother's death are entitled to inherit her. The will left her estate, equally divided, to the child or children of her son and daughter and about $1 million was left in trust to grandchildren "who shall survive me and attain the age of 25 years". The Court was asked to determine whether two frozen embryos, and their live siblings, should share in their grandmother's estate. The court concluded that while it was highly unlikely that the grandmother did not wish to benefit grandchildren born after her death, he would take the traditional definition of "survive" – that one had to be alive at the time of the grandmother's death. That excluded all the embryos, including the two children who have since been born.

This example suggests that frozen embryos, sperm, and more recently also frozen oocytes, may eventually lead to birth of a child, sometime long after the death of family member and thus could delay the distribution of the heritage. As the example given above suggests, such strange cases do occur. Whereas in the past, blood or legal marital ties seemed sufficient to document important relationships, currently, the existence of a pre-conception life is fully recognized, at least by legal terms.

Epilogue

This chapter discusses several examples of how ART-related circumstances changed the concept of fatherhood, motherhood, and parenthood. Some of these cases are obviously unique and by all means do not represent the vast majority of ART pregnancies and parentage. Nonetheless, these cases have a message. For example, several chapters in this book suggest that the baby is considered as part of the 'self' of the pregnant woman. How is this related to pregnancies following egg donation? How does the surrogate mother consider that 'self' when the embryo was created from heterologous gametes? How do these factors influence the decision about the mode of delivery? How does the male partner react to the entire pregnancy created by donor sperm and to the 'coming into the world' process, i.e., birth?

These cases, to a certain extent, point to the need for change in the traditional way of thinking and calls for open-mindedness to the unnatural way and new definition of parenthood: Praeter Naturam.

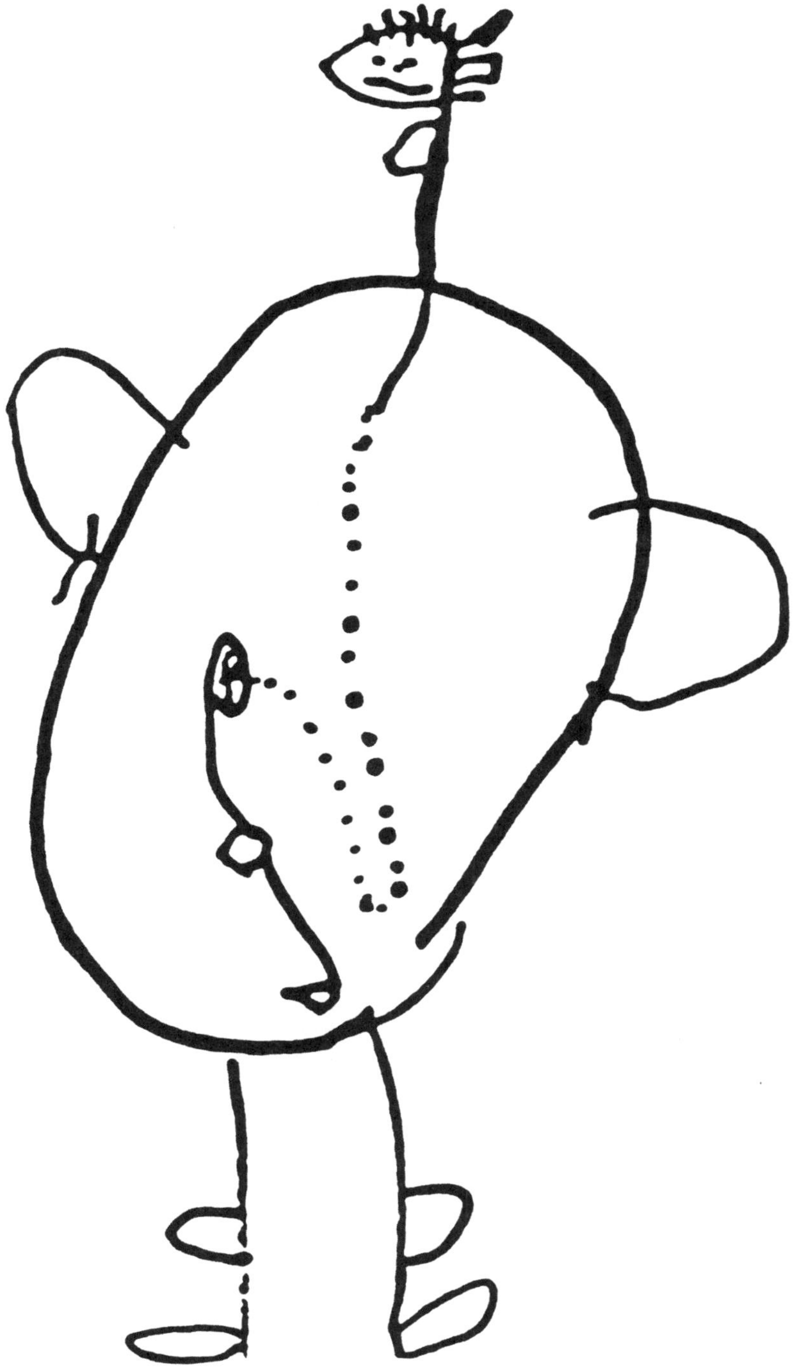

(Luca, 4 yrs. 3 mos.)
A baby grows in the mother's tummy because the mother eats and the baby eats the crumbs.

4. Self and dyadic expansion of consciousness, meaning-making, open systems, and the experience of pleasure

Ed Tronick; Departments of Pediatrics and Psychology,
Harvard Medical School Cambridge, Massachusetts, USA;
School of Psychology, Fielding Graduate University,
Santa Barbara, California, USA

There is a connection between experience, including the experience of pleasure, creativity and development, which has to do with individuals making new meanings as well as their experience when making them. This perspective is based on the first principles of dynamic systems governing the operation of open biological systems, of which we, humans, are but one example (Tronick, 2005). These first principles assert that as an open complex system individuals seek energy in the service of maximizing their organizational complexity, including its coherence, integration and flexibility. Bridging between the principles of system theory and experience requires finding concepts that relate the principles governing the operations of *any* kind of biological system to the operation of *humans* as complex open systems. For me, such a concept is provided by Bruner's (1990) beguiling simple assertion that humans are *meaning* makers, a concept easily linked to dynamic systems' principles (Stengers, Prigogine, 1997). Humans, when thought of as meaning-making open systems, utilize energy to create complexly organized, coherent, integrated and flexible states of consciousness. States of consciousness are psychobiological states that contain the private meanings an individual gives to their place in the world. In the language of systems theory, states of consciousness are attractor states.

These states are organized moment-by-moment by the individual and function to organize and anticipate the future based on the immediate present and updated past; that is, to organize the whole individual's movement into the world. An individual's states of consciousness generate intentions and actions. Meanings, the elements assembled into states of consciousness may be in, or more likely out of awareness. In fact, meaning may only come into awareness when it is violated. Few of us walk around with an awareness of our belief in the existence of things until we confront a magician who makes things disappear. Indeed, though typically out of awareness, a state of consciousness has always an impelling certitude that the world ***is*** this way. An 8 month-old in one moment is absolutely certain that a hidden object is gone and in the next moment when the object is brought into view the infant is absolutely certain that it exists. The two certitudes do not fit together but they are impelling in each moment.

States of consciousness are generated by self- and social- meaning-making processes of an embodied mind as individuals engage their own private meanings and the world of things and people. One of the most robust ways of expanding the complexity of an individual's state of consciousness is to create what I call a dyadic state of consciousness. Like Vygotsky's zone of proximal development, these states are a joint creation of two embodied minds bringing together elements from each of their own states into a shared dyadic state. As participants in this dyadic state, individuals appropriate new elements into their own state of consciousness and, as a consequence, the complexity of each individual's state of consciousness grows. Paradoxically, though systems principles suggest that the organism strives to maximize the coherence of their sense of the world, and even though these states have an impelling certitude, the states produced are always unpredictable and messy, and may be contradictory and incoherent.

The messiness is inherent to the process of meaning-making because of the large number of different kinds of meaning that must be integrated, limitations in the capacity of meaning-making systems, and the different kinds of a large number of meaning-making processes including affective, cognitive, memorial, linguistic, and bodily processes and psychodynamic meaning-making processes such as a dynamic unconscious, projective identification and transference. Nonetheless, the messiness of meanings is the stuff from which new meanings are created. Were states of consciousness are fixed, nothing new could be created and complexity could not be increased. An implication is that humans are more attracted to making meaning with others, as contrasted to objects, because messiness is always greater for the meanings made with people than with things or events in the world. Dyadic states of consciousness are joint creations and as such bring together the messy, unpredictable and inchoate features of each individual's state of consciousness. By contrast, most events in the inanimate world are predictable and simple by comparison, such that while new meanings may be created, the process is one of diminishing returns. Thus making meaning with others presents a greater possibility of the emergence of new meanings.

Returning to the principles of open systems, systems that successfully gain energy and become more complex and integrated. By contrast, when sufficient energy is not obtained, systems lose complexity and coherence, dissipate and move toward chaos and death. Thus organisms, human or otherwise as open biologic systems, are always engaged in a struggle against chaos.

But the term energy is too generic for humans. All systems struggle to gain particular forms of energy that they can utilize to increase their complexity; that is, not any form of energy for any given species will do. The food prey eat to provide energy for growth is not in an appropriate form for predators, though once it is formed in the body of the prey it can now be utilized by predators for growth. Humans, too, are always engaged in this struggle against chaos, and the struggle is for energy in many forms but its most critical form is in the form of meaning.

When meaning is made – humans grow, and when it is not made – humans dissipate, even if other energetic needs are fulfilled. This assertion is exactly the opposite of reductionism often seen in the neurosciences and psychology. Following Freeman (2000) it as an assertion of downward causality with the highest level of the hierarchical system (e.g., states of consciousness) affecting processes lower down in the system (e.g., metabolism).

The effects of a failure to make meaning on the utilization of other forms of energy is seen in the chronic "deprivation" of infants in orphanages described by Spitz (Spitz, Cobliner, 1965). These infants were in an extremely pathological state in which there was a reduction of their attempts to act on and make sense of the world. Such a failure is to fail to fulfill the basic system principle. The resemblance of these deprived infants to the infant monkeys raised by surrogates has often been noted. It is easy to think how compromising the food intake would lead to "malnourished" behavior, body, and brain. But in many cases we know that the nutrition and other 'necessities' were adequate. The general consensus is that the absent "necessity" was social stimulation. But stimulation is a too dispassionate and too general a term.

For me, these children were deprived of meaning-making, that is, they were unable to form dyadic states of consciousness with others. The Spitzian infants were open human systems that, deprived of meaning-making, could neither increase the complexity of their states of consciousness nor could they even maintain their complexity. They were failed open systems. When these "Spitzian systems" are viewed as the little experiencing humans they in fact were, we can see that they had lost their capacity to engage with others or even the world of things to make meaning. Their self-organizing and dyadic capacities were so stunted and compromised that they could not make coherent sense of their place in the world. Perhaps more accurately, and even more insidiously, their impelling certitude was that they had no place in the world.

To further explore meaning-making I have created an experiment to disrupt meaning-making in infants, children and adults: the Face-to-Face Still-face Paradigm. The Still-face creates a situation in which there is a failure to create a dyadic state of consciousness which leads to dissipation of the complexity of the individual's state of consciousness. (Adamson, Frick, 2000; Tronick et al., 1978). With young infants we ask the mother to 'freeze' while *en face* with her infant – to hold a Still-face and refrain from talking or gesturing. The (in)-action of the Still-faced mother precludes the formation of a dyadic state of consciousness because there is no exchange of meaningful affect and action with the infant, no creation of meaning. The infants are forced to make meaning with their own self-organizing abilities, and though they can do it for a while, their self-organizing abilities are limited and quickly fail. Initially in response to the Still-face, infants act to re-instate their exchange of meaning by smiling at and gesturing to their mothers. But with the mother's continued lack of response the infants disengage, look away, become sad and engage in self-organized regulatory behaviors such as thumb sucking to maintain their coherence and complexity, to avoid the dissipation of their already achieved complexity level of their state of consciousness.

Figure 1 shows an infant during the Still-face who literally loses postural control, turns away, has a sad facial expression, and is self-comforting with his hands in his mouth. Indeed, what we are seeing is a failed attempt to make meaning and a collapse of a whole set of systems including motor and attention systems and the deployment of self-regulatory maintenance systems. Though we cannot truly know the age-possible impelling certitude of the infant's state of consciousness in the face of the still-faced mother, it must be something like, "[this is] threatening," or perhaps "I no longer exist." As the Still-face continues, the infant's state of consciousness is likely to change to something like, "I must try to hold myself together." If one doubts these or similar interpretations, simply consider that the infant could apprehend the Still-face mother in other ways

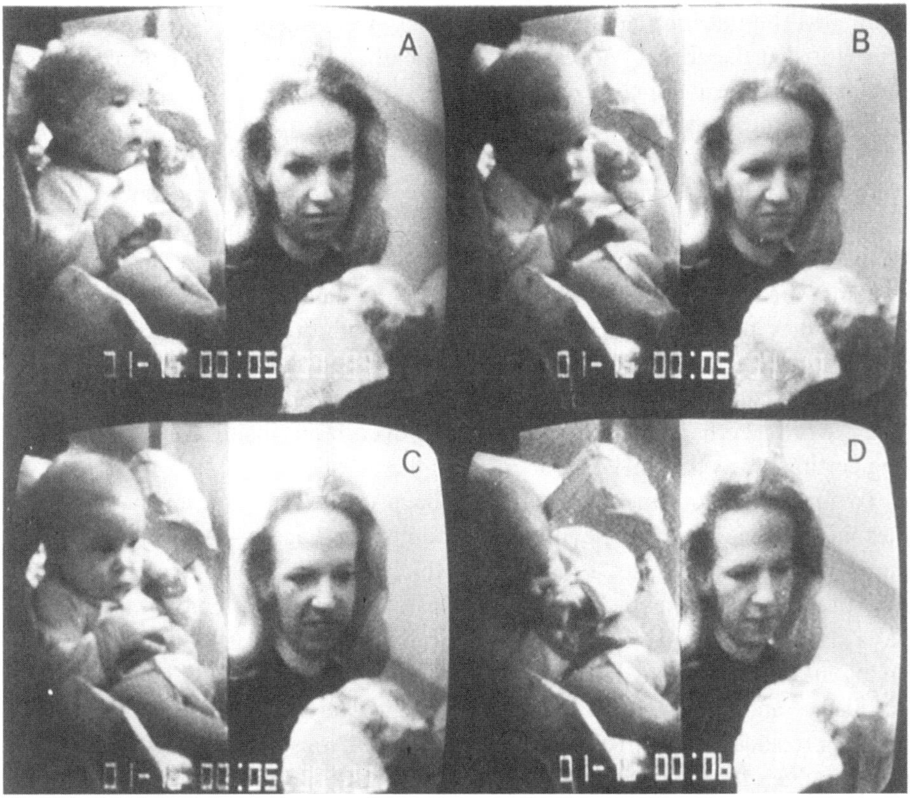

Figure 1. An infant losing postural control and turning to self-comforting behaviors in response to the mother being still-faced.

– as boring, playful, or novel – all of which would result in different forms of organized infant behaviors, behaviors which are *not* seen during the Still-face. Thus for the infant in the still-face there is meaning and certitude made *by* and expressed *in* his or her posture, actions and affects but the meaning is one that precludes gaining complexity.

More recent work on the Still-face with young children and adults makes it even clearer how the Still-face is a failure to co-create meanings and form dyadic states of consciousness. In my laboratory we have developed a procedure for using the Still-face with children 18 to 54 months of age (Weinberg et al., 2002; Tronick 2005). In the first episode of this procedure the child and the adult are seated on the floor and play with toys. This episode is followed by a Still-face episode in which the mother 'freezes" and does not respond to the infant. In the third episode the mother resumes her normal play. The findings are as striking as our original Still-face findings with infants. Young children respond to the maternal Still-face with heightened negative affect and expressions of confusion and demands for change. Toddlers ask, "Why don't you talk to me?" or command, "Talk to me!", while simultaneously soliciting the mother's interactive behavior (e.g., pointing at her eyes, tapping or almost hitting the mother, making repeated louder and louder demands). In the end they may distance themselves from her and even appear to be in an internally focused engagement with their own internal thoughts about what to make of what is going on.

Importantly and in keeping with their greater meaning-making capacities compared to infants, toddlers attribute states of mind to the mother (e.g., "Are you sleeping? Wake up!" or "Don't be afraid of the [toy] alligator!"). There is meaning in their words, in their affect and actions that reflects their capacities for pretend play, cognition, language, mentalization (Fonagy, Target, 1998), and complex affects, capacities not available to infants. Their impelling certitude is one of fearfulness and confusion at the break in connection. But the need for making sense of the world is so great that when play is resumed, some of the toddlers ask questions that attempt to make coherent sense of what happened with the mother (e.g., "Why didn't you talk to me?") even though it brings back the painfulness of the experience.

In further extension of the Still-face to adults, one of my research assistants, Lisa Bohne (unpublished) interviewed college students after they participated in an experimental role-play of an adult version of the Still-face. In this procedure, one student role-played an unresponsive mother and the other simulated being "in the mind of an infant." The "infant-persons" reported feeling anxious and vulnerable, angry, frustrated, sad, afraid, confused, even "panicky." The Still-faced, "mother-person" reported feeling guilty, distressed, anxious, depressed, shamed, vulnerable, and confused. One reported, "It felt terrible to be so closed off from the infant. It made me feel depressed and I'm sure the "infant" did too after our interaction." Preventing an exchange meaning and the formation of a dyadic state of consciousness disorganized each adult's own state of consciousness and generated a fearful, confused and less coherent sense of the world. Importantly, these adults did not try to step away from their negative experience, but in more sophisticated ways than the toddlers, continued to try to make coherent sense of what they had experienced after the procedure was terminated. They talked with each other about their experience and some of them actually apologized for what they had done.

The still-face experiments serve as a contrast to what happens during normal social engagement when making meaning is successful. The contrast is needed because meaning-making is like the fish not noticing the water because meaning-making like the water is an ongoing and continuous process of the self- or co-creation of new meaning. Self-organized meaning-making can be observed in the smile of the infant when she grabs hold of an object that had been out of reach or the exuberance of the newly walking toddler as he moves upright into the world, or the announcement by the 5 year-old that "I did it" when they put the last puzzle piece in place. There are also the "I did its" that continue throughout life when finally the sense of something is made of what up to that moment had been insensible. The *co*-creation of meaning is seen in the mutual smiling and cooing of mother and infant in face-to-face interactions. Their exchange is an example of a dyadic state of consciousness in which there is a mutual creation of new meanings of what they can do together. So too is the pretend play of the toddler with another person and the all night conversations of adolescents. Social referencing (i.e., looking at other's reactions to an event to understand one's own reaction) by infants, children and adults is a way to gain meaning that leads to a new impelling certitude about an event's meaning (Campos, Lucariello, 2000).

By co-creating a dyadic state of consciousness, individuals experience a growth in the coherence and complexity of their state of consciousness. As should be clear from the work on the Still-face and on normal interactions, meaning does not only exist in words and narrative. Meanings are age-possible, an idea that harks back to Bruner's idea that children of any age could learn anything in their own way. The concept of "age-possible" states of consciousness is needed to take into account the developmentally possible sense of their place in the world that individuals are capable of making, given their meaning-making processes. Young infants' states of consciousness are moment-by-moment assemblages of affect and actions. The meaning is in what their body and brain do. It is *of* and *in* the moment, though the moment soon integrates personal experience and lengthens with development.

The toddler and young child have qualitatively different states of consciousness from those of the infant. Their meaning-making tools include language and symbols, and complex body skills (e.g., fine finger movements to running) and body micro-practices (e.g., false coyness). In pretend play toddlers assemble fantasy, reality, and their age-possible memories into new states of consciousness. They hardly are only in the moment, but their meanings are disjunctive assemblages of illogical narratives. That is, their states of consciousness of toddlers have an "*and ___, and ____, and ___,...*" form of organization of apprehension that places no demand for the possible or the logical. Think only of a toddler's impelling certitude when he loudly demands to have the identical berries that fell from a branch back on the tree exactly the way they were and his utter distress when he says a different branch is bad and he does not want it... ever! (A. Bergman, personal communication). Children's states of consciousness have concrete meanings and here and now language. Adolescents have impossibly abstract states of consciousness with annoying impelling certitude.

There is little need to further elaborate the idea that states of consciousness are age-possible and qualitatively different for older children, adolescents and adults. Nonetheless it is worth noting, because developmental and neuroscientists tend not to attend to it, that at some point in development, states of consciousness assemble meanings from psychodynamic processes including a psycho-dynamic unconscious and transference. These dynamic processes are not equivalent to the passionless non-conscious or implicit processes invoked by developmental psychologists, cognitive neuroscientists or even some psychoanalytic writers. I believe that unconscious dynamic processes are inherent to the states of consciousness of children and adults. While I would not, Kleinians would assert they are present in infants. Dynamic unconscious processes make one person's knowing what is in another person's state of consciousness cryptic and as problematic as knowing the state of consciousness of the infant, even though children and adults use language. Thus, only explicitly knowing the other's sense of the world is not sufficient for truly knowing another person's state of consciousness. It is barely the tip of the iceberg of their sense of their place in the world. Further, the concept of age-possible makes explicit that the dyadic states of consciousness made between an infant and adult versus a child and adult are qualitatively different. Thus states of consciousness are not of one kind but are dynamically changing with development.

What, then, is the link between the open systems theory, meaning-making and experience, in particular the experience of pleasure? After all, other species make meaning in the world and are also governed by first principles of systems theory. But what do humans exclusively do, or at least do more of compared to other species that makes pleasure a consequence of their meaning-making as open systems. Humans, like other biologic systems, strive to utilize energy to expand the complexity of their states of consciousness. However, I believe that humans always implicitly and sometimes explicitly have an *experience* of the extent to which their meaning-making fulfills systems principles. Thus, when humans are seen as *experiencing* meaning-making systems, the systems phenomenon of the dissipation or of the increase of complexity of their systems have powerful *experiential* consequences.

Dissipation, the losing of complexity, occurs in all open systems. In humans dissipation occurs when there is a failure to make meaning. There is a loss of complexity of the individual's state of consciousness and the loss has experiential consequences. When it occurs, the individual experiences shrinkage, anxiety, a loss of self and a fear of annihilation. One's self in the world begins to come apart. Spitz's infants were chronically deprived of the possibility of making meaning and every level of their system literally failed to grow and expand, and their experience was one of apathy, fearfulness and sadness. This experiential state further amplified their failure to make meaning. Infants, children, and adults, when confronted with a non-meaning-making partner in the Still-face, initially experience disappointment and confusion but eventually experience anger, sadness and withdrawal. They also feel helpless and panicky in the face of the threat they experience to their on-going self-organization. I think it is noteworthy that in the adult Still-face study these experiential effects occurred in *role playing* adults who knew that the situation was set-up and unreal. Nonetheless, the effects were powerful because the experiment taps into a basic primordial experience of failing to make a connection and experiencing a dissipation of self-organization. In these situations pleasure is not possible.

The increase of the complexity of a system also occurs in systems and in humans it too has experiential consequences. When new meanings are self-created or co-created, the individual experiences an expansion of her own state of consciousness, a feeling of being bigger and a connectedness to the action, idea or person on which or with whom the new meaning was made. In contrast to a blockage of meaning-making, individuals – infants, children, adults – when creating new meanings, grow in every possible way and experience joy, interest, curiosity, and exuberance. Ultimately I believe there is a primordial embodied experience of fulfilling a basic life governing principle: the success of making sense of one's place in the world and becoming more complexly organized. Often this feeling of wholeness, completeness, safety and exuberance is out of awareness. Occasionally it is in awareness, and when it is, it is special indeed. But whether in or out of awareness, it is the experience of pleasure, a deep abiding pleasure.

Humans as meaning makers have no option but to strive to increase the complexity of our states of consciousness. Were we to stop we would perish, dissipate and experience the terror of annihilation. Successfully striving to create new meanings increases our complexity and brings pleasure. However, it is not as simple as either strive or fail, because striving to create something new requires taking apart some of the old. But when taking apart the old organization to create something new, complexity is actually reduced and the reduction is experienced as anxiety, and the anxiety is further increased because there is no guarantee of success of the creative effort. An apparent way to prevent the anxiety is to remain fixed and not change, but of course such fixedness precludes the pleasure of expanding and the fulfillment of systems principles. Thus the dilemma of striving to be a system that grows in complexity and simultaneously risks dissolution is to experience pleasure tinged with terror or to not strive to grow and never experience pleasure. Healthy humans choose pleasure and terror. For example, in Carol Gilligan's recounting of the myth of Psyche and Cupid, Psyche has all the pleasure one could imagine, yet chooses to look at Cupid because she *must* strive for the deep pleasure of expanding her knowing of him and her relation to him, even at the risk of dissolution of the complexity she has already achieved. It is something she must do to be human, and she is, indeed, human. Her greatest pleasure comes when the old dissolves and she expands her state of consciousness. Thus the myth captures the momentous and the everyday nature of meaning-making, the experience of pleasure and, yes, even systems principles: to create the new is to risk the old for the possibility of a greater pleasure, but to not create the new is surely to perish.

References

Adamson L, J Frick: Research with the Face-to-Face Still-Face paradigm: A review. Infancy 4, 4 (2000) 451–73

Bruner J: Acts of Meaning. Harvard University Press, Cambridge, MA 1990

Campos JJ, J Lucariello: Origins and consequences of social signaling. 2000

Fonagy P, M Target: Mentalization and the changing aims of psychoanalysis. Psychological Dialogues 8 (1998) 87–114

Freeman WJ: How Brains Make Up Their Mind. Columbia University Press, New York 2000

Gilligan C: The birth of pleasure. Knopf, New York 2002

Spitz RA, WG Cobliner: Emotional deficiency diseases of the infant. In: The First Year of Life. A Psychoanalytic Study of Normal and Deviant Development of Object Relations. International Universities Press, Inc., New York 1965

Stengers I, I Prigogine: The End of Certainty. Simon & Schuster, New York 1997

Tronick EZ, H Als, L Adamson, S Wise, TB Brazelton: The infant's response to entrapment between contradictory messages in face-to-face interaction. Journal of the American Academy of Child & Adolescent Psychiatry 17 (1978) 1–13

Tronick EZ: Interactions that effect change in psychotherapy: A model based on infant research. Infant Mental Health J 19 (1998) 1–290

Tronick, EZ. Why is connection with others so critical? The formation of dyadic states of consciousness: coherence governed selection and the co-creation of meaning out of messy meaning making. In: J. Nadel and D. Muir (eds). Emotional Development. Oxford University Press, Oxford, 2005, 293–315

Weinberg MK, M Beeghly, KL Olson, EZ Tronick: Preschoolers' reaction to their still-faced mother. International Conference on Infant Studies, Toronto 2002

Vygotsky L: Mind in Society. Harvard University Press, Cambridge 1978

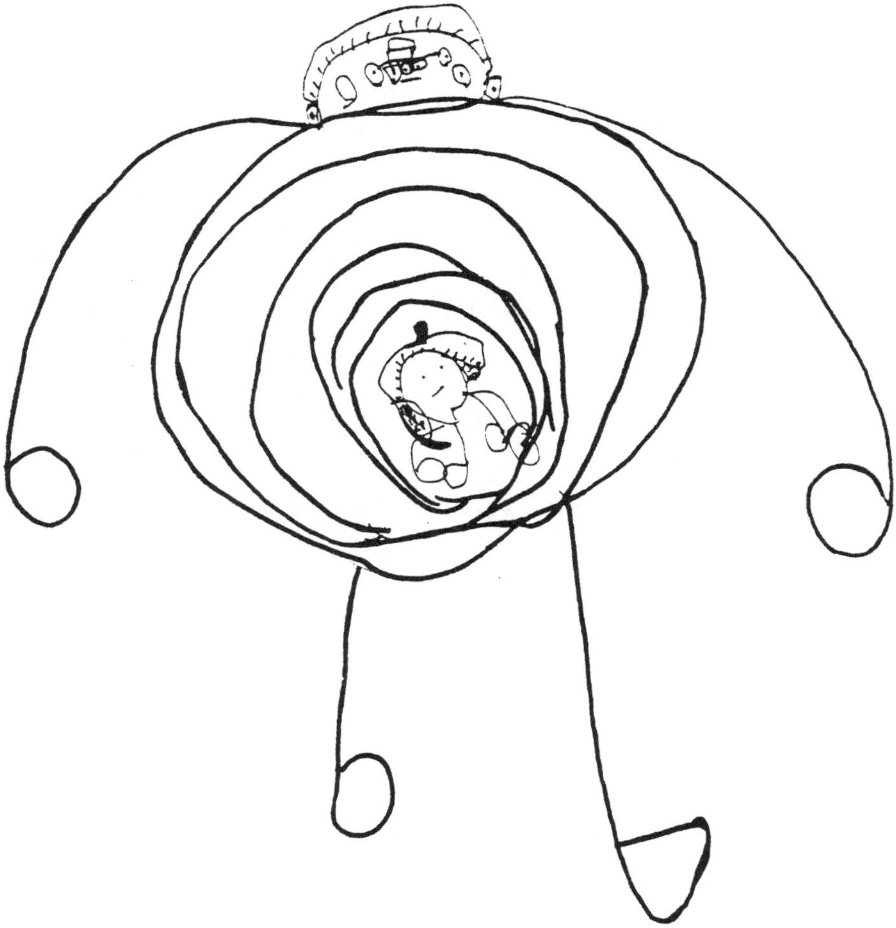

(Maddalena, 3 yrs. 8 mos.)
I was all wet, I was in water inside a balloon… I didn't ask them if I had a bathing suit on.

5. Birth: Between medical and human science

Vanna Iori; Family Pedagogy, Catholic University of Milan and Family Observation, Reggio Emilia, Italy

The 'naturalness' and the complexity of birth

Being born is the most *natural* and, at the same time, the most *complex* event. It is natural because it is a biologically defined event which belongs to human nature and, with its continuation, guarantees the very prolongation of life and human history. It is thus natural if we understand it as a *biological* and *spontaneous* event (and it is not by chance that this very word should indicate a delivery where no 'artificial' intervention is required); it is natural, because it is *normal*, that is to say, ordinary, usual, common; and because it can be identified with the '*beginning*', the *original* event which marks the beginning of life.

To these *natural* aspects, however, there correspond equal assumptions of *complexity*.

First of all, birth is not simply the 'normal' *beginning* of our presence in the world; it is the very origin to which we go back every time we look for our beginning: it represents the insuppressible need to grasp the roots of personal and relational identity, to discover the meaning of our existential condition, to plan the time of life. This return to the *place of personal origin* is characterized by the never-allayed fears and uncertainties related to the very origins of humanity, a powerful archetype which has found an expression in every society through various myths of origin.

Secondly, the experience of being born (and of giving birth) is lived, every time, as an extraordinary, exceptional, unique, and unrepeatable event which storms into ordinary, everyday life and forever modifies people's relationships and their personal biographies.

Even when birth is anticipated, prepared, and even planned, it always assumes unforeseen characteristics. Life is marked by a 'before' and an 'after', and entrance into parenthood represents an irreversible turning point. Birth is therefore an *event* (a 'happy event', as the saying goes), which, while being seemingly characterized by naturalness, coincides nonetheless with the very core of a great complexity. The couple is invested with new roles and duties which are connected to the 'creation of a space' for the newcomer, not only on a physical level (within the mother's womb), but, more fundamentally, on an emotional one, and this will change life as the couple knows it forever.

Consequently, even the *spontaneity* of the *biological* dimension becomes increasingly complex because of the very presence of the 'delivery scene', the various ways this is conceived (which express the different cultures in which this natural event inscribes itself), and the different ways in which it is interpreted and supported. In ancient times, for instance, childbirth used to take place at home, and the only protagonists of the event were women. In contrast, hospitalization has progressively assigned a prominent role to doctors and health services (Pizzini, 1985). Therefore, the rates of maternal, perinatal and infant mortality have decreased, but there has been a loss of meaning – that meaning which was once expressed in the rituals and symbolic gestures which used to accompany the female protagonists during the lived experienced of giving birth. Furthermore, the development of biomedical science intersects today with ambivalent feelings towards motherhood and fatherhood: the refusal of procreation and, at the same time, the opposite desire for maternity at all cost. In this context, the heated bioethical debate concerning the different techniques of medically assisted procreation confirms the complexity of the relationship with the body.

Furthermore, we should also bear in mind another complexity, which is linked to the many cultures we inhabit: during a period characterized by inter-culturality, what is conceived as 'natural' is becoming more and more heterogeneous and polysemic, because we interpret and experience procreation differently.

We can therefore conclude that 'childbirth' is simultaneously an intense and complex experience, dominated by violent and contrasting passions: hope and fear, love and aggressiveness, happiness and pain. Although these passions are part of every birth, their intensity depends on many variables (Finzi, 1992). The ambivalent contraposition nature-culture (here referred to childbirth), recalls other dichotomies: mind-body, masculine-feminine, identity-difference, acceptance-rejection, desire-impossibility, technique-arts, imaginary-real, conditioning-projection, private-public, care-carelessness, life-death and other multiple cultural factors which assign a character of 'complexity' even to the normal spaces and times of *childbirth.*

These antonyms assume very important symbolic values and express cultural stratifications.

Medical and human science

In order to separate the existing conceptions of birth from the socio-cultural repressions which have conditioned the possibility of achieving a systematized knowledge founded on a dialogue between different disciplines, we should investigate many aspects.

Hence the innovative connotation of this conference, which focuses on those meeting-points where technical-scientific competence meets that 'existential knowledge' which, within the context of the health system, is not actually taken into consideration, in spite of the fact that it is acknowledged from a theoretical point of view.

The need for a significant scientific dialogue between the various fields of knowledge which focus on childbirth from a variety of perspectives should be by now common knowledge. However, this is not so, and the reasons for this lack of dialogue can be traced to the history of the various scientific fields and their epistemological guidelines.

No single phenomenon (and even less so childbirth) can be legitimately connected to a particular and exclusive field. Indeed, only the mutual recognition of various competences can respect the complexity of this event. The inherently human experience of childbirth therefore appears less and less circumscribable to the sole area of medical science. Indeed, it appears increasingly necessary to retrieve the strong bond with human science.

The boundaries between humanistic and medical-scientific fields that were very neatly drawn during the nineteenth century (which was characterized by a positivist attitude), are now less marked: with the crisis of classical positivism, the meaning of 'scientific' has become increasingly problematic and articulated, raising issues of rigor and complexity in the articulation of any problem.

The drawing of neat boundaries has become increasingly difficult because of the complex network of cross-references. When talking about childbirth, the divide between medical and human science becomes untenable, and we cannot disregard its existential aspect as far as the meaning of birth is concerned.

The progressive medicalization of birth has led to a decreased interest in the experiences which accompany it. Focusing on the delivery and the way it is conducted from a technical and an instrumental perspective has often suggested that no thought is given to the fact that childbirth is much more than a simple delivery. "In any society, childbirth is a revelatory event which highlights, first of all, the 'place' women occupy in that society; it is as if the delivery scene represented the relationship between men and women [...] thereby achieving the personification of nature and culture, whose boundary coincides with social order, that is to say, the *locus* where human beings can express their humanity" (Pizzini, 1985).

The many views provided by various disciplines cannot offer a complete *explanation* of the feeling of 'becoming hollow' which procreation entails, or of the physical transformations and intense emotions which follow the separation of childbirth, feelings which can find a verbal expression only with some difficulty. Indeed, if the astonishment felt by the mother when she realizes that she is the guardian of life, can take her breath away, and can certainly 'freeze' her words. Withdrawing from the anxiety and the desire to communicate in words what cannot, in fact, be expressed verbally, means to grant oneself the liberty to live the experience at a different level, through the intelligence of the heart (Musi, 2005).

Hence, a new qualification of the culture and the practices connected to childbirth requires, first of all, the retrieval of the fundamental relationship between *medical and human science*. The former maintains of course its distinct identity, but cannot be separated from a reflection on the prerequisites of gnoseology and the input of philosophy, psychology, pedagogy, sociology, cultural anthropology, ethics, history, as well as other fields, from politics to architecture.

Legitimacy related to the separation between human and medical science naturally raises an epistemological issue. Our reply basically coincides with a critique of the attempted objectification of the richness typical of childbirth and its constraint within the narrow limits of technical procedures. The epistemological issue refers to a network of conceptual cross-references whose boundaries (by definition rather tortuous), intersect and then separate, but, most of the time, do not meet. Although in this context it is not possible to analyze all the themes concerning the epistemology of birth, it might be nonetheless useful to indicate some basic epistemological aspects, putting them in relation to a phenomenological matrix which can enable the creation of a bridge between medical and human science.

For an epistemology of birth

An epistemology of birth appears particularly necessary because current medicine runs the risk of pursuing a scientific model which is mainly concerned with sophisticated techniques (which are of course necessary), rather than investigating various other issues. I am not simply referring here to the issues raised by bioethics, but to the more general ones relating to the *fundamentals* and the *significance* of any medical procedure.

Various techniques, which effectively make life easier, can sometimes supersede the stimulus to reflect and think about that *epistème* which derives from the verb *epì-histànai*, literally, 'to stay' on things, think about them. Sergio Nordico, an expert in medical pedagogy, says that when you ask final-year and graduate students in medicine what they mean by epistemology, very often they answer that *they do not know what it is* and that they consider it a superfluous philosophy of science. "Everybody says that you have to be scientific in the medical science, but many do not feel the need to discuss the notion of science and the scientific aspect of medicine" (Nordico, 1994).

In the attempt to obtain a greater scientific status, medical science has undoubtedly developed a great deal. However, it has very often confined itself to the models derived from positivism, which tend (often in a programmatic way) to assume anti-philosophical positions. On the contrary, the re-qualification of scientific rigor should always posit itself within the context of a critical resumption of the relationship between 'philosophy' and 'science'. In particular, any discussion of childbirth requires praxis based on both *philosophy* and *science.*

It is important to remember that Hippocrates's ancient maxim "*iatròs philòsophos isòtheos*" (the doctor who becomes a philosopher becomes a sort of god) suggests that the doctor, by becoming a philosopher, can achieve a different awareness of the common existential condition and of his own actions. Karl Jaspers, a doctor who later became a professor of philosophy at Heidelberg, remembers this view well and, in fact, affirms that "the doctor's practice is a practical philosophy". By so doing, he suggests the epistemological necessity for a dialogue between philosophy and science. "The kind of philosophy which does not have, as its momentum, the spirit of science, today becomes, in its entirety, untrue. Despite the accuracy of specific data, science without philosophy becomes globally uncritical." But, Jaspers immediately underlines, "philosophy does not mean abstraction [...]. It becomes the vital breath of existence (*Existenz*). This is the only way existence can talk of a meaningful origin" (Jaspers, 1991). Even when they exhibit a great medical-scientific knowledge, many doctors do not confront these *existential* components, mainly because university and professional education is strongly influenced by a positivist vision, and consequently focuses on the body-as-organism rather than the body-as-person.

The irreversible turning point can be placed in the seventeenth century, with Descartes *Discourse on Method*: it is in fact in this work that the body-as-thing (*res extensa*) is born as separate from the mind (*res cogitans*) which can conceive it, "a body as it is thought of by the intellect, and not as it is experienced by and during life, the idea of a body, not a body in flesh and blood, a body which has a disease, not a body that feels pain, an anatomic body and not a subject of life [...] This way, *modern medicine* is born, a medicine which would have never been possible without the reduction of the 'body' to an 'organism'" (Galimberti, 2002).

The body-mind antithesis is already present in Greek mythology (where Athena is born out of Zeus's head), and is recalled by the connection of the terms 'conception' and 'to conceive', 'concept' and 'conceiving' (Winnicott, 1990). The mind and the body belong to the same substance, in the same way that emotion and feeling are part of the same process. This is what neuroscientist Antonio Damasio (1995) claims, when he identifies "Descartes mistake" with the separation of body and mind.

On the basis of what Pascal maintained, Descartes' rationalist procedure (*ésprit de géométrie*) does not lead to a certain knowledge but to an illusionary and superficial knowledge of reality; a sort of knowledge which lacks both essence and foundation. In order to overcome Descartes' cognitive modules, Pascal confronts the central core of human condition; through *l'ésprit de finesse*, 'intelligent intuition' becomes possible, and enables us to go beyond the mere analysis of data, in order to achieve the perception of fundamental truths. Yet, Nordico wonders "how much *esprit de finesse* can we detect nowadays in a medical world that is pervaded by a quantitative and calculating mental attitude, a world that converges on empirical data and that can be described as technological and technocratic?"

Medical science is increasingly characterized by this objectifying, quantitative and 'mathematizing' attitude, which focuses on empirical data and whose predominance runs the risk of turning medicine (which is both art and science), into mere technique.

According to Karl Jaspers, the modern scientist/doctor has lost his humanity. In spite of the incredible conquests achieved by technical and scientific progress, an individual can really become a doctor only when he takes on the philosophical implications of this praxis. His actions, in fact, should "rest on two pillars: on the one hand his scientific knowledge and technical ability, on the other, his humanitarian *ethos*." The path is of course difficult, and today very few doctors embark on it. While the first pillar has seen enormous advances in the acquisition of new competences, the second has not been cultivated. Modern medicine has privileged more and more the objectivity of clinical data which can be inferred thanks to the equipment at hand. As such, however, the clinical view has lost all understanding of the human element. This *ethos* "cannot be simply reduced to the mere 'respect' for the patient, but should assume a larger meaning, leading to a 'patient-oriented' attitude. It is like this that ethos becomes meaningful, in that it qualifies not only clinical actions, but also [the doctor's] empathy, his listening ability and his affective resonance" (Parma, 1994).

It therefore clear that it is impossible to reduce the existential relevance of childbirth to a purely biological reality. This principle is also emphasized in the field of medical science. Yet, in this context, it does not automatically lead to the recognition of the fact that it is necessary to go beyond that objectivism which is often considered a prerequisite of science.

A new episteme: subjectivity and objectivity

The predominance of objectivity has concealed the demand for meaning put forth by life itself, which implies a sort of epistemological Copernican revolution. In fact, the questioning of the dominance of the objectivity of knowledge over its subjectivity, reverses the paradigms on which scientific knowledge (including the medical one), has until now relied.

Our scientific culture is dominated by the idea that science should coincide with neutrality and the interposition of some distance between the subject and the object of study. Even in ordinary language, we define an affirmation as 'objective' when we think it is irrefutable, ascertained and shared by everybody; while everything that is defined as 'subjective' is devaluated, because it represents an uncertain, debatable, and unsubstantiated point (Iori, 1988).

This contraposition between what is *subjective* (therefore unscientific), and *objective* (thus scientific), has led to the exclusion of any knowledge which is not based on the object itself. Galileo, with his mathematization of the natural world, has deleted subjectivity. Because of the Cartesian division and the contraposition between the subject and the world of things, scientific knowledge has focused on the object. Because this dominance accorded to objectivity, *external* reality and factual data, scientific culture has separated completely from humanistic culture.

But Descartes' paradigm has influenced Western thought to such an extent that it is considered the measure for science even when it comes to the *subject*, to whom procedures and methods inferred by the 'exact sciences' are now applied. This heuristic attitude has even produced an 'objectifying knowledge' of what pertains to the human sphere. Positivism, in fact, has led even human science (whose *object* is the study of the *subject* him/herself), to appropriate naturalistic and objectifying methodologies: the subject is thus de-humanized and stripped of properly human traits.

Science which focuses on the human being (thus also medical science) needs a rigor and a scientific capability of avoiding the reduction of the subject to a 'thing'. As Heidegger (1976) states, "the person is not a thing, not a substance, and not even an object. This is what Husserl himself means when he says that the unity of the person needs an essentially different constitution from that of natural things."

This phenomenological science pursues a type of knowledge which, by investigating *meaning*, retrieves the intentional relationship between the subject and his/her world, rather than investigating the object in itself, merely as 'data'. By so doing, it opens up a new and unexplored space of experience, that of intentional consciousness, which allows a link between experience and meaning (Husserl, 1987). Phenomenology does not conceive itself as the refusal of the empirical-objectifying method or as a critique of certain possibilities offered by mathematical, physical, and biological science; rather, it pushes into problematic status their pretension to *absoluteness* and exhaustiveness.

To retrieve the scientific dignity of subjectivity means to identify *rigor* and *objectivity* as the essential requirements of any kind of science. However, it also means emphasizing that the physical-mathematical model cannot be extended to the study of all aspects of human life, in so far as not every aspect can be *explained* on the basis of that paradigm. In the pursuit of a new *episteme*, the effort made to bring back "science to its subject" (in Husserl's sense of the expression), is assumed as fundamental. Even though this might appear paradoxical, this new episteme should posit itself simultaneously as both *subjective* and *objective*. Taking into account the double need of both rigor and signification, the phenomenological method (and the development it underwent during Existentialism), opens new paths to a new form of science which, rather than *explain* childbirth from a causal point of view, tries to *understand* its meaning, connecting it to the existential and historical situation, thereby guarding its complexity.

The distinction between *erklären* (that is, explaining causally from the exterior, using logical-rational tools) and *verstehen* (that is, understanding through a meaningful and significant knowledge) dates back to Wilhelm Dilthey (1985), who tries to free the cognitive task from the kind of thinking which divides, categorizes, and analyses. This Diltheyanian concept opened a path which was later to become fundamental for Husserl and Jaspers, and their search for a science which knows how to extend the boundaries of naturalistic empiricism. Thus, *Erlebnis* (the lived experience) can be considered a particularly helpful category for a science which does not want to reduce human beings to a mass of objectified elements, thus enabling us to understand them from within, that is to say, from the lived experience itself (*erlebt*).

However, subjective elements such as lived experience and intuition do not simply coincide with a form of subjectivism that cannot be expressed, but they are made comprehensible and expressible amongst subjects through different kinds of *explanations*. The view of *understanding* is fundamental, as it allows to ask and to be asked questions of meaning during one of the most intense experiences of life, namely at a time when doctors and obstetricians are required not to render the process of coming into the world unnatural by taking away its symbolic and existential value.

To be born to life

The objectification of childbirth often leads to a defensive attitude, meant to protect doctors from the emotions which the event of procreation entails, and hiding, behind the operations carried out in an aseptic hospital room, the possibility to express the way we experience the *unknown* which procreation always represents. This "readiness to face the unknown" (Arcidiacono, 1985) coincides with the acceptance of the mysterious nature of an uncontrollable and astonishing process in front of which the word 'to *explain*' seems utterly inadequate.

Childbirth, in a similar way to death, expresses a *separation.* The Italian term for 'to give birth', namely *partorire*, derives, in fact, from the Latin *perere*, which shares the same Indo-European root of *parens* (that is, parent) but is in the past participle (*partus*), and recalls the same root of *pars* and *partiri,* meaning 'to separate' and 'divide' from one another. Delivery (in Italian, 'parto') is therefore conceived, first of all, as a separation and a loss which, for the female body, coincides with the loss of a part of itself.

In spite of the inauthentic attitude which tends to conceal these questions by hiding them behind the use of impersonal forms (the Italian *Si*, the German *Man*, the French *On* etc.), birth, in a similar way to death, raises important issues of meaning. The statements 'one' is born' or 'one' dies, do not offer answers to the questions raised by birth and death, because the focus moves somewhere: delivery and death itself, namely, *moments* which can be described as the functional mechanisms of a body-machine. But separation leaves in the dark a sort of existential anxiety. The retrieval of human subjectivity legitimates the expression of those inexplicable aspects of this event: "being the subject of childbirth means to be the protagonist of the process, also in its dark part" (Arcidiacono, 1985).

From the beginning of humanity, the highest number of myths and rituals relating to human experience has been dedicated to birth and death: both are, in fact, enveloped in the very mystery which envelops the presence of human beings in our world. Mythical thought, with its wisdom, tried to pursue a type of knowledge which does not ask the immediate reason of these events or their cause (*aitìa*), but, rather, questions their original meaning and their foundation (*arkè*).

Being born to life is an event which does not question solely the immediate causes of fecundation, the various stages of pregnancy, breast-feeding and puerperium: these are always etiologies which belong to the *aitìa* logic. In contrast, 'being born to life' attentively investigates the meaning of being *thrown* into life. (Heidegger, 1976) This natural and, at the same time extraordinary event, concerns the meaning of human existence itself.

'Being born' is the vital foundation of existence; it is an event which can be connected to the moment of delivery, but it is an *act*, not a *fact*. If we understand 'being born' in terms of 'fact', then the lived experiences which accompany it (the expectations, the projects, the anxieties, the pain and the joy it provokes) cannot render it comprehensible, in so far as in this instance, it remains outside personal and social history, positing itself within an extra-temporal 'fixity'. Understood as an 'act', on the other hand, 'being born' is conceived as a *dynamic* event which posits itself within *temporality* and is founded on a *project*.

According to Martin Heidegger (1976), the human subject, understood as a being-there (*Dasein*), is in the world because it has been 'thrown into life'. The condition of *Geworfenheit* (translated as 'dejection' or 'thrown-ness'), is therefore a constitutive aspect of human nature, which appears in all its distressing and fascinating 'effectivity' at the moment of birth.

If we consider various etymological correspondences, we can detect, in the concept of *project*, the past participle *proiectum*, from the Latin *proicere* (to throw, to hurl), and the past participle *geworfen* of the German *werfen* (to throw, to hurl): these obvious consonances reveal how the condition of being 'thrown' and the condition of 'project' are indissoluble. Thus, 'being thrown into life' can always be understood as a project. From the very moment we are born, every 'existential history' gives support to a project, in so far as human beings are enabled to *ex-sistere*, that is to say, go beyond and transcend the 'factuality' of the situation they are 'thrown into'.

Birth, therefore, coincides with the actual beginning of the subject's *biography*: the initial project which others have conceived in relation to the future child, thus meets the project which every newborn begins to pursue in relation to him/herself from the very moment s/he is born.

If we circumscribe childbirth to its immediate causes, then we deprive this process of its projectuality, and, therefore, of all the emotions which are face-to-face with a new life can trigger. If they want to let themselves be affected by this *joyful anxiety*, doctors must in the first instance achieve an 'existential competence'.

The meeting between medical and human science becomes significant when it allows us to investigate the meaning of *being born to life*. It is precisely this question that medical science must constantly ask, being brave enough to query its own epistemological paradigms and accepting the consequences of this question completely, thereby discovering the fragility of all the certainties propounded by natural science.

From the body-as-thing to the body-as-existence

Issues of meaning are potentially disruptive for the health system and the medical practice, as they refer to "Husserl's distinction between the objectified body of science, which offers itself to the anatomic-physiologic examination (*Körper*), and the individual's body as it is actually experienced in life (*Leib*)" (Galimberti, 1983). When medical science refers to the reality of the body in a merely naturalistic sense, it considers it an organism or a machine, a body-as-thing, deprived of all humanity.

The difference between *homo natura* and *homo existentia* elaborated on by Ludwig Binswanger (1989), derives from the distinction Husserl views (1989) in the fifth of his *Cartesian Meditations*, which reads: "I then find *my body* in its unique peculiarity, that is to say, as a body which is not merely a physical entity (*Körper*), but a living body (*Leib*)." Phenomenology has thus enabled us to free the body from its objectification (and reification), in order to retrieve its radically human foundation (Borgna, 2001).

In a perspective according to which "medical view does not meet the patient but his/her illness, and in his/her body does not read a *biography* but a *pathology*, where subjectivity disappears behind the objectivity of symptoms" (Galimberti, 1985), even the woman who is giving birth disappears as a subject which is generating life; her world-of-life (*Lebenswelt*) with its relations and its meanings, breaks in order to be replaced by a case history, which is felt to be more adequate to the hospital environment.

Childbirth cannot be a mere physiological event because the body is not simply a body-machine but a body-*Leib*. Within an indissoluble psychosomatic and existential entirety, we do not *have* a body, but *we are a body*. Before any other intuition might be formed, every subject perceives his/herself as a corporeal entity. As Merleau-Ponty (1980) emphasizes, "I am not in front of my body, I am inside my body, better still, I am my body".

The notion of *having* a body is very different from *being* a body; this difference entails a drastic reversal of the way subjectivity is understood in terms of a *lived corporeity*. Gabriel Marcel (1974) stated that "the category of *having* is not suitable to the notion of corporeity". By emphasizing that we do not *have* a body, but that we *are* a body, a body-as-existence, conceived beyond any naturalistic reduction, we *preserve* the awareness of, and the *responsibility* for, the body that lives and 'speaks' in our relationships.

Being a body represents the first 'effectiveness' of our existence, the first rooting which characterizes 'being thrown' into human existence. Simultaneously, however, it coincides with the first place where the common 'world-of-life' (*Lebenswelt*) can be expressed, thus allowing the existential communication of life; "we communicate with our body: a living and lived body; and we communicate through our body in an unexplored vortex of meanings." (Borgna, 1992)

Being-there (in the world) is also, always, being-with: in this situation of 'being thrown' we are not alone; indeed, in order to accomplish our journey, we need others, and from this relationship, we can achieve an understanding of birth from the standpoint of *intersubjectivity*. Every experience, in fact, posits itself in the *world of us all*, the world of co-existence. (Husserl, 1986) Eugenio Borgna (1992) states: "what makes life 'emotional', that is, affectivity, the essential prerequisite for any cure, is the fact that life always consists of relationships, and as such it allows the construction, albeit fragile and fragmentary, of a form of dialogue, made of silences and contacts: of intersubjectivity."

The maternal body

Human life as a whole is born from a body: a woman's body. It is therefore easy to conceive this origin of 'birth' as the fundamental element in the relationship between human and medical science, an element which is most significant from both a symbolic and a cultural point of view.

The hospitalization of childbirth has led to the objectification of the female body and the depreciation of both '*feeling*' and that kind of knowledge which is connoted in terms of gender. This knowledge is actually characterized by its matrilineal transmission, and by the fact that it did not sever the lived experience (*Erlebnis*) from the accompanying practices of the expectant mother.

Before the medicalization of childbirth, up to the eighteenth century (and, in many cultures, until a few decades ago), birth and early infancy was considered part of a woman's knowledge. From this perspective, women were considered the depositary of life, both from a corporeal and a symbolic point of view. As such, "women felt they were adding a link in the chain of different generations, thereby safeguarding the future of their family and their lineage, ensuring the perpetuation of the species" (Gelis, 1985).

Recent transformations have also led to a progressively decreasing number of midwives and the constant presence of doctors and obstetricians: the knowledge which used to be transmitted in the form of an oral heritage belonging to a feminine culture (with all its superstitions and inadequacies, but also with its symbolic rituals, which did nothing to destroy the central role played by women in childbirth), has been supplanted by institutionalized practices and scientific procedures. These, while reducing the mortality rate and granting better health to both the mother and the child, have also disrupted the relationship which the common experience of giving birth used to create among women, marginalizing the lived experience of the female body and emphasizing what can be seen ('examined') by the doctors' view. (Pizzini, 1999)

The subjectivity of the interior experience becomes irrelevant to the objectivity of scientific knowledge: the female body is assigned to biology. The set goal, namely the well-being of mother and child, determines the way women are assisted during childbirth, leading to a detachment from their 'body-as-person' and to a misuse of their 'body-as-thing'. Women introject the untrustworthiness of their lived and corporeal experience, "immediately assigning the interpretation of their symptoms to technicians" (Regalia, 1997): it is the woman herself who now asks the doctor what she can no longer ask her own body.

The paradoxical 'extraneousness' of women to their body (on which others intervene and make decisions), turns the mother from an active subject into a passive object. Childbirth becomes an event which is always monitored from the exterior and can therefore be induced, augmented, and regulated. By relying on mere technique, the woman (understood here both as a body and as a person), loses the continuity between 'before' and 'afterwards', interior and exterior, her home as the locus of affections and significant relationships, and the hospital, a neutral and alien place. This fracture leads to fragmentation of the self, in relation to both the already difficult constitution of a maternal identity and the relationship the woman establishes with her child.

The mother-to-be who is taken care of within a technical-specialist apparatus, according to external standard procedures, progressively loses her role as the authoritative referent for the transformations occurring during pregnancy and the lived experience of her own corporeity. Having lost the possibility to interpret childbirth in terms of the postures and movements they freely wanted to assume and make, women in labor have been increasingly obliged to submit to the tools of science: at first, the tool kits of obstetricians, whose formation was the result of a specific school and whose *scientific* role was publicly acknowledged; afterwards, the structures of the delivery room.

The meeting of medical and human science should encourage us to recognize that in order to 'assist' well, we should also try to create the conditions for an emotive participation in the event, thus avoiding its reduction to a mere mechanical fact which has been purged of all emotional value.

From early ultrasound scans, the modes typical of *listening* are suppressed and replaced by the modes of *seeing*. The woman's *biography*, the subjective and unique history which determines the way every woman lives maternity and childbirth, are not listened to; it is the woman who, often in awe, *listens* to the doctor; but "what the woman brings the doctor is not a body that wants to be examined and palpated, but a whole history which has become flesh." (Duden,

1994) The anamnesis process must therefore be based more on listening, so that doctors can welcome and accompany the birth as a biography, rather than simply assigning it to monitors and examinations.

The ethics of care

Finally, I would like to emphasize the necessity for the doctors and other staff present in the delivery room, not to reject the emotional dimension. Stop trying to disperse it by relying solely on technical instruments, but be open to the relationship with (and the emotions of) both the woman herself and the couple. Is the exclusion of emotions from the relationship established during care, legitimate, especially when we are dealing with apical moments of human existence such as life and death? The habit, typical of medical culture, of ignoring or hiding its emotional dimension, precludes an involvement which is seen as a 'threat' to scientific and professional behavior. Defense from emotionality which could burst in, finds an expression in the detachment of doctors who, in order to protect themselves, reject any relationship with the woman and the couple (Regalia, 1997).

Doctors' (apparent) imperturbability, prevents them from establishing an authentic relationship during care, rejects 'understanding' (*verstehen*), in favor of 'explaining' (*erklären*) and 'offering a service', without actually listening to 'feeling'. This attitude entails a reduced attention to *care*, at the very moment when care for life should be at its highest. Even those performances which, from a medical and technical perspective, can be considered perfect, become merely 'secure' (that is, *sine cura*), while what is necessary is precisely the attention for the life being born. *Taking care* thus becomes essential, which implies the willingness and the ability to go beyond the role identified by the white coat, the uniform which 'divides' those who withhold scientific power/knowledge from those who are in their hands.

Jaspers wonders whether "it is this apparent imperturbability that doctors, who are mostly exposed to emotions, actually need." (Jaspers, 1991) Why shouldn't doctors feel free to be moved by birth? Why shouldn't they accept emotions, listen to them, let them be? Emotion, during 'care', does not represent a threat for professionalism. On the contrary, it coincides with one of its components, and not even a secondary one. The 'taking care', however, is not an 'innate' dimension and cannot be improvised; quite the opposite, it requires a long apprenticeship which, according to Hippocrates's maxim quoted above, should be based on philosophical wisdom as well.

The sharing of emotions requires a preparation that should be able to teach doctors how to 'be there' and 'be close', reaching a proximity created not simply by diagnostic tools but also by words, looks and the ability to listen,. "A genuinely original understanding […] depends on the willingness to take notice of what this new knowledge *un-veils* which, once we free ourselves from prejudice, appears as if it were seen and heard for the first time". (Jaspers, 1991) The art of taking care requires us to be ready to 'feel', without being frightened, and to find, in every different situation, that 'correct distance' which can prevent us from running away when confronted with emotions and, at the same time, from being submerged by feelings. In the particular context of childbirth, we can say that "what helps us find the right measure from the point of view of self-presence in the relationship of 'care' is the quality of the feelings that occupy our thoughts" (Mortari, 2003).

In health institutions, the difference between '*to care* or *care about*' someone, and '*to cure* or *care for*' someone, emphasizes the divide between daily life, with its lived experiences, and the approach of the institutions, where the 'cure' often takes place without any 'care' for the person. The health institution appropriates the *body-as-thing* and 'cares' for it, without 'caring' about the *body-as-person*, with its concerns, its hopes, its habits, its memories, namely, its history, which is not only 'anamnesis' but also a way to be in the world.

Caring for without caring about is the paradox to which the separation of science and the subject has led, thereby rendering the institutions themselves more and more anonymous and making them follow often incomprehensible rules which are imposed onto, and are endured by, the patients. These rules break the rhythms of life, to make them conform to the institution, and rather than favor family relationships, they render them emotionally difficult.

Entrance into the trail of medical science and its techniques pretends to be impersonal in order to 'keep a distance' and allow doctors not to put themselves at stake. In addition, because doctors have only few occasions to grow emotionally, they run the risk of being unprepared when faced with issues of meaning and the *ethics of 'caring about'*. Although the attempt not to acknowledge one's feelings might give the impression that one is actually keeping the feelings under control, it certainly leads to their manifestation in forms which might not always be correct or compatible with doctors' professional function and, above all, with their emotional resources (Iori).

When the ethics of 'care' governs childbirth and help is provided in the process, 'thoughts' and 'feelings' cannot be separated. Indeed, this is the only way we can elude total ignorance of the language which can only be expressed by tears of joy or suffering, especially in an environment where it appears absolutely necessary to get rid of all masks.

A psychological and human character capable of relating to another person at the moment when she is becoming a mother will not damage medical competence but, quite the contrary, will enrich it. Recent medical history has assumed a very defensive position: human science can help it come out of its fortress and open up to the experience of inter-human encounters.

Becoming a parent

My final remarks on childbirth concern the support and the assistance provided during the assumption of the parental roles.

Birth is the fundamental human experience of renovation and, simultaneously, of continuity, of projected hope and irreversibility (Iori, 2001). The parental relationship represents the assumption of a responsibility which *never ends*, even if the couple should break up. The relational complexity of any generative encounter expresses the close connection of the lived experiences which intersect in this event: a body that changes in order to make space for a new life and the months spent in a woman's womb: an experience which leaves a mark for the rest of our lives (Rich, 1996). Gender differences render this experience *shared* but *different* for mothers and fathers. Although procreation is a *dual* process, childbirth only concerns the woman's body. Consequently, the modalities and developments of maternity and paternity are necessarily different.

Women receive biological signs and educational orientations which have always indicated maternity as a possibility/predestination (whether it is later accepted or rejected). In contrast, for men the idea of virility is constructed outside the notion of paternity. Furthermore, whereas women set up a dialogue with their child during pregnancy, fathers assume a paternal role much later. When the woman-mother tells her partner that she is pregnant, the father-to-be begins a slow process towards the assumption of his parental role, even though this is generally experienced in terms of extraneousness. Despite the fact that they might participate, men actually become *fathers* only when they hold the baby in their arms, and sometimes not even then. In addition, for a long time the elaboration of paternity remains a rational, rather than emotional, fact. To the participation in the delivery room there does not always correspond an educational involvement, especially when it does not express gender differences, with their respective specificities and partialities.

The traditional educational 'absence' of fathers is slowly turning into an increasing awareness of their formative role, which is all the more important in those situations where fathers manage to remain 'loyal' to their gender in the encounter with the Other/child: "Good and heroic men are generations in formation: cuddled in the hearts and cradled in the arms of fathers who were in their turn cuddled in the hearts and initiated in the arms of their own fathers" (Keen, 1993).

The *birth of the first child* represents a critical and extremely complex moment which involves a relational reorganization and a redefinition of one's identity. The real history of the family begins with the transition to the procreative phase, a crucial event which marks the boundary between youth and adulthood. This existential turning point is lived as a divide from a past, during which the couple communicated on the basis of paradigms which now appear inadequate.

If the relationship of the couple is fragile and immature, these changes can bring to the surface either new or latent relational instabilities. Nowadays, fathers and mothers express the experience of becoming parents in rather different ways from the past. Very often, young couples feel unprepared and need some support in order to face this moment, which entails the assumption of a permanent responsibility. If this is so, it is also because the models represented by earlier generations are considered inadequate for the reality of the new families.

Parenthood can assume a transformational characteristic of *growth* in the life of a couple that knows how to welcome a child as an enrichment of their previous relationship. But mutuality is not always exempt from ambiguous symbiotic connections or unconscious refusals. Furthermore, the ego-alter rivalry which characterizes father-child and mother-child relationships, has never been unproblematic: suffice to think of all the parricides, infanticides and exoricides already present in Greek mythology and in the tragedies of Orestes, Oedipus and Medea.

The first requirement of parenthood is the ability to see the Other – who with his/her new life enters a whole network of consolidated relationships – as the 'you' of a new personal encounter, rather than, as it often happens, perceiving him/her as another Self, an instrumental presence or, not so rarely, an 'intruder'.

Every family, when a child is born, becomes in fact a relational system, but it is not a system in itself, as it constantly interacts with its context. In addition, this system is constantly changing, and in fact during a single generation the structure of the family unit has drastically changed and new typologies of family types have formed. As a consequence, even the cycle of family life, female and male roles, parental duties, and educational styles have become increasingly complex.

Procreation places itself within this complex *system*, which is in constant connection with other social systems (beginning with the health system which materially hosts childbirth). This complexity organizes on the basis of the relationship between the subjects that compose the family and their relationship with the external world. Every birth thus activates a system of systems, a structure of material and imaginary elements which depend on each other. As a consequence, by modifying one element, we modify the entire system (Von Bertalanffy, 1976).

By connecting multiple factors concerning reproduction, this complexity enables us to know, understand and, somehow contextualize them, thereby retrieving the social, symbolic and cultural dimension of birth. In particular, mothers represent a solid link between different generations, a medium of communication and *care*. It is up to them to create life and knowledge, thus assuming a much greater function than the biological one: to reproduce humanity, i.e., to *bring the world into the world* (Cavarero, 1989), to reproduce human beings and, as Edith Stein states, "to protect, guard and help develop real humanity" (Stein, 1987).

Acknowledging the value of this *culture of care* means to reactivate critically the history, the knowledge, and the relationships amongst subjects and to become aware both of those feminine connotations which have been reduced to invisibility and of the often *subversive* (Gilligan, 1987) character of the knowledge involved in care.

Reproduction can thus be understood as a biological and symbolic process that embodies and defends the larger notion of the *ethics of care*. Caring for childbirth therefore forms a new solidarity, in that it potentially founds and nourishes a social culture based on the diffusion of responsibility and on the idea of caring about.

The meeting between medical and human science thus posits itself as an occasion to re-evaluate the efficiency we assign to techniques, in order to favor a perspective based on an increasing humanization of the 'coming into the world' process, in order to find, from the very beginning, those relationships between newborns and their families that the procedures of progressive medicalization seem to have disrupted.

The health of the newborn baby should of course be *protected*, but at the same time, s/he should also be *welcomed*. Childbirth can retrieve its humanity only if we acknowledge the value of the human relationships entailed by the 'normal complexity' of coming into the world, and if we establish our practice on this knowledge.

References

Arcidiacono C: Oltre il tabù del dolore: la fatica e il piacere di esistere e far nascere. In: Oakley A, P Romito et al.: Le culture del parto. Feltrinelli, Milano 1985

Bateson G: Verso un'ecologia della mente. Adelphi, Milano 1976

Binswanger L: Per un'antropologia fenomenologia. Feltrinelli, Milano 1989

Borgna E: I conflitti del conoscere. Feltrinelli, Milano 1992

Borgna E: L'arcipelago delle emozioni. Feltrinelli, Milano 2001

Cavarero A: Dire la nascita. In: Diotima. Mettere al mondo il mondo. La Tartaruga, Milano 1989

Dilthey W: Idee per una psicologia descrittiva e analitica. In: Dilthey W: Per la fondazione delle scienze dello spirito. Angeli, Milano 1985

Duden B: Il corpo della donna come luogo pubblico. Bollati Boringhieri, Milano 1994

Finzi SV: Il romanzo della famiglia. Mondatori, Milano 1992

Galimberti U: Il corpo. Feltrinelli, Milano 1983

Galimberti U: Psiche e techne: l'uomo nell'età della tecnica. Feltrinelli, Milano 2002

Gélis J: Il parto e l'evoluzione della coscienza del corpo nell'epoca moderna (XVI–XIX sec.). In: Oakley A, P Romito et al.: Le culture del parto. Feltrinelli, Milano 1985

Gilligan C: Con voce di donna. Feltrinelli, Milano 1987

Heidegger M: Essere e tempo. Longanesi, Milano 1976

Husserl E: Idee per una fenomenologia pura e una filosofia fenomenologia, vol II. Einaudi, Torino 1986

Husserl E: La crisi delle scienze europee e la fenomenologia trascendentale. Il Saggiatore, Milano 1987
Husserl E: Meditazioni cartesiane. Bompiani, Milano 1989
Iori V: Essere per l'educazione. La Nuova Italia, Firenze 1988
Iori V: Il sapere dei sentimenti. In: ID, (a cura di), Emozioni e sentimenti nel lavoro educativo e sociale. Guerini, Milano 2003
Iori V: Fondamenti pedagogici e trasformazioni familiari. La Scuola, Brescia 2001
Jaspers K: Il medico nell'età della tecnica. Raffaello Cortina, Milano 1991
Keen S: Nel ventre dell'eroe (trad. dall'inglese). Frassinelli, Como 1993
Marcel G: Être et avoir. In: Giornale Metafisico. Abete, Roma 1974
Merleau-Ponty M: Fenomenologia della percezione, 1945. Il Saggiatore, Milano 1980
Mortari L: Per un'etica della cura a partire dalla relazione materna. In: Musi E, M Toscani: Theuth e Thamus. Unicopli, Milano 2003
Musi, E: Per una pedagogia della nascita. In: La Famiglia (2005) 230
Nordio S: Epistemologia della e nel'educazione medica. In: Bertolini G: (a cura di) Diventare medici. Guerini, Milano 1994
Parma E: La medicina generale: un ponte tra la medicina come scienza della natura e come scienza umana. In: Bertolini G: (a cura di) Diventare medici. Guerini, Milano 1994
Pizzini F: (a cura di) Sulla scena del parto: luoghi, figure, pratiche. Angeli, Milano 1985
Pizzini F: Corpo medico e corpo femminile. Parto, riproduzione artificiale e menopausa. Angeli, Milano 1999
Regalia A: La medicalizzazione della nascita. In: Binda W: (a cura di) Diventare famiglia. La nascita del primo figlio. Angeli, Milano 1997
Rich A: Nato di donna. Milano, Garzanti 1996
Stein E: La donna. Città Nuova, Roma 1987
Von Bertalanffy L: Teoria generale dei sistemi. ILI, Milano 1971
Winnicott DW: Dal luogo delle origini. Raffello Cortina, Milano 1990

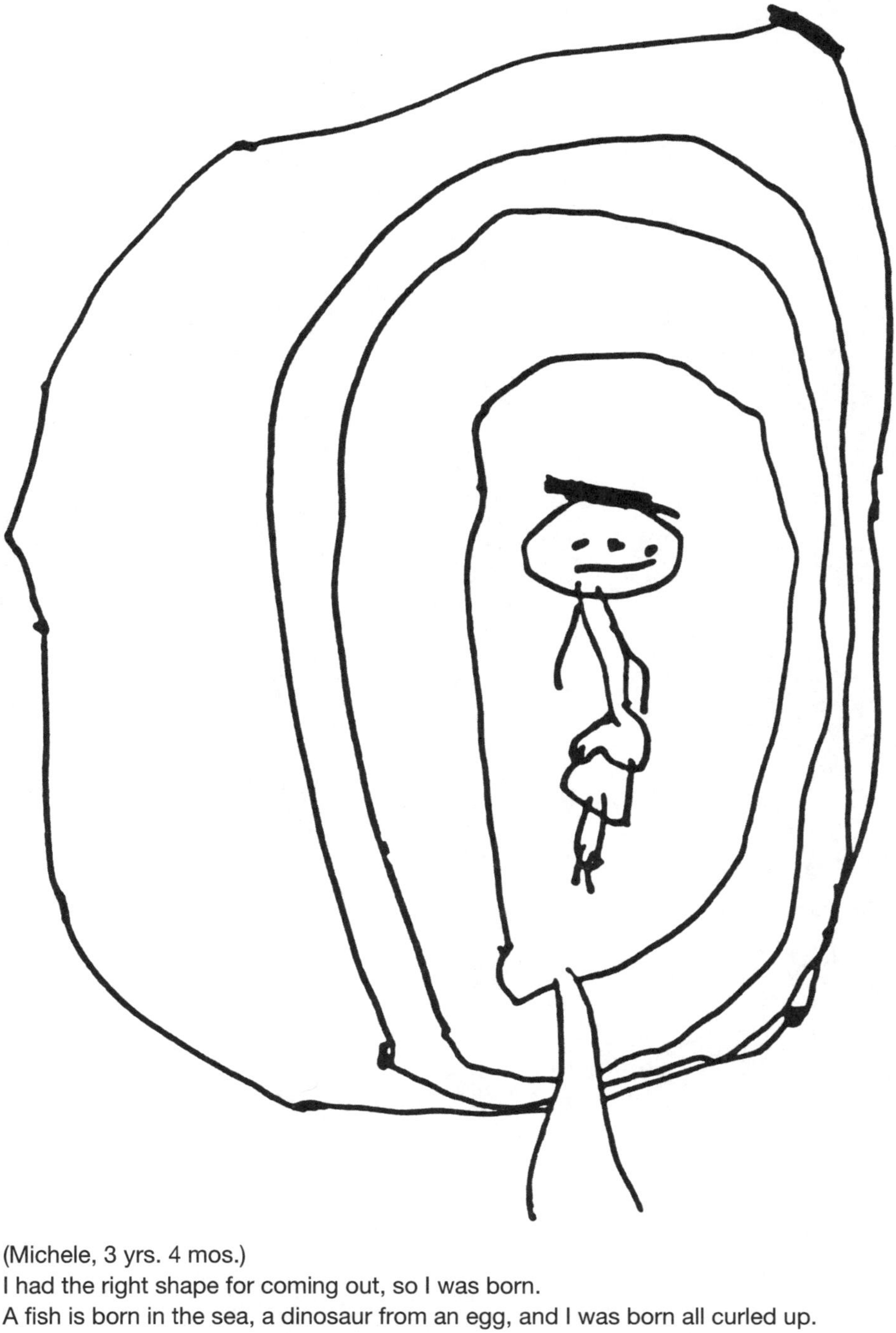

(Michele, 3 yrs. 4 mos.)
I had the right shape for coming out, so I was born.
A fish is born in the sea, a dinosaur from an egg, and I was born all curled up.

6. Intentional attunement: Mirror neurons, inter-subjectivity, and autism

Vittorio Gallese; Department of Neuroscience, Physiology Department, University of Parma, Italy

Introduction

The relationship between social complexity and cognition is well established in primates. Humphrey (1976) originally suggested that the intelligence of primates primarily evolved to solve social problems and this view is supported by empirical data. Several studies revealed the unique capacity of non-human primates to understand the quality of the relationships within their social group, not only in terms of kin, but also in terms of coalitions, friendship and alliances. The capacity to understand co-specific behaviors as goal-related provides considerable benefits to individuals, as they can predict actions of others. The advantage of such a cognitive skill would allow individuals also to influence and manipulate behavior (see the Machiavellian Intelligence hypothesis (Whiten, Byrne (1997)), or to achieve better social cooperation within a group.

As pointed-out by Tomasello and Call (1997), primates can categorize and understand third-party social relationships. The evolution of this cognitive trait seems to be related to the necessity to deal with social complexities that arose when group-living individuals had to compete for scarce and patchily distributed resources. Dunbar (1992) suggested a relationship between primates' group size and the degree of expansion of the neo-cortex. The increase of social group complexity exerted a powerful pressure for the development of more sophisticated cognitive skills.

The problem of intentionality in primates was almost simultaneously and independently raised by Humphrey (1978, 1980) and Premack and Woodruff (1978). The traditional view in the cognitive sciences holds that human beings are able to understand the behavior of others in terms of their mental states by exploiting what is commonly designated as "Folk Psychology". The capacity for attributing mental states – intentions, beliefs and desires – to others has been defined as the theory of mind (ToM; Premack, Woodruff 1978). The attributes of "Folk Psychology" have been thus basically identified with the view of Theory of Mind (Carruthers, Smith 1996). A common trend on this issue has been to emphasize that non-human primates, apes included, do not rely on mentally based accounts for others' behavior (Hayes, 1998; Povinelli et al., 2000). According to this perspective, social cognition becomes almost synonymous of mind reading abilities.

The dichotomous account of primate social cognition based on a sharp evolutionary discontinuity between species of behavior readers (non-human primates) and one species of mind readers (humans) appears, however, over-simplistic.

As recently pointed out by Barrett and Henzi (2005), this traditional approach is "…heavily oriented toward a particular model of cognition that focuses solely on internal mental representations, whereas recent work in cognitive science and neurobiology argues for a more distributed and embodied approach".

In the present paper I propose a different approach. I submit that social cognition is not only "social meta-cognition", that is, *explicitly* thinking about the contents of someone else's mind by means of abstract representations. There is also an experiential dimension of interpersonal relationships, which enables a direct grasping of the *sense* of the actions performed by others, and of the emotions and sensations they experience. This dimension of social cognition is embodied in such a way that it mediates between the multimodal experimental knowledge we hold of our living body, and the experience we make of others.

I proposed that our capacity to share experiences with others rests on the constitution of a shared meaningful interpersonal space. This "shared manifold" (Gallese, 2001, 2003, 2005) can be characterized at the functional level as embodied simulation (Gallese, 2005), a specific mechanism by which our brain/body system models its interactions with the world (for a similar account of the mechanisms at the basis of empathy, see Preston and De Waal, 2002). I submit that embodied simulation constitutes a crucial functional mechanism in social cognition.

The self/other distinction in my opinion is not the most difficult problem in social cognition, neither from a theoretical, nor from an empirical point of view. The "hard problem" in social cognition is to understand how the epistemic gulf separating single individuals can be overcome. The solipsistic attitude inspired by Folk Psychology and purported by the approach of classic cognitive science, leaves this difficult problem unsolved. Recent neuro-scientific evidence suggests alternative answers. Here I discuss this evidence and provide a theoretical framework for its interpretation. Before doing so, I want to briefly discuss the problem of social cognition from an ontogenetic point of view.

The ontogenesis of social cognition

The idea of "social cognition" sounds almost as a pleonasm, since from an ontogenetic point of view the relationship between cognition and the social dimension is intrinsically tight.

At the very onset of our life, interpersonal relations are established when a full-blown self-conscious subject of experience is not yet constituted. However, the absence of a subject does not preclude the presence of a primitive "we-centric space". The infant shares this space with others. At a few hours after birth, neo nates display facial imitation (Meltzoff, Brooks, 2001). Furthermore, empirical research has shown that mothers and infants systematically engage in mutually coordinated activities during which their movements, facial expressions, and voice intonation synchronize in time (Reddy et al., 1997). From 4 months of age onwards, infants and mothers show proto-dialogic behaviors in which they time their behavior in a bi-directional coordinated way (Trevarthen, 1979). Approximately at the same age, infants become sensitive to social contingencies (Striano et al., 2005). According to Daniel Stern (1985/2000), this evidence suggests that such proto-dialogic behaviors enable mother and infant to establish an affective attuning by means of which inner feeling states can be shared.

According to my hypothesis, the shared we-centric space enables the social bootstrapping of cognitive and affective development because it provides a powerful tool to detect and incorporate coherence, regularity, and predictability in the course of the interactions of the individual with the environment. The we-centric space is likely paralleled by the development of perspective spaces defined by the establishment of the capacity to distinguish self from other, as long as self-control develops. Within each of these newly acquired perspective spaces, information can be better segregated in discrete channels (visual, somato-sensory, etc.) making the perception of the world more finely grained. The concurrent development of language possibly contributes to further segregate single characters or modalities of experience from the original multimodal perceptive world. Yet, the more mature capacity to segregate the modes of interaction, together with the capacity to carve out the subject and the object of the interaction, do not obliterate the shared we-centric space.

In fact, the establishment of a self-centered perspective is paralleled by the creation of an epistemic gap between self and others. The gulf separating self from non-self poses a challenge to any account of inter-subjectivity and social cognition. I suggest that the inter-subjective we-centric space may provide the individual with a powerful tool to help overcome such epistemic gap. If my hypothesis is correct, social identity, the "selfness" we readily attribute to others, the inner feeling of "being-like-you" triggered by our encounter with others, are the result of a preserved shared we-centric space.

The proposition that self-other physical and epistemic interactions are shaped and conditioned by the same type of body and environmental constraints sounds almost like a truism. Less trivial, in my opinion, is the fact that this common relational character of inter-subjectivity is underpinned, at the level of the brain, by shared neural networks, the mirror neuron systems, compressing the "who-done-it", "who-is-it" specifications into a narrower content state. This content specifies what kinds of interaction or state are at stake. A concise overview of the evidence supporting the existence of such shared neural mechanisms will be the focus of the next sections.

The mirror neuron system for actions in monkeys and humans: empirical evidence

About ten years ago, a new class of premotor neurons was discovered in the ventral premotor cortex of the macaque monkey brain. These neurons discharge not only when the monkey executes goal-related hand actions like grasping objects, but also when observing other individuals (monkeys or humans) executing similar actions. They were called "mirror neurons" (Gallese et al., 1996; Rizzolatti et al., 1996). Neurons with similar properties were later discovered in a sector of the posterior parietal cortex reciprocally connected with area F5 (Gallese et al., 2002; Rizzolatti, Craighero, 2004; Fogassi et al., 2005).

Action observation causes in the observer the automatic activation of the same neural mechanism triggered by action execution. It has been proposed that this mechanism could be at the basis of a direct form of action understanding (Gallese et al., 1996; Rizzolatti, Craighero, 2004; Rizzolatti et al., 2001).

Further studies carried out by our research group at the Department of Neuroscience of the University of Parma corroborated and extended the original hypothesis. In a paper by Umiltà et al. (2001) it was shown that F5 mirror neurons are also activated when the final critical part of the observed action, that is, the hand-object interaction, is hidden. In a second study, Kohler et al. (2002) showed that a particular class of F5 mirror neurons, "audio-visual mirror neurons", could be driven not only by action execution and observation, but also by the sound produced by the same action.

More recently, the most lateral part of area F5 was explored where a population of mirror neurons related to the execution/observation of mouth actions was described (Ferrari et al., 2003). The majority of these neurons discharge when the monkey executes and observes transitive, object-related ingestion actions, such as grasping objects with the mouth, biting, or licking. However, a small percentage of mouth-related mirror neurons discharge during the observation of intransitive, communicative facial actions performed by the experimenter in front of the monkey ("communicative mirror neurons" (Ferrari et al., 2003)). Thus, mirror neurons seem also to underpin aspects of the monkeys' social facial communication.

Several studies using different experimental methods and techniques have demonstrated also in the human brain the existence of a mirror neuron system matching action perception and execution. During action observation there is a strong activation of premotor and parietal areas, the likely human homologue of the areas in which mirror neurons were originally described in the monkey (Rizzolatti, Craighero, 2004; Rizzolatti et al., 2001; Gallese et al., 2004). Furthermore, the mirror neuron matching system for actions in humans is coarsely organized in a somatotopic fashion, with distinct cortical regions within the premotor and posterior parietal cortices being activated by the observation/execution of mouth, hand, and foot related actions (Buccino et al., 2001).

The involvement of the motor system during observation of communicative mouth actions in humans is shown by the results of recent fMRI and TMS studies (Buccino et al., 2004; Watkins et al., 2003). The observation of communicative, or speech-related mouth actions, facilitate the excitability of the motor system involved in the production of the same actions.

A recent study carried out by Buxbaum et al. (2005) on posterior parietal patients with ideomotor apraxia has shown that they were not only disproportionately impaired in the imitation of transitive as compared to intransitive gestures, but they also showed a strong correlation between imitation deficits and the incapacity to recognize observed goal-related meaningful hand actions. As argued by the authors of this study, these results further corroborate the view that the same action representations support both action production and action understanding. In the next section I will introduce new empirical results suggesting that embodied simulation may play a role even in more complex social cognitive abilities.

Mirror neurons and the understanding of intentions

Monkeys may utilize the mirror neuron system to optimize their social interactions. As we have seen in the previous section, audio-visual mirror neurons can be driven not only by action execution and observation, but also by the sound produced by the same action (Kohler, 2002). This mirroring mechanism can support social facilitation in monkeys. It has been recently shown that the observation and hearing of noisy eating actions facilitates eating behavior in the pigtailed macaque monkeys (Macaca nemestrina) (Ferrari et al., 2005).

Another recently study showed that pigtailed macaque monkeys recognize when they are imitated by a human experimenter (Paukner et al., 2005). Pigtailed macaques preferentially look at an experimenter imitating the monkeys' object-directed actions compared with an experimenter manipulating an identical object but not imitating their actions. Since both experimenters acted in synchrony with the monkeys, the monkeys based this preference not on temporal contingency, but took into account the structural components of the experimenters' actions.

It may well be the case, as repeatedly argued, that macaque monkeys are not capable of motor imitation – though recent evidence shows that they are capable of cognitive imitation (Subiaul et al., 2004). The study by Paukner et al. (2005) nevertheless shows that macaque monkeys do have the capacity to discriminate between very similar observed goal-related actions on the basis of their degree of similarity with the goal-related actions the monkeys themselves have just carried out. This capacity seems to be cognitively quite sophisticated, in that it implies a certain degree of meta-cognition relative to the domain of goal-related action.

I suggest that macaque monkeys might have a rudimentary form of "teleological stance", a likely precursor to a full-blown intentional stance. This hypothesis extends to the phylogenetic domain as the ontogenetic scenario proposed for human infants (Gergely, Csibra, 2003). New experiments are being designed in my laboratory to test this hypothesis. Monkeys certainly do not have a full-blown *explicit* mentalization. Thus, what makes humans different? Language certainly plays a key role. Though, at present, we can only make hypotheses about the relevant neural mechanisms underpinning the mentalizing abilities of humans, still poorly understood from a functional point of view. In particular, we do not have a clear neuro-scientific model of how humans can understand the intentions promoting the actions of others they observe.

When an individual starts a movement in order to attain a goal, such as picking up a pen, she/he has clear in mind what he/she is going to do, for example, write a note on a piece of paper. In this simple sequence of motor acts, the final goal of the whole action is present in mind and is somehow reflected in each motor act of the sequence. The action intention, therefore, is set before the beginning of the movements. This also means that when we are going to execute a given action we can also predict its consequences. But a given action can originate from very different intentions. Suppose one sees someone else grasping a cup. Mirror neurons for grasping will most likely be activated in the observer's brain. The direct matching between the observed action and its motor representation in the observer's brain, however, can only tell us what the action is (grasping) and not why the action occurred. This has led to arguing against the relevance of mirror neurons for social cognition, and in particular, for determining the intentions of others (Jacob, Jeannerod, 2005).

But what is an action intention? Determining why action A (grasping the cup) was executed means determining its intention and can be equivalent to detecting the goal of the still unexecuted and impending subsequent action (say, drinking from the cup). In a recently published fMRI study (Iacoboni et al., 2005), we tried to address these issues experimentally. Subjects watched three kinds of stimuli: grasping hand actions without a context, context only (a scene containing objects), and grasping hand actions embedded in contexts. In the latter condition the context suggested the intention associated with the grasping action (either drinking or cleaning up). Actions embedded in contexts, compared with the other two conditions, yielded a significant signal increase in the posterior part of the inferior frontal gyrus and the adjacent sector of the ventral premotor cortex where hand actions are represented. Thus, premotor mirror areas – areas active during the execution and the observation of an action – previously thought to be involved only in action recognition – are actually also involved in understanding the "why" of action, that is, the intention that promotes it.

Another interesting result of this study is that being or not being explicitly instructed to determine the intention of the observed actions of others makes no difference in terms of the activation of the premotor mirror areas. This means that – at least for simple actions as those employed in this study – the attribution of intentions occurs by default and is supported by the mandatory activation of an embodied simulation mechanism.

The neuro-physiological mechanism at the basis of the relationship between intention detection and action prediction was recently unveiled. Fogassi et al. (2005) described a class of parietal mirror neurons whose discharge during the observation of an act (e.g., grasping an object), is conditioned by the type of a subsequent act (e.g., bringing the object to the mouth) specifying the overall action intention. This study shows that the inferior parietal lobe of the monkey contains mirror neurons discharging in association with monkey motor acts (grasping) only when they are embedded in a specific action aimed at different goals. For example, a neuron discharges when the monkey grasps an object only if the aim of grasping is to bring the object into the mouth and not aimed to place it in a cup. It appears therefore that these neurons code the same motor act differently depending on the distal, overarching action goal. Single motor acts are dependent on each other as they participate in the overarching distal goal of an action, thus forming pre-wired intentional chains, in which each next motor act is facilitated by the previously executed one.

The visual response of many of these parietal mirror neurons is similar to their motor response. In fact, they discharge differentially depending on whether the observed grasping is followed by bringing the grasped object to the mouth or by placing it in a cup. It must be emphasized that the neurons discharge before the monkey observes the experimenter starting the second motor act (bringing the object to the mouth or placing it into the cup). This new property of parietal mirror neurons suggests that in addition to recognizing the goal of the observed motor act, they distinguish identical motor acts according to the action in which these acts are embedded. Thus, these neurons not only code the observed motor act but also seem to allow the observing monkey to predict the agent's next action, henceforth his/her overall intention. It is possible to interpret this mechanism as the neural correlate of the beginning of the sophisticated mentalizing abilities characterizing our species.

The mechanism of intention understanding just described appears to be rather simple: depending on which motor chain is activated, the observer is going to activate the motor scheme of what, most likely, the agent is going to do. How can such a mechanism be formed? At present we can only make speculations. It can be hypothesized that the statistical detection of what actions most frequently follow other actions, as they are habitually performed or observed in the social environment, can restrict preferential paths chaining together different motor schemes. At the neural level, this can be accomplished by the chaining of different populations of mirror neurons coding not only the observed motor act, but also those that in a given context would normally follow.

Ascribing simple intentions would therefore consist in predicting a forthcoming new goal. According to this perspective, action prediction and the ascription of intentions are related phenomena, suggested by the same functional mechanism – embodied simulation. In contrast with what mainstream cognitive science would maintain, action prediction and the attribution of intentions – at least of simple intentions – do not appear to belong to different cognitive realms, but both pertain to embodied simulation mechanisms suggested by the activation of chains of logically related mirror neurons (Fogassi et al., 2005; Iacoboni et al., 2005).

If this is true, it follows that one important difference between humans and monkeys could be the higher level of recursion attained by the mirror neuron system for actions in our species. A similar proposal has been recently put forward in relation to the faculty of language by contrasting our species, capable of mastering hierarchically complex "phrase structure grammars", with other non-human primate species, confined to the use of much simpler "finite state grammars" (Hauser et al., 2002; Hauser, Fitch, 2004). A quantitative difference in computational power and degree of recursion could produce a qualitative leap in social cognition.

Mirroring emotions and sensations

As already suggested by Charles Darwin (1872) the coordinated activity of sensory-motor and affective neural systems results in the simplification and automatization of the behavioral responses that living organisms are supposed to produce in order to survive. Emotions constitute one of the earliest ways available to the individual of acquiring knowledge about its situation, thus enabling a reorganization of this knowledge on the basis of the outcome of the relations shared with others. The integrity of the sensory-motor system indeed appears to be critical for the recognition of emotions displayed by others (Adolphs, 2003), because the sensory-motor system appears to support the reconstruction of what it would feel like to be in a particular emotion, by means of simulation of the related body state. The implication of this process for empathy should be obvious.

In a recently published fMRI study we showed that experiencing disgust and witnessing the same emotion expressed by the facial mimicry of someone else, both activate the same neural structure – the anterior insula – at the same overlapping location (Wicker et al., 2003). When we see the facial expression of someone else, and this perception leads us to experience a particular affective state, the other's emotion is constituted, experienced and therefore directly understood by means of an embodied simulation producing a shared body state. It is the activation of a neural mechanism shared by the observer and the observed that enables direct experiential understanding. A similar simulation-based mechanism has been proposed by Goldman and Sripada (2005) as "unmediated resonance".

Let us now examine somatic sensations as the target of our social perception. As repeatedly emphasized by phenomenology, touch has a privileged status in making possible the social attribution of lived personhood to others. "Let's keep in touch" is a common phrase in everyday language, which metaphorically describes the wish of being related, being in contact with someone else. Such examples show how the tactile dimension can be intimately related to the interpersonal dimension.

As predicted by the shared manifold hypothesis (Gallese, 2001, 2003, 2005), empirical evidence suggests that the first-person experience of being touched on one's body activates the same neural networks activated by observing the body of someone else being touched (Keysers et al., 2004; Blakemore et al., 2005). This double pattern of activation of the same somato-sensory-related brain regions suggests that our capacity to experience and directly understand the tactile experience of others could be mediated by embodied simulation, that is, by the externally triggered activation of *some* of the same neural networks underpinning our own tactile sensations. The study by Blakemore et al. (2005) actually shows that the *degree of activation* of the same somato-sensory areas activated during both the subjective tactile experience and its observation in others could be an important mechanism enabling the subject to sort out *who* is being touched. In fact, what this paper shows is that the difference between empathizing with someone else tactile sensation, and actually feeling the same sensation on one's body (as in the case of synesthesia) is only a matter of degrees of activation of the same shared brain areas. These data support the concept that differentiating who is who (patient vs. observer) does not pose a problem to my hypothesis.

I suggest that a similar embodied simulation mechanism underlies our experience of the painful sensations of others. Single neuron recording experiments carried out in neurosurgical patients who are awake (Hutchison et al., 1999), and fMRI (Morrison et al., 2004; Singer et al., 2004; Botvinick et al., 2005; Jackson et al., 2005), Empathy, and TMS experiments (Avenanti et al., 2005) carried out in healthy subjects, all show that the same neural structures are activated both during the subjective experience of pain and the direct observation, or symbolically mediated knowledge that someone else is probably experiencing the same painful sensation.

It should be noted that the results of the fMRI (Morrison et al., 2004; Singer et al., 2004; Botvinick et al., 2005; Jackson et al., 2005) and TMS (Avenanti et al., 2005) studies show that the overlap of activation in the self/other experience conditions can be modulated in terms of the brain areas involved by the cognitive demands imposed by the type of tasks. When subjects are required to simply watch the painful stimulation experienced by some stranger's body part (Avenanti et al., 2005), the observer extracts the basic sensory qualities of the pain experienced by others mapping it somatotopically onto his/her own sensory-motor system. However, when subjects are required to imagine the pain suffered by their partner out of their sight (Singer et al., 2004), only brain areas mediating the affective quality of pain (the anterior cingulate cortex and the anterior insula) are activated. In particular, the anterior cingulate cortex (ACC) appears to mediate the affective dimension of pain processing and the motivational aspects of response selection. Thus, in the context of the perception of pain, the ACC could play a role in linking events with outcomes, allowing the prediction and avoidance of noxious stimuli (Singer et al., 2004). As it has been convincingly argued (Singer, Frith, 2005), one can conclude that the particular mental attitude of individuals could be the key variable determining the degree and quality of the activation of shared neural circuits when experiencing the sensations of others, as in the case of pain.

Intentional attunement, embodied simulation, and empathy

Some functional mechanism must mediate between the multimodal experimental knowledge we hold of our living body, and the experience we make of others. Such body-related experiential knowledge enables a direct grasping of the sense of the actions performed by others, and of the emotions and sensations they experience.

When confronting the intentional behavior of others, we experience a specific phenomenal state of "intentional attunement". This phenomenal state generates a peculiar quality of familiarity with other individuals, produced by the collapse of the intentions of others into the observer's ones. This seems to be one important component of what being empathic is about (Preston, De Waal, 2002). Of course, self-other identity is not all there is in empathy. Empathy, with respect to emotional contagion, entails the capacity to experience what others do experience, while being able to attribute these shared experiences to *others* and not to the self. The quality of our lived experience of the external world and its content are constrained by the presence of other subjects that are intelligible, while preserving their altered character. This altered character is in fact also evident at the sub-personal level, instantiated by the different neural networks coming into play, and/or by their different degree of activation, when *I* act with respect to when others act, or when *I* experience an emotion or a sensation with respect to when others do the same.

When we observe the intentional behavior of others, according to my hypothesis, embodied simulation, a specific mechanism by means of which our brain/body system models its interactions with the world, generates a specific phenomenal state of "intentional attunement". This phenomenal state in turn generates a peculiar quality of familiarity with other individuals, produced by the collapse of the others' intentions into the observer's ones. Embodied simulation constitutes a crucial functional mechanism in social cognition, and can be neuro-biologically characterized. The different mirror neuron systems represent its sub-personal instantiations. By means of embodied simulation we do not just "see" an action, an emotion, or a sensation. Alongside the sensory description of the observed social stimuli, internal representations of the body states associated with these actions, emotions, and sensations are evoked in the observer, "as if" she/he were doing a similar action or experiencing a similar emotion or sensation.

Any intentional relation can be mapped as a relation between a subject and an object. The mirror neuron matching systems described in this paper map the different intentional relations in a fashion that is neutral about the specific quality or identity of the agentive/subjective parameter. By means of a shared functional state realized in two different bodies that nevertheless obey the same functional rules, the "objective other" becomes "another self".

Embodied simulation is probably not the only functional mechanism behind social cognition. The meaning of social stimuli can also be decoded on the basis of the explicit cognitive elaboration of their contextual perceptual features, by exploiting previously acquired knowledge about relevant aspects of the situation to be analyzed. Our capacity to attribute false beliefs to others, our most sophisticated meta-cognitive mind reading abilities, are likely to involve the activation of large regions of our brain, certainly larger than a putative and domain-specific Theory of Mind Module. These brain sectors certainly encompass the sensory-motor system. In fact, it has been shown that brain areas reportedly active during mind reading tasks, such as the Superior Temporal Sulcus (STS) region and the paracingulate cortex, also are activated in a simple action prediction task (Ramnani, Miall 2004).

It must be stressed that the use in social transactions of the belief-desire propositional attitudes of Folk Psychology is probably overstated (Hutto, 2004). As emphasized by Bruner (1990), "When things *are as they should be*, the narratives of Folk Psychology are unnecessary". Furthermore, recent evidence shows that 15 month-old infants understand false beliefs (Onishi, Baillargeon 2005). These results seem to suggest that typical aspects of mind reading, such as the attribution of false beliefs to others, can be explained on the basis of low-level mechanisms, which develop well before fully developed linguistic competence.

The idea put forward by Gergely and Csibra (2003) that the intentional stance can be anticipated by a much earlier developed "teleological stance" is consistent with this view. It should be added, though, that non-mentalistic accounts of the so-called "teleological stance" displayed by young infants are possible (e.g. by relying on mechanisms such as attention, physical causality, stimulus relevance, and the like), thus corroborating the notion that the role of propositional attitudes in social cognition is exaggerated, and that they are much less frequently employed than was assumed by classic cognitive science. A target for future research will be to determine how embodied simulation, which is experience-based, and probably the most ancient mechanism from an evolutionary point of view, may support more sophisticated, language-mediated forms of mind reading.

It is possible that embodied simulation mechanisms might be crucial in the course of the long learning process required to become fully competent in how to use propositional attitudes, as during the repetitive exposure of children to the narration of stories (Hutto, 2004). In fact, embodied simulation is certainly operative during language processing (Gallese, 2005; Rizzolatti, Craighero, 2004; Gallese, Lakoff, 2005).

If intentional attunement does indeed play a crucial role in inter-subjectivity, one should expect its deficiency to cause problems at various levels in social cognition. In the next section I explore the possibility of applying the intentional attunement hypothesis to interpret pathological aspects of social cognition, such as those exemplified by the Autistic Spectrum Disorder.

The mirror neuron hypothesis of autism

The Autistic Spectrum Disorder (ASD) is a severe and chronic developmental disorder characterized by social and communicative deficits and by a reduced interest in the environment, towards which restricted and often stereotyped initiatives are taken (Dawson et al., 2002). To be an autistic child means, with variable degrees of severity, to be unable to establish meaningful social communications and bonds, to establish visual contact with the world of others, to share attention with others, to imitate behavior of others or understand their intentions, emotions, and sensations.

Let us briefly focus on some of the early onset symptoms. Towards the end of the first year of life, autistic children experience difficulties or even the impossibility of orienting on the basis of cues provided by others. They are incapable of sharing attention with others and of reacting in a similar fashion to others' emotions. They are also highly impaired in recognizing human faces or in displaying imitative behaviors. All of these early manifestations of autism share a common root: the cognitive skills required to establish meaningful bonds with others are missing or seriously impaired.

My hypothesis is that these deficits, like those observed in the related Asperger Syndrome, are attributed to a deficit or malfunctioning of "intentional attunement", because of a malfunctioning of embodied simulation mechanisms, in turn produced by a dysfunction of the mirror neuron systems. If this is true – as held throughout this paper – that at the basis of our social competence is *in primis* the capacity to constitute an implicit and directly shared we-centric space, enabling us to establish a link with the multiple intentional relations initiated by others, then it follows that a disruption of this shared multiplicity and the consequent incapacity to develop a full and comprehensive intentional attunement with others, could be the core of the problems of the autistic mind.

The lack of a fully developed intentional attunement will produce various and diverse cognitive and executive deficits, all sharing the same functional origin: a lack or malfunctioning of embodied simulation routines, likely resulting from impairments in connectivity and/or functioning of the mirror neuron system. If my hypothesis is correct, the suggested intentional attunement deficit should become manifest at the various levels of social cognition it normally underlies. A series of experimental data seems to suggest this to be the case.

A recent study investigating postural adjustments in autistic children has shown that compared to healthy individuals, they use motor strategies basically relying on feed-back information, rather than on feed-forward modes of control. Such disturbance of executive control strategies prevents autistic children from adopting anticipatory postural adjustments (Schmitz et al., 2003). Given the functional characterization of embodied simulation as an anticipatory mechanism, it is difficult not to interpret these data as evidence of a simulation deficit. Such postural deficits are not intrinsically social; however, they could stem from a disruption within the executive control domain of a functional mechanism – embodied simulation – which I proposed to be at the root of the constitution of the we-centric experiential interpersonal space.

Two recent studies employing different techniques such as EEG (Oberman et al., 2005) and trans-cranial magnetic stimulation (Theoret et al., 2005) show that individuals with ASD might be suffering an action simulation deficit induced by a dysfunction of their mirror system for action. The study by Oberman et al. (2005) showed that ASD individuals, with respect to with healthy controls, did not show any mu frequency suppression over the sensory-motor cortex during action observation. The study by Theoret et al. (2005) showed that, again with respect to healthy controls, ASD individuals did not show TMS-induced hand muscle facilitation during hand action observation.

A further indication of embodied simulation deficits in ASD is exemplified by imitation deficits. Autistic children have problems in both symbolic and non-symbolic imitative behaviors, in imitating the use of objects, in imitating facial gestures, and in vocal imitation (Rogers, 1999). These deficits characterize both high- and low-functioning forms of autism. Furthermore, imitation deficits are apparent not only in comparison to the performances of healthy subjects, but also to those of mentally retarded non-autistic subjects. According to my hypothesis, imitation deficits in autism are determined by the incapacity to establish a motor equivalence between demonstrator and imitator, most likely due to a malfunctioning of the mirror neuron system, and/or because of a disrupted emotional/affective regulation of the same system. Imitation deficits thus can be hypothesized to be further examples of a disrupted shared manifold.

Let me now briefly turn to emotional-affective deficits. Several studies reported the severe problems which autistic children experience in the facial expression of emotions and its understanding in others (Hobson et al., 1988; Snow et al., 1988; Hobson et al., 1989; Yirmiya et al., 1989). In a recent fMRI study, Dapretto et al. (2005) specifically investigated the neural correlates of the capacity to imitate the facial expressions of basic emotions in high-functioning ASD individuals. This study showed that during observation and imitation, autistic children did not show any activation of the mirror neuron system in the pars opercularis of the inferior frontal gyrus. It should be emphasized that activity in this area was inversely related with symptom severity in the social domain. The authors of this study concluded, "...a dysfunctional mirror neuron system may underlie the social deficits observed in autism". Furthermore, McIntosh et al. (2005) recently showed that individuals with ASD, as compared to healthy controls, do not show automatic mimicry of the facial expression of basic emotions, as revealed by EMG recordings. Hobson and Lee (1999) reported that autistic children score much worse than healthy controls in reproducing the affective qualities of observed actions.

I suggest that all these deficits can be explained as instantiations of intentional attunement deficits produced by defective embodied simulation, likely caused by a malfunctioning of the mirror neuron systems. This hypothesis is further corroborated by the recent finding that the brains of ASD individuals show abnormal thinning of the grey matter in cortical areas known as being part of the mirror neuron system (Hadjikhani et al., 2005), such as ventral premotor, posterior parietal, and superior temporal sulcus cortices. Interestingly, cortical thinning of the mirror neuron system correlated with ASD symptoms severity.

My hypothesis to interpret the ASD as an intentional attunement deficit diverges noticeably from many of the mainstream ideas concerning the origin of this developmental disorder. One of the most credited theories, in spite of its different – not always similar – articulations, suggests that ASD and the related Asperger syndrome are caused by a deficit of a specific mind module, the Theory of Mind module, selected in the course of evolution to build theories about the mind of others (Baron-Cohen et al., 1985; Baron-Cohen 1988). This theory is at present totally untenable, even more so in the light of recent empirical results. A recent study carried out on a patient who suffered a focal bilateral lesion of the anterior cingulate cortex (ACC), previously identified as the candidate site for the Theory of Mind Module, showed no evidence of mind reading deficits (Bird et al., 2004).

A further problem of the mainstream theory of ASD as a deficit Theory of Mind is that it can be hardly reconciled with what we learn from the reports of high functioning autistics or Asperger individuals like Temple Grandin (1995). They claim that in order to understand how they supposedly should feel in given social contexts, and what others supposedly feel and think in those same contexts, they must rely on theorizing. What these reports seem to suggest is that, as I have argued elsewhere (Gallese, 2001), theorizing about the others' mind is not quite the basic deficit of ASD or of Asperger syndrome, but the only compensating strategy available in the absence of more elementary and basic cognitive skills enabling a direct experiential contact with the world of others.

Conclusions

The shared diversity of inter-subjectivity and the intentional attunement it generates constitute a general hypothesis on many aspects of social cognition (Gallese, 2005; Gallese 2005a), which as we have seen, has already empirical grounds at multiple levels, both in healthy and sociopath individuals. Furthermore, this theory and the approaches it generates can establish a more perceptive therapeutic bonds with patients suffering impairments in social cognition, and more generally, in any psychotherapeutic setting.

The appeal of such a scenario consists not only in its parsimony, but also in providing for the first time a neuro-physiological mechanism at the basis of the activation of many of the cortical regions involved in social cognition. We cannot be satisfied with merely knowing that a given cortical area is active during social cognitive tasks. In doing so, we face the risk of resurrecting phrenology. Social cognitive neuroscience must seek to know *why*, *how*, and because of *which functional mechanism* a particular brain area or cortical network happens to be activated in a particular social cognitive task.

It is obvious that embodied simulation and its neural cause fall short of providing a thorough account of what is implied in our sophisticated mentalizing skills. What the results presented here indicate, however, is that embodied mechanisms, involving the activation of the sensory-motor system, seem to have a major role in social cognition. This should persuade us that the automatic translation of the tenets of Folk Psychology into brain modules or circuitries specifically dedicated to mind reading abilities should be carefully scrutinized as it might be a very poor epistemic strategy for revealing what social cognition really is.

Acknowledgments

This work was supported by MIUR, and as part of the European Science Foundation EUROCORES Programme OMLL, was supported by funds to V.G. from the Italian C.N.R.

References

Adolphs R: Cognitive neuroscience of human social behaviour. Nat Rev Neurosci 4(3) (2003) 165–178

Avenanti A, D Bueti, G Galati, SM Aglioti: Transcranial magnetic stimulation highlights the sensorimotor side of empathy for pain. Nat Neurosci 8 (2005) 955–60

Baron-Cohen S: Social and pragmatic deficits in autism: Cognitive or affective? Journal of Autism and Developmental Disorders 18 (1988) 379–402

Baron-Cohen S, AM Leslie, U Frith: Does the autistic child have a "theory of mind"? Cognition 21 (1985) 37–46

Barrett L, P Henzi: The social nature of primate cognition. Proc. Royal Soc. Biol. 272 (2005) 1865–1875

Bird CM, C Castelli, O Malik, U Frith, M Husain: The impact of extensive medial frontal lobe damage on 'Theory of Mind' and cognition. Brain 127 (2004) 914–928

Blakemore S-J, D Bristow, G Bird, C Frith, J Ward: Somatosensory activations during the observation of touch and a case of vision–touch synaesthesia. Brain 128 (2005) 1571–1583

Botvinick M, AP Jha, LM Bylsma, SA Fabian, PE Solomon, KM Prkachin: Viewing facial expressions of pain engages cortical areas involved in the direct experience of pain. Neuroimage 25 (2005) 315–319

Bruner J: Acts of Meaning. Harvard University Press, Cambridge, MA 1990

Buccino G, F Binkofski, GR Fink, L Fadiga, L Fogassi, V Gallese, RJ Seitz, K Zilles, G Rizzolatti, H-J Freund: Action observation activates premotor and parietal areas in a somatotopic manner: an fMRI study. European Journal of Neuroscience 13 (2001) 400–404

Buccino G, F Lui, N Canessa, I Patteri, G Lagravinese, F Benuzzi, CA Porro, G Rizzolatti: Neural circuits involved in the recognition of actions performed by nonconspecifics: An fMRI study. J Cogn. Neurosci. 16 (2004) 114–126

Buxbaum LJ, KM Kyle, R Menon: On beyond mirror neurons: Internal representations subserving imitation and recognition of skilled object-related actions in humans. Cog. Brain Res. 25 (1) (2005) 226–39

Carruthers O, PK Smith (eds.): Theories of Theories of Mind. Cambridge University Press, Cambridge 1996

Dapretto L, MS Davies, JH Pfeifer, AA Scott, M Sigman, SY Bookheimer, M Iacoboni: Understanding emotions in others: mirror neuron dysfunction in children with autism spectrum disorders. Nature Neuroscience 9 (2005) 28–30

Darwin C: The expressions of the emotions in man and animals. Albemarle, London 1872

Dawson G, S Webb, GD Schellenberg, S Dager, S Friedman, E Aylward, T Richards: Defining the broader phenotype of autism: Genetic, brain, and behavioral perspectives. Dev. and Psychopathol. 14 (2002) 581–611

Dunbar RIM: Neocortex size as a constraint on group size in primates. J Hum. Evol. 20 (1992) 469–493

Ferrari PF, V Gallese, G Rizzolatti L Fogassi: Mirror neurons responding to the observation of ingestive and communicative mouth actions in the monkey ventral premotor cortex. European Journal of Neuroscience 17 (2003) 1703–1714

Ferrari PF, C Maiolini, E Addessi, L Fogassi, E Visalberghi: The observation and hearing of eating actions activates motor programs related to eating in macaque monkeys. Behav. Brain Res. 161 (2005) 95–101

Fogassi L, PF Ferrari, B Gesierich, S Rozzi, F Chersi, G Rizzolatti: Parietal lobe: From action organization to intention understanding. Science 302 (2005) 662–667

Gallese V: The "Shared Manifold" Hypothesis: from mirror neurons to empathy. Journal of Consciousness Studies 8 N° 5–7 (2001) 33–50

Gallese V: The manifold nature of interpersonal relations: The quest for a common mechanism. Phil. Trans. Royal Soc. London B. 358 (2003) 517–528

Gallese V: Embodied simulation: from neurons to phenomenal experience. Phenomenology and the Cognitive Sciences 4 (2005) 23–48

Gallese V: "Being like me": self-other identity, mirror neurons and empathy. In: Hurley S, N Chater (eds.): Perspectives on Imitation: From Cognitive Neuroscience to Social Science. MIT Press, Cambridge, MA 2005(a)

Gallese V, G Lakoff. The Brain's Concepts: The Role of the Sensory-Motor System in Reason and Language. Cognitive Neuropsychology 22 (2005) 455–479

Gallese V, L Fadiga, L Fogassi, G Rizzolatti: Action recognition in the premotor cortex. Brain 119 (1996) 593–609.

Gallese V, L Fogassi, L Fadiga, G Rizzolatti: Action Representation and the inferior parietal lobule. In: Prinz W, B Hommel (eds.): Attention and Performance XIX. Oxford University Press, Oxford 2002

Gallese V, C Keysers, G Rizzolatti: A unifying view of the basis of social cognition. Trends in Cognitive Sciences 8 (2004) 396–403

Gergely G, G Csibra: Teleological reasoning in infancy: the naive theory of rational action. TICS 7 (2003) 287–292

Goldman A, CS Sripada: Simulationist Models of Face-based Emotion Recognition. Cognition 94 (2005) 193–213

Grandin T: Thinking in Pictures. Doubleday, New York 1995

Hadjikhani N, RM Joseph, J Snyder, H Tager-Flusberg: Anatomical differences in the mirror neuron system and social cognition network in Autism. Cerebral Cortex. Advanced Online access, Nov. 23 2005

Hauser MD, WT Fitch: Computational constraints on syntactic processing in a non human primate. Science 303 (2004) 377–380

Hauser MD, N Chomsky, WT Fitch: The faculty of language: What is it, Who has it, and How did it evolve? Science 298 (2002) 1569–1579

Hayes CM: Theory of mind in nonhuman primates. Behavioral Brain Sciences 21 (1998) 101–148

Hobson RP, J Ouston, A Lee: Emotion recognition in autism: Coordinating faces and voices. Psychological Medicine 18 (1988) 911–923

Hobson RP, J Ouston, A Lee: Naming emotion in faces and voices: Abilities and disabilities in autism and mental retardation. British Journal of Developmental Psychology 7 (1989) 237–250

Hobson RP, A Lee: Imitation and identification in autism. Journal of Child Psychology and Psychiatry 40 (1999) 649–659

Humphrey NK: The social function of intellect. In: Bateson P, RA Hinde (eds.): Growing points in ethnology. Cambridge University Press, Cambridge 1976

Humphrey NK: Nature's Psychologists. The New Scientist, 29 June 1978

Humphrey NK: Nature's Psychologists. In Josephson BD, VS Ramachandran (eds.): Consciousness and the Physical World. Pergamon, Oxford 1980

Hutchison WD, KD Davis, AM Lozano, RR Tasker, JO Dostrovsky: Pain related neurons in the human cingulate cortex. Nature Neuroscience 2 (1999) 403–405

Hutto DH: The limits of spectatorial Folk Psychology. Mind and Language 19 (2004) 548–573

Iacoboni M, I Molnar-Szakacs, V Gallese, G Buccino, J Mazziotta, G Rizzolatti: Grasping the intentions of others with one's owns mirror neuron system. PLOS Biology 3 (2005) 529–535

Jackson PL, AN Meltzoff, J Decety: How do we perceive the pain of others: A window into the neural processes involved in empathy. NeuroImage, 24 (2005) 771–79

Jacob P, M Jeannerod: The motor theory of social cognition: a critique. Trends in Cog. Neurosci. 9 (2005) 21–25

Keysers C, B Wickers, V Gazzola, J-L Anton, L Fogassi, V Gallese: A Touching Sight: SII/PV Activation during the Observation and Experience of Touch. Neuron 42 (2004) 1–20

Kohler E, C Keysers, MA Umiltà, L Fogassi, V Gallese, G Rizzolatti: Hearing sounds, understanding actions: Action representation in mirror neurons. Science 297 (2002) 846–848

McIntosh DN, A Reichman-Decker, P Winkielman, J Wilbarger: When the Social Mirror Breaks: Deficits in Automatic, but not Voluntary Mimicry of Emotional Facial Expressions in Autism. Developmental Science 3 (2006) 295–302

Meltzoff AN, R Brooks: "Like Me" as a building block for understanding other minds: Bodily acts, attention, and intention. In: Malle BF, LJ Moses, DA Baldwin (eds.): Intentions and intentionality: Foundations of social cognition. MIT Press, Cambridge, MA 2001

Morrison I, D Lloyd, G DiPellegrino, N Roberts: Vicarious responses to pain in anterior cingulate cortex: Is empathy a multisensory issue? Cognitive, Affective, and Behavioral Neuroscience 4 (2004) 270–278

Oberman LM, EH Hubbard, JP McCleery, E Altschuler, VS Ramachandran, JA Pineda: EEG evidence for mirror neuron dysfunction in autism spectrum disorders. Cog Brain Res 24 (2005) 190–198

Onishi KH, R Baillargeon: Do 15 months-old understand false beliefs? Science 308 (2005) 255–258

Paukner A, JR Anderson, E Borelli, E Visalberghi, PF Ferrari: Macaques (Macaca nemestrina) recognize when they are being imitated. Biol. Lett. 1 (2005) 219–222

Povinelli DJ, JM Bering, S Giambrone: Toward a science of other minds: escaping the argument by analogy. Cognitive Science 24 (3) (2000) 509–541

Premack D; G Woodruff: Does the chimpanzee have a theory of mind? Behav. Brain Sci. 1 (1978) 515–526

Preston SD, FBM De Waal: Empathy: its ultimate and proximate bases. Behavioral and Brain Sciences, 25 (2002) 1–72

Ramnani N, CR Miall: A system in the human brain for predicting the actions of others. Nature Neurosci 7 (2004) 85–90

Reddy V, D Hay, L Murray, C Trevarthen: Communication in infancy: mutual regulation of affect and attention. In: Bremner G, A Slater, G. Butterworth (Eds.): Infant development: recent advances. Psychology Press, East Sussex 1997

Rizzolatti G, L Craighero: The mirror neuron system. Ann Rev Neurosci 27 (2004) 169–192

Rizzolatti G, L Fadiga, V Gallese, L Fogassi: Premotor cortex and the recognition of motor actions. Cog. Brain Res. 3 (1996) 131–141

Rizzolatti G, L Fogassi, V Gallese: Neurophysiological mechanisms underlying the understanding and imitation of action. Nature Neuroscience Reviews 2 (2001) 661–670

Rogers S: An examination of the imitation deficit in autism. In. Nadel J, G Butterworth (eds.): Imitation in infancy. Cambridge University Press, Cambridge 1999

Schmitz C, J Martineau, C Barthélemy, C Assaiante: Motor control and children with autism: deficit of anticipatory function? Neurosci. Lett. 348 (2003) 17–20

Singer T, C Frith: The painful side of empathy. Nature Neurosci 8 (2005) 845–846

Singer T, B Seymour, J O'Doherty, H Kaube, RJ Dolan, CF Frith: Empathy for pain involves the affective but not the sensory components of pain. Science 303 (2004) 1157–1162

Snow ME, ME Hertzig, T Shapiro: Expression of emotion in young autistic children. Annual Progress in Child Psychiatry & Child Development (1988) 514–522.

Stern DN: The interpersonal world of the infant. Basic Books, New York 1985/2000

Striano T, A Henning, D Stahl: Sensitivity to social contingencies between 1 and 3 months of age. Developmental Science 8 (2005) 509–518

Subiaul F, JF Cantlon, RL Holloway, HS Terrace: Cognitive imitation in Rhesus macaque. Science 305 (2004) 407–410

Theoret H, E Halligan, M Kobayashi, F Fregni, H Tager-Flusberg, A Pascual-Leone: A. Impaired motor facilitation during action observation in individuals with autism spectrum disorder. Curr Biology 15 (2005) 84–85

Tomasello M, J Call: Primate Cognition. Oxford University Press, Oxford 1997

Trevarthen C: Communication and cooperation in early infancy: a description of primary intersubjectivity. In: Bullowa M (ed.): Before Speech: The Beginning of Interpersonal Communication. Cambridge University Press, New York 1979

Umiltà MA, E Kohler, V Gallese, L Fogassi, L Fadiga, C Keysers, G Rizzolatti: "I know what you are doing": a neurophysiological study. Neuron 32 (2001) 91–101

Watkins KE, AP Strafella, T Paus: Seeing and hearing speech excites the motor system involved in speech production. Neuropsychologia 41(8) (2003) 989–94

Whiten A, RW Byrne: Machiavellian Intelligence 2: Evaluations and Extensions. Cambridge University Press, Cambridge 1997

Wicker B, C Keysers, J Plailly, J-P Royet, V Gallese, G Rizzolatti: Both of us disgusted in my insula: The common neural basis of seeing and feeling disgust. Neuron 40 (2003) 655–664

Yirmiya N, C Kasari, M Sigman, P Mundy: Facial expressions of affect in autistic, mentally retarded and normal children. Journal of Child Psychology & Psychiatry & Allied Disciplines 30 (1989) 725–735

7. Becoming a parent: What parental writings teach us

Véronique Francis; University Teachers Training Centre of Orleans-Tours, University of Paris-X-Nanterre, Bourges, France

Following the publication in 1960 of the work by the historian Philippe Ariès *L'enfant et la vie familiale sous l'Ancien Regime* [*Centuries of Childhood. A social history of family life, 1962*] (Ariès, 1960), important research has taken place. This has allowed historians to single out an "increase in emotion in front of the child" (Rouche, 1981) observable from the middle ages onwards in different domains from which derive the discussion on education. Around 1256, the Dominican Vincent de Beauvais made reference to the *Protagoras* of Plato to persuade his readers that education begins from the first years of life. Expressing the ideas current at the time, Guillaume de Tournai considers that parents are very important in the education of their children (Rouche, 1981). The collection of advice by Philippe de Novare (1888) which appeared in 1265, insists on the methods of fore-arming young children against the great dangers which lurk around every corner: suffocation in the family bed, water, and fire. *La Civilité Puérile* by Erasmus, published for the first time in 1530, became the object of translations and numerous re-editions which inspired anonymous authors whose texts spread throughout the country through the literature of travelling booksellers (Andries, Bollème, 2003). Witness the title, published in 1599 by the Bibliothèque Bleue – *La Civilté puérile à laquelle avons ajouté la discipline et l'institution des enfants. Aussi la doctrine et l'enseignement du père de famille à la jeunesse* [*The 'Civilité Puerile' to which we have added the discipline and institution of children. Also the teachings of the pater familias to youth.*] (S.N, 1599). From the end of the 17th century, in a period marked by a significant rate of infant mortality and by the development of wet-nursing the newborn, which extended through all social classes in the urban areas, the treatises by doctors and midwifes, the advice of moralists, the recommendations of pedagogues, philosophical writings, multiplied. In the 18th century, in the decade 1760–1770, two or more works on childhood appeared (Parias, 1981), among which was the famous *Émile ou de l'Éducation* by Jean-Jacques Rousseau. These have, as a common objective, the diffusion of knowledge on ways of caring for and educating children. They are aimed principally at parents: to help them to put into into practice, to inspire them or even to be consulted in order to choose and determine the roles of wet-nurses and masters. This specialized literature on maternity, childhood, and education certainly contributed in shaping the role of the parents; however, to approach what becoming a parent means in different ages, it is necessary to explore the domain of family writings.

Some testimonies of parental experience

Family writings and parenthood

The memoirs of families in Florence in the 14th and 15th centuries allow us to approach what being a parent could represent in accordance with each milieu (Klapisch-Zuber, 1998). These family annals were above all intended to record the management of the patrimony. In a period where communal administration was strengthening its control over the citizens, certain fathers reported therein the date of birth, particulars of the rituals which accompanied it or of the expenses occasioned by a wet-nurse or by the salaries of the masters. The formulas used by fathers to register the birth or death of a child, testify above all to the devotion with which they undertook paternity. The texts concerning boys can be more wordy, the child representing the hope of seeing a name or family lineage perpetuated. From these paternal writings, a concept emerges which can be considered as also revealing the feelings of the mothers: bringing children into the world and educating them was considered the chief duty of adults united by marriage; as the "task" of married women (Opitz, 1991). The tenderness of the parents was certainly far from being negligible. It is expressed here by their concern for the well-being of the neonate in the care accorded to the choice of the wet-nurse. This can be seen in the writings of the notary Etienne Borelly (Sauzet, 1996) who follows with great vigilance his children being wet-nursed since his wife cannot breastfeed them. When they reached maturity, expenses, often considerable, were adopted for their education. Despite the constant presence of death and the religious approach to it – the neonate or the infant are recalled by the will of God – adults do not assume their role as parents with the indifference we might have granted them (Shorter, 1970).

In contrast with the writings of the family annals and ledgers, often laconic due to their end, private chronicles and epistolary practices better permit us to approach what "becoming a parent" means. These "writings about myself" – notes jotted in a diary, personal journals, . . . – and those "writings for others" – correspondence, birth journals, . . . – of the "register of intimacy", started to spread in the 18th century (Dufief, 2000). They illuminate the experience of parents at a period when a family model centered on the child and on the place of affection within the bourgeoisie was emerging. Thus, the "Journal of paternity" published by Charles-Etienne Coquebert de Montbret (s.d.), from before the birth of his first child attests to the sentiments of the parents. This French diplomat, who wrote in the name of the couple between 1781 and 1784, describes the behavior of their son, their choices and hopes as parents, their hesitation before decisions as important as that of having their child inoculated to protect him from smallpox. The mother will take her role upon the birth of their daughter Cécile, born in 1784. She will write, for her, and for Eugène, born in 1788, some letters where she tells them of the care she lavishes on them, the activities she performs with them, and the attitudes she adopts to "forge their character".

Assuming the role of parent, a heavy charge but "sweet and useful"

Some decades later, while the period was exalting maternity (Kniebielher, Fouquet 1977), Madame Fabre d'Olivet explained the practices and maternal feelings to her young friend Victorine who had just become a mother. In 1820, she gathered her correspondence in "a work without any pretensions, dealing only with the part of education which one is accustomed to regarding as indifferent" (Kniebielher, Fouquet 1977). Madame Fabre d'Olivet, who presents herself as a mother having a low level of instruction, assumes herself the functions of wet-nurse and tutor for her three children. Just like Charles-Etienne Coquebert de Montbret, she has read "L'Émile of Jean-Jacques [Rousseau]" but she considers herself convinced, even after a second reading, that that manner of raising a child is an impracticable thing in its ensemble" (Kniebielher, Fouquet 1977). She therefore describes her manner of caring for, feeding, sending to sleep, and waking her neonate. She followed on in 1819 by presenting her manner of acting to favor the development of young children. Madame Fabre d'Olivet realized that from the moment that the parent takes charge of the child, they are confronted by various unexpected situations. They are led to outline some responses, to adjust them to the situation, adapt them to the child, to validate them or construct new ones. Despite the complexity of the task, we are dealing with "the most agreeable, sweetest and most useful of occupations" (Kniebielher, Fouquet 1977).

It is a useful occupation since only a parent can assiduously carry out the thoughtful observations indispensable to find the responses best adapted to the most complex situations. It is "the sweetest of occupations" because the care, which mothers dispense themselves, contributes to engendering trust and love of children for their parents. However, Madame Fabre d'Olivet underlines the constant commitment of the adult in some functions ,which highlight as much the household function – knowing how to make a soup which will not provoke colic in the child – as intellectual and moral education – learning obedience to protect them from domestic danger. This text, which preceded by about fifty years the epoch where, in the bourgeois milieus numerous epistolary exchanges "sound like nursery-rhymes" (Perrot, 1987), reveals an ambition which is located far beyond the methods of being and doing to care for, raise and educate children. The aim of this "reflective chatting" (Perrot, 1987) is not solely to advise young parents. It is also to reassure the mothers, to lead them to conduct a thoughtful constraint in their ways of acting: "I believed that [the publication of the correspondence intended for my friend] could serve mothers by showing them what perhaps they had already established by themselves, furnishing them with the occasion to reflect on their own observations" (Kniebielher, Fouquet 1977).

Parenthood and writing practices: a triple tradition

During the 20th century, the writings produced by parents concerning their child were to become little by little a common practice, the birth of a child often occupying one of its parents in consigning the events to a "baby journal" or an "album of the first year". Compiling or composing the journal immediately from the first months or the first years, such are the commonplace writings done today by numerous parents. What do these writings teach us on what it is to "become a parent"? We will examine this question starting from the study of the journals of birth, albums of childhood, baby books, etc, kept by parents. This corpus comprises the material of these productions and the discussions of the parents who presented them to us. It is completed by the most recent forms of writing, those of the journals in the form of 'blogs' kept by parents.

The heritage of medical surveillance documents

Whether as paper version or posted on the web, these writings on birth and childhood are inscribed in a triple tradition: above all that of medicine and child-welfare (Fine et al., 1993). Parents are invited to complete some indexes, close neighbors of those used in pediatrics to follow the health of the child: they mention its weight and size, its sleep rhythms, its alimentary regime or childhood diseases. They report the first murmurs, the first smiles or the first steps, etc. The first document of this type was done with a plethora of details, by the doctor of Louis XIII. From the day of the Royal Infant's birth in 1601, Jean Héroard produced a true journal of his health (Foisil, 1989). His medical surveillance rests on scrupulous written work and he reports daily in his book indications on the infant's sleep, his meals, growth, the development of his motor skills and speech.

These schemes recall those of a document which is today officially ascribed to the child from the moment of birth – the medical card. From the end of the 19th century, in France, the objective of sanitary and social control led to establishing different reports in order to follow certain populations. These documents were published while quite particular attention was being paid to the rationalization of the activity (Rollet-Echalier, 1990). The chronological order which was progressively imposed in commercial activity starting from the 17th century, extended to all sectors of social activity. Instruments for measuring time, such as clocks and watches, but also those such as calendars and diaries, foresaw, fixed, and recorded the course of daily time and familial events. In this process, writing practices played an important role. By permitting the activities of classification and ordering, they influenced the relationship which individuals maintained with time (Goody, 1979).

In the 19th century, Marc-Antoine Julien, author of an educational treatise inspired by Pestalozzi and theories on the employment of time, considered that it was essential that everyone exercised strict control over their own time (Simonet-Tenant, 2001). The reports which he conceived to teach individuals to organize themselves have an objective of "moral mirror", of "moral compass" (Lejeune, Bogaert, 2006). Medical cards also have the aim of prescribing, controlling, rationalizing, and moralizing the care of children. Used since the 1880s, these cards were destined to assure the surveillance of those children who depended on the wet-nurse or public assistance. A French doctor proposed them to the mothers themselves with the aim of guiding them and improving their diagnosis in the case of the child becoming ill (Rollet, 2005). The medical file entered definitively into practice at the beginning of the 1950s. Today, this file is held by the Health Service and registers the developmental stages of the child but it can also include blank pages reserved for the comments of the parents.

Apart from the medical file, birth albums were inspired by another medical document: the Medical File of Maternity whose objective was to follow the pregnancy of mothers-to-be, distributed in France after 1989. In fact, in birth albums, certain indexes refer to the period before birth. Including the months of expecting, these invite the parents to introduce themselves, the mother is invited to note her first sensations or the transformation of her body month by month. Some spaces dedicated to photographs and ultrasound images appear here and there. The indexes also include the description of the material transformations of home: the preparations carried out to welcome the child, the preparation of the paraphernalia for the child.

The fashion for autobiographical writings

Birth albums also come from another tradition, dating back to before the existence of official medical documents: chronicles, log books, and travel journals whose use spread from the 15th century. These "journals of beyond", testimonies of the everyday observed by their writers, contributed to the development of personal writings such as memoirs or the biography, a literary genre fashionable during the 18th century (Lejeune, Bogaert, 2006). According to the terminology of M. Leleu (Leleu, 1952), the journal is above all an *aide-mémoire* dedicated to recording the "acta", the "cogitata" and the "sentita". However, personal journals have different forms and functions (Simonet-Tenant, 2001). In fact, in the intimate journal, which was inspired by epistolary writings, the writer dialogues no longer with his dearest correspondent, but with himself. While certain journals were destined to remain confidential, others include the reader, warranting a reader who can play the role of interlocutor, guide, even director of conscience. In the 19th century, the journal was particularly recommended in the education of young women, where it was used, and sometimes even prescribed, so that the young could, alone or under the supervision of the persons charged with their education, note down their weaknesses and their good resolutions. At the age of about ten, little Marie Bonaparte would compile, in the 1880s, five note-books, whose texts would be re-read, and in certain periods, corrected and critically annotated, by the adults charged with her education (Becchi, 1998). Claire P. de Chateaufort describes in her *livre pour anniversaires* – constructed on the model of English 'birthday books' – her life as a young girl and high-society spouse. After the birth of her baby in 1903, the writing "*marks time with the growth and raising of the child*" (Martin-Furgier, 1987).

These are the points of view, conjointly inspired by the memoir writer, biographer and adventurer which the first baby journals adopted. At the beginning of the 20th century, the major brands of baby food were assuring their promotion by being distributed free of charge. While France was at war, infant mortality increased. The childhood section of the American Red Cross (*Children's Bureau*) launched an intensive campaign to educate mothers from the lower classes by spreading booklets and strip cartoons (Kniebielher, Fouquet, 1977). After 1914, the firm Nestlé offered "*to mothers who want to miss nothing of the beginnings of their baby's life*" a journal in which to convey the growth, the stages of progress, the events marking its existence. The introductory text to the *Baby Journal Kept by Daddy and Mummy*, re-published by Grasset in 1980, considers that we are dealing with a "*good habit in which father and mother can interchange*".

The portrait, painted and photographic

Finally, the third source of inspiration for childhood journals joins the previous tradition, although older, of elaborating biographical traces, not written yet but somewhat iconographic. To conserve the memory of the individual is to give him or her a physical and social representation, and since antiquity, this has been done by making a sculpted or painted portrait. As the considerable collections of drawings and pictures in Western museums testify, the pictorial genre of the portrait, which responded to various social functions, has considerable importance starting from the 16th century, when it became secular (Beyer, 2003). Placed in the center of aristocratic social practices, the portrait did not solely assure the perpetuation of the memory of the departed. It played a precise role alongside epistolary writings: it strengthened the presence of the living; it was used in matrimonial negotiations and also acted as health bulletin. When the children were depicted beside their parents, they represented the certain prolongation of the family lineage. In the course of the 17th and 18th centuries, the art of portraiture imposed itself little by little and the official portrait gave way to the intimate portrait. We encounter the peak of this genre in the 19th century, where the affluence of the leaders in bourgeois milieus attests, on the one hand, to their social ascent, and on the other, to novel representations of family and childhood. Mothers and children united constitute at one and the same time testimonies of maternal love and proof of paternal pride (Martin-Furgier, 1987). But the child alone became more and more the exclusive subject, as shown by the work of the painter Carolus-Duran who realized numerous portraits of children between 1875 and 1900 (Catalogue d'exposition, C. Duran, 2003).

With the invention of photography in 1836, the pictorial portrait was dethroned by the photographic portrait. From the second half of the 19th century, the spread of photographic techniques caused the emergence of a new genre of representation among the aristocracy and bourgeoisie: the family album, where the configurations of intimacy and the grand rituals of familial life were given value for future generations. Its development placed amateur photography at the very heart of grand familial ceremonies and everyday situations. From the 1960s, this practice allowed the great majority of families to capture 'live' the small and great events of family life. A central position was reserved for the portrait and, among its variables – self-portrait, portrait of the couple, group portrait – the portraits of children occupied a growing position and served as a way of preserving the memory of the successive transformations of childhood. A new breath of life was given in the 2000s with the emergence of digital photography. With these types of technology where the clichés are 'live', the adult does not content himself with memorizing the extraordinary in the child's history. He records the ordinary until he distills it.

This increase of photographs ends in the creation of specialized albums: the birth album, for example. Children's journals can thus be considered as a specialized and augmented variant of the photo-album: specialized variant since the objective is focused on the child; augmented variant because writing is given a prime position, to the point that sometimes it occupies pride of place. The predilection for the amateur photographic portrait, where "the boundaries between 'posed' portrait and instantaneous 'stolen moment' are quickly surpassed, which doubtless explains the choice position reserved for the writing that gives a date to or comments on the image. The writing says what the image alone cannot show: it accompanies these biographical visual crumbs with the emotions surrounding them. With storage, the writing assures a second life to those objects which have common a transient existence: ultrasounds, birth bracelets, and above all, the first piece of writing realized by the parents, seal of the social birth: the birth announcement of the child.

Parenthood and "ordinary" writing practices
Keeping the journal of your child

Whether they are abridged or abundant, it is rare that a family does not posses archives of the family memoirs. The time dedicated to the organization of these reservoirs of memories is variable. From a box where some objects of the past are gathered, to the creation of a journal of the first years or photo-albums, there exists a broad sweep of practices to comfort and nourish familial intimacy, strongly structured around childhood and its rituals, already at the beginning of the 19th century in bourgeois families, and in the second half of the 19th century in the middle classes. Today, it seems more than all the others, the event of birth and the period of infancy that engenders practices of conservation and the classifying of familial memoir documents, and stimulate writing practices. On the specialized shelves of large bookshops, an abundance of albums and birth journals is available. Certain albums invite parents to comment on the different stages of the child's life : *Le livre de mon bébé* (Hachette), *Journal de mon bébé* (Marabout). Others want him or her to pick up the pen in the name of his or her child: *Mon Journal de bébé* (De Vechi), *Me Voilà* (Hurtubise).

Parents, who often receive a journal of birth as a gift, sometimes choose to abandon the "square writing" practices of these commercialized journals. Their preference then tends towards an object chosen for its aesthetic or practical aspects: a bound notebook, hardcover book, diary, or photo-album.

Finally, we must underline a third type of journal. Entering the field of new writing customs, the numerous online journals spread through the Web show original textual forms where personal tales may mix with collective writing experiences.

If it is chronological organization which structures the writings, then a certain liberty of expression prevails in the journals created by parents. The parents speak therein of their experience as parent in the first person singular, or in the first person plural if they write in the name of the couple. When they address the child they make use of the familiar "tu". "*Tu as 1 an aujourd'hui*" ["*You are 1 today*"]. The journal sometimes manifests their twofold presence in front of the child: in their direct contact, and in a written dialogue. Thus, while her son is seven months old, Sandra describes his crying in a text of fifteen lines and finishes with these words : "*What's more I hear you arguing so I'll leave you now to take care of you*". In commercialized journals, the space accepted by the parents depends on the style imposed. This can differ from one book to another. But the parents take a distance from it and willingly adopt a liberty of tone. Thus, in *Mon Journal de bébé* (De Vechi, 1988), under the heading, "*My Daily Life*" a mother writes in her name "*Today, the 20th of April 2002, you ate with a spoon for the first time*" while only a few pages further on, she speaks in the name of the child "*I adore playing with my rubber giraffe!*".

Writing and "finding oneself parent"

Writings on birth and infancy often hark back to an ideal model, an idealized image of both the family and the child (Segalen et al., 2002). If the more liberal writing of personal journals, on paper or on the Web, seems closer to a real family, it is the discussions of the parents on these writing practices which allow us to assume what they represent. The choice of keeping a journal responds to the desire to live the intensity of birth and early infancy: the writing records the emotions, allows "living twofold that intense period which flies so quickly". It can transcribe the feelings of separation of those early moments when, as a mother who had begun her journal during pregnancy writes, "*at birth, it was hard to come to terms because as I noticed you are yourself and meanwhile you are another*". The texts reveal the tensions between patience and impatience, gaiety and gravity, confidence and anxiety. Objective indications on the child, his date of birth, his weight and size for example, accompany passages which give liberal expression to the feelings of the parent. The expression of joy, "*You have finally arrived my darling!*"; of wonder – "*You are so beautiful, you are more beautiful than I had dreamed*", can give way to the need to understand and interpret the baby's signals – "*But why do you cry so much? Tell me*!". The time of writing and that of observation can be almost simultaneous. Certain parents say they collect "*the evolution, step by step*" of the child. They try to "*cope with the rapidity of the evolution*", to profit by each of those instants which appear to them so brief. Fixing the present is also to adapt to it. It means being able to measure the way traveled along: that of the child but also that which retraces one's own itinerary as a parent, from the fears felt before the all-too-small, to the acquired ease. Sandrine notes four months after the birth of her son: "*I re-read the first days when you were here! The fears I had at the start are finished, that's how much I have learned from you!*". The journal returns to past experience. Once written, it becomes material inclined to being explored, distant, or even examined with an ironic gaze. "*When I think that I was worried that you weren't eating enough while the doctor says that you are too fat now!*", writes Salouah.

Sharpening the sense of observation

If writing is considered as a method of "*better taking advantage of each novelty*" it is because it considers the observation as much as the feeling of it. The act of writing "*makes me sensitive to the smallest changes, to the smallest developments. As I write in Stéphanie's notebook, I notice better all she does*" explains her mother. Delivering remarks means having discerned trends or noticed developments. These are not always immediately perceived as important. The indexes proposed in pre-prepared journals encourage the parent to center his attention on aspects which he would not have noticed himself or which he would have perhaps observed only later on. "*When I wanted to fill in the part about her favorite toy, I told myself that Houria didn't really have one, but afterwards watching her better in her play-pen, I realized that she returned more often to a blue rabbit*". Writing has a "*projector effect*". This dimension is also underlined when there are many children, in particular in re-composed families. The attention accorded to each child seems more similar when one has developed a "*habit of observation*". Writing is far from conveying everything. But the process of selection operated sometimes makes tendencies appear "sunken" and leads to questioning and seeking solutions or responses. A father underlines "*you end up by noticing some things which don't immediately strike the eye and which can be important*".

In the professional life, managing familial intent and parental activity, writing "*marks a pause*". The mother of Estelle, who has been looking after her daughter in alternation with her father since she was thirteen months old, explains that she notes her observations during the fortnight when she is in her care. The journal is a large format diary which serves to record the activities and meetings planned. She notes therein in a concise form, and practically day by day, the moments shared with her daughter, progress in her speech and motor skills. Always insisting on the importance for her of keeping track of Estelle's progress, she also emphasizes the need to better organize the time which she devotes to her when she is at her side. The pages on the periods when Estelle is absent are occupied by photographs of the child. One can find here a divergence in the use of the diary observed in different circumstances: used also for bookkeeping, the diary is completed by some notes which are transforming it little by little into a journal.

Coping with adversity

When the parent is confronted by a dramatic event, writing represents the anxiety and the joy linked to the presence of the child. The journal of Sandra, started at the beginning of her pregnancy, reveals her numerous difficulties: absence of a home due to a recent divide with her mother, lack of resources deriving essentially from her seasonal work in agriculture, violence and departure of her partner. At the moment of birth, this young mother of nineteen expresses her solitude, her grief faced with the absence of the father: "*I would so much love him to be here to see how beautiful you are! It's not so serious, we'll find a way out!*" Sandra notes the objective reasons to reassure herself, to discern the positive elements in a situation which leaves her disarmed: "*I don't know what I'm going to do but the main thing is that you have arrived in good health*". She expresses her fear of "*not knowing*" of "*not being up to it*". Put up at home after birth, she keeps a daily chronicle with the details of her small victories, her isolation, her exhaustion, the organization of her time, her ways of treating the baby. Here the journal has the function of a mirror. It reflects the difficulties which the parent experiences but also her initiatives and the obstacles surpassed, whether they are trivial or more important. It draws, through the inventory of the responses given, the outlines of her new skills.

In dramatic circumstances, writing can have a role of focusing and support, it is "*a way of keeping your head above water*". This double dialogue, carried out with oneself and the child, appears as a means of re-grasping at life, coping with adversity. "*My journal is what allowed me to hold on*" says Sandra, "*I noted everything, from one day to the next, that helped me to see the positive things*". In the string of words written and re-read, the cortège of "little joys" seems to facilitate the perception of resources. Because writing about one articulates reading about oneself. The divergence through reading calls forth different approaches to the situation. Some points of balance are lost between the discouragement in experimenting and the hopes raised by the presence of the child, bouts of anxiety and periods of serenity. Today Sandra considers that this journal has been her "*life-jacket*". Even if numerous passages concern the child, its introspective and confidential dimension makes it say it is "*hers*". She does not show it to her son. "*Later perhaps,*" she says.

In contrast to Sandra, other parents make the choice of "*rubbing out*" the accidents of life. Philippe had two daughters of six and three years, and a little boy of four months when his wife died in a road accident. In each of the journals of his children, which his wife had regularly updated, he noted down "*Your mummy left us on the 3rd March 1996*". It is he who from now on will pick up the pen even if he had not filled in the indexes where the father was invited to record his impressions after the birth. He considers that "*for the children it's important. Later on, they will be able to see that there are still many things in their childhood which resemble what other children live*". We find also that the same concern to fabricate and "*to offer the image of a happy childhood*" in the testimony of Cindy who completes regularly and copiously her son's notebook. He was three when his father left them. The father has not been heard from since. She noted the day of his departure "*many weeks later, when I understood I would never see him again,*" but she followed up by applying herself to describing her son's first return to school, his favorite activities, the re-organizing of their life, their house-moving. This continuum in the writing seems like defiance, as if the interruption of the journal should not be added to the break provoked by death or separation.

By testifying, we are supported

With the possibility of appearing on the Web, journals leave the private sphere. Child journals have not escaped from this movement of spreading personal writings. They are often accompanied by photographs, even short video clips. The objective declared by a certain number of these journals is, as a father writes, "*to allow our families and our friends to participate 'live' in the TV-fiction of the first years*" of his son. In some cases, the journal also corresponds to the need to communicate with other parents. With the commentaries that readers can add, the journals produced and diffused on the Web become productions of several hands.

These writing practices and the distribution of the texts allow us to witness parental practices, to accumulate experience. The exchanges of points of view, knowledge, and practices seem to be exhibited more easily in this context where the anonymity of the Web protects everybody's intimacy. Thus on the 'blog' which she has named *Mamansoupeu*, Eliette describes, as frequent as two or three times a week, the approach of birth, her joys, her fears. When she elicits some testimonies on breastfeeding, her interlocutors bring forth their commentaries and retrace their experiences. They describe step by step their difficulties, their moments of doubt, their ventures, their mistakes. Some of them direct her to relevant sites on the same theme. These testimonies favor comparisons where the pitfalls are to be avoided and where practices that work appear. The parents do not hesitate to comment on each other's propositions, to mutually encourage one another. The discussions which ensue do not content themselves with replying to the questions asked: they also open up new perspectives, such as the parent who explains "*how much he participated in the breastfeeding even as a father*".

The objective of certain journals is clearly to "*be as useful to parents confronted by the same difficulties*" as those who keep them. Thus, on her 'blog' Célia seeks advice for her daughter of thirteen months who has never once slept a whole night. Some journals, kept regularly for several years, describe the everyday life of parents of children affected by an illness or handicap. The chronicles take up the calendar of events. They deploy day after day the multiple situations where the parents accomplish their daily acts. In the correspondence exchanged between net users, we can identify the mutual support that parents bring to each other, whether they have a child in the same situation or not. In the communications on the Web, the balance between distance and confidentiality encourages the adults to express what is still probably too timidly affirmed in the environment of a parent: the difficulty, the energy, the will, even the tenacity and courage needed to be a parent. This correspondence hinging on the sharing of testimonies, the exchange of experiences and simple suggestions, the expressions of encouragement and support, seem to contribute to an explicit identification of those resorts of the parental function which, whether for modesty or tradition, are often implicit. In this "*network intimacy*" of the 'blog', adults proclaim the joy of being a parent and of being the parent of a child who is different. They also express without deviating the discouragement, the sense of being in limbo, the fatigue or exhaustion which await parents exposed to difficult situations. The paradoxical feelings often experienced by parents are here posted, described and discussed.

The parent as a biographer of the child

Offering one's past to the child

The journal is above all a "keeper of memories" (Simonet–Tenant, 2001) for the parent and for the child. One of its goals is "*to give some souvenirs to the child*". Saïda admits that this choice comes from her regret of knowing so little about her own past. The choice of writing a journal can also be linked to the fact of possessing one's own childhood. Before the birth of his son, Frédéric's parents had removed from a wardrobe the journal they had compiled when he was a child. The emotion he felt on reading each of the stages of his childhood made him decide to "*keep the memory of life's good moments for us the parents and for our baby*". He writes the first times instead of the "last times": the last breastfeed, the day when the child threw away his dummy, . . . These passages were socialized in other ways by village or familial rituals in certain regions: thus, the end of breastfeeding, for example, occasioned the endowment of presents by the godfather and godmother, while the neighbors were invited to a toast when the child took his first few steps (Brékilien, 1978). Frédéric took some photographs and filmed the child. Meanwhile, with his wife, he attributes another value to writing: "*we note your emotions, the funny situations, those which form part of a life which doesn't belong to anyone else, but to Manuel, and to us!*". These writing practices emerge as duty of transmission, especially when the family ties are not so stable, few propitiations to the construction of family reminders. "*When I was a child, with my brothers, the place for souvenirs was my grandmother's house, my brother's children and my own don't really have such a place*". Whether he keeps the birth bracelet from the maternity ward or takes note of the first words, the parent conserves the trace of privileged moments. This trace is a witness for the child of "his first steps in life". It describes his evolving personality and notes his reactions before the events: "*tell me, mummy, when will Anatole go back inside your stomach?*" Manuel asks when his brother is only a few days old.

Writing attempts to capture the unique character of these episodes of infantile experience. The parent poses as a witness, primarily of the first years, those which cannot be memorized by the child. In keeping photographs and texts, these traces of strong affective and commemorative value, whose absence is sometimes perceived of as "*the index of defective filial relation*" (Parenté, 2002), the parent weaves familial memory. As Maurice Halbwachs has shown, this is a social construction and it is built in a context where everyone seeks to construct his/her own identity (Halbwachs, 1925).

The child, invited reader

The studies performed on intimate journals show that some of them are characterized by writing to and for oneself, where the diarists address themselves and exclude all other potential readers (Simonet-Tenant, 2001). This is not prevalent in a child journal. An inherent component in the writing of journals kept by parents is to integrate as an emblem the child as recipient when they are not writing in his name. With the desire to retain the memory of the significant times of childhood, parents combine their desire to be discovered by the child when older. In proceeding with this work as memoir writer, the parents project themselves from the moment of birth in a very different role from the one they occupy when they highlight these crumbs of biography. As they are collecting these souvenirs, they place them at the core of interchanging situations. The child is designated as the invited reader of these writings, the listener of his own exploits, and the interlocutor of future conversations. Thus Philippe is writing, "*in order to share these good times with his children later on*". Sandra pays attention "*to discuss difficult moments with her son and above all share the best memories*". This collection of chosen moments from childhood completes a project for the future where the parent and child find themselves reunited. A relational project of this type was already present in the mind of Charles-Etienne Coquebert de Montbret, who in 1781, expressed, formulating it in the terms of the time, his joy at being a father and the happy perspectives which offered themselves to him: "*So here is the friend Heaven has given to me, he who is to be the charm of my life, my study companion, my confidant.*" The historians and sociologists who have retraced the transformations in the family have shown that the relational family model, which replaced the moral family, rests in part on the resources used by the parents to retain the happy moments of childhood and to perpetuate their memory (Muxel, 1996 ; Martin-Furgier, 1987). These moments of exchange around the child's first experiences sometimes take place very early, when journals and albums are made available to the young child. Estelle's mother explains: "*When she was three or four years old, my daughter often looked at her album all alone or even asked me to tell her history: she adored it when I spoke to her of the day she ate alone for the first time, for example!*". These returns to the past go beyond the evocation of the joyous moments of early infancy. They accord the parent a privileged role, living witness of the child's growth. They bring to the fore their role as vigilant chaperon as much as the relationship of love between the parent and child. On a Quebec site a woman writes: "*These books or notebooks are likewise fragments of love to transmit to them.*"

Writing and consulting these journals can be placed among the new familial rituals. "*At every birthday I bring out the album, we look at it and we read it together*" explains Saïda. These traces where the best moments of childhood are collected become the "*federal treasure*" of the family (Lejeune, 1986). If this "portable memorial" rebinds the child to an extended family network, it also rebinds the parent to the child's infancy and to the functions which they assured him/her otherwise: changing, carrying, feeding. This past written and directed by the parents, provides a collection of common references capable of fertilizing present relations, of realizing this relational and affective family which characterizes the contemporary family (Perrot, 1991). Is is founded on the communication between members, and especially on the communication between parents and children. These souvenirs, writings and images, symbolic markers of familial history, contribute in organizing the sentimental and emotional history of the family and in building what we can call "*an affective family identity*" (Bertaux-Wiame, Muxel, 1996).

*****

As with every ordinary writing practice, the writings on birth and infancy record "the minor or major events which weave the net of everyday life" (Chartier, 2001). The history of memoirs on paper, dedicated to evoking the period of childhood, clarify that stage of life where the adult becomes a parent. They also witness to the antiquity of questioning the parental role. While these writing practices on the everyday are often placed at the edge of legitimate social practices, numerous studies demonstrate that they are instruments of thought (Barré-De Miniac, 1995). They engage the persons in appropriation behavior in the situations being lived. They favor the processes of distancing and being objective (Lahire, 1993). These journals can be situated at the boundary between "writings about myself" and "writings for others", but generally they have a designated recipient: the child. The writing transcribes images of birth and childhood – disturbing, happy, tender, anxious; kept with the future in mind and thus taking the form of a narration. Jérôme Bruner (1983) has shown the importance of the biographical narrative in the building of oneself. This process by which we construct reality links us to the world of others. Narrative gives a sense of human interaction. It permits equally to rebind past, present, and future, it helps in understanding the sense of experience. Autobiographical narratives, brief or developed, oral or written, reveal an "I" who becomes or has become another (Bruner, 1983).

The place which these texts on childhood occupy in numerous Western families, marked by a writing culture anchored in the school tradition (Francis, 2002), must not lead to neglecting or obscuring the importance of the traces kept in the memory and given back orally in other families. Thus Soudjata, of Indian origin, who arrived in France in 2001 and is mother of two little daughters born since, explains: "*I have some photos which my daughters look at when I show them to my guests. But the talismans which protected them when they were young, the locks of hair, . . . I offered them to the temple when I went to India, because these gifts to the temple protect my daughters*". In the multicultural context in which we live now, we must consider that the scenario of the past, which draws these stories under construction, is far from being constituted only by the keeping of objects and writings. Similarly, the ideal image, often proclaimed in parental writings, of a blossoming parenthood and a happy childhood, must not erase a marked reality, in every country of the world, by the numerous forms of violence and exploitation suffered both by children and their parents.

References

Andries L, G Bollème: La Bibliothèque bleue. Littérature de colportage. Laffont/Bouquins, Paris 2003

Ariès Ph: L'Enfant et la vie familiale sous l'Ancien Régime. Plon, Paris 1960/Centuries of childhood. A social history of family life. Vintage, New York 1962

Barré-De Miniac C: La Didactique de l'écriture : nouveaux éclairages pluridisciplinaires et état de la recherche. Revue Française de Pédagogie 113 (1995) 93–133

Becchi E: Ecritures enfantines, lectures adultes. In: Becchi E, D Julia: Histoire de l'enfance en Occident, 2. Du XVIIIème siècle à nos jours. Seuil, Paris 1998

Bertaux-Wiame I, A Muxel: Transmissions familiales: territoires imaginaires, échanges symboliques et inscription sociale. In: De Singly F, C Martin, A Muxel et al. (eds): La Famille en questions. Etat de la recherche. Syros, Paris 1996

Beyer A: L'Art du portrait. Citadelles et Mazenod, Paris 2003

Brékilien Y: La Vie quotidienne des paysans bretons au XIXème siècle. Hachette, Paris 1978

Bruner J: Child's talk: Learning to use language. Oxford UP, Oxford 1983

Carolus-Duran 1837–1917. Catalogue d'exposition Lille, palais des Beaux-Arts, 9 mars-9 juin 2003; Toulouse, musée des Augustins, 27 juin–29 septembre 2003. Éditions de la Réunion des Musées Nationaux, Paris 2003

Chartier R: Culture écrite et littérature à l'âge moderne. Annales 4–5 (2001) 787

Coquebert de Montbret Charles-Etienne: Journal de la vie d'Ernest (1781–1784) suivi des Lettres à Cécile (1784-an VII) et des Lettres à Eugène (1788). Cahier couverture cuir, Bibliothèque municipale de Rouen

De Novare Ph: Les Quatre âges de l'homme; 1265. M. de Fréville, Paris 1888

Dufief J-P: Introduction. In: Actes du colloque de Brest, 23–25 octobre 1997. Les Écritures de l'intime, La Correspondance et le journal. Champion, Paris 2000

Fabre d'Olivet. Conseil à mon amie sur l'éducation physique et morale des enfans par Madame Fabre d'Olivet. Lefebvre, Paris 1820

Fine A, S Labro, C Lorquin: Lettres de naissance. In: Fabre D: Écritures ordinaires. POL-Centre Georges Pompidou, Paris 1993

Foisil M: Journal de Jean Héroard, médecin de Louis XIII. Fayard, Paris 1989

Francis V: Créer un répertoire de textes: un encouragement à «l'art du bricolage». Les Actes de Lecture, Revue de l'Association Française pour la Lecture 78 (2002) 57–63

Goody J: La Raison graphique, la domestication de la pensée sauvage. Éditions de Minuit, Paris 1979

Halbwachs M: Les cadres sociaux de la mémoire. PUF, Paris 1925

Klapisch-Zuber C: L'Enfant, la mémoire et la mort. In: Becchi E, D Julia D (eds): Histoire de l'enfance en Occident, 1. De l'Antiquité au XVIIème siècle. Seuil, Paris 1998

Kniebielher Y, C Fouquet: Histoire des Mères du Moyen-Age à nos jours. Montalba, Paris 1977

Lahire B: La Raison des plus faibles. Rapport au travail, écritures domestiques et lectures en milieux populaires. PUL, Lyon 1993

Lejeune Ph, C Bogaert: Le Journal intime, Histoire et anthologie. Textuel, Paris 2006

Lejeune Ph: Moi aussi. Seuil, Paris 1986

Leleu M: Les Journaux intimes. PUF, Paris 1952

Martin-Furgier A: Les Rites de la vie privée bourgeoise. In: Ariès Ph, G Duby (eds): Histoire de la vie privée, Tome 4. De la Révolution à la grande guerre. Seuil, Paris 1987

Muxel A: Individu et mémoire familiale. Nathan, Paris 1996

Opitz C: Contraintes et libertés (1250–1500). In: Klapisch-Zuber C, (ed.): Histoire des femmes en Occident, 2. Le Moyen-Age. Plon, Paris 1991

Parenté MB: Des biens et des liens. In: Dortier J-F (coordinateur): Familles: permanence et métamorphoses. Sciences Humaines, Paris 2002

Parias L-H: L'Enseignement et l'éducation en France, Tome II. De Gutemberg aux Lumières (1480–1789). Nouvelle Librairie de France, Paris 1981

Perrot M: Figures et rôles. In: Ariès Ph, G Duby (eds): Histoire de la vie privée, Tome 4. De la Révolution à la grande guerre. Seuil, Paris 1987

Perrot M: Les échanges à l'intérieur de la famille. Approche historique. In: De Singly F (ed): La Famille, l'état des savoirs. La Découverte, Paris 1991

Rollet C: Pour une histoire du carnet de santé de l'enfant: une affaire publique ou privée? Revue française des affaires sociales 3 (2005) 131–156

Rollet-Echalier C: La Politique à l'égard de la petite enfance sous la IIIème République. INED-PUF, Paris 1990

Rouche M: L'Enseignement et l'éducation en France. Des Origines à la Renaissance. Nouvelle Librairie de France, Paris 1981

S.N: La civilité puerile a laquelle avons adjousté la discipline et institution des enfans. Aussi la doctrine et enseignemans du pere de famille a la jeunesse. Jean Micard, Paris 1599

Sauzet R: Une Éducation nîmoise au XVIIème siècle. In: Actes du colloque des 15 et 16 mars 1996 organisé par le Centre d'Histoire Moderne et Contemporaine de l'Europe Méditerranéenne et de ses périphéries (XVIème–XIXème siècles): Naissance, enfance et éducation dans la France méridionale de XVIème au XXème siècles. Hommage à Mireille Laget. Université Paul-Valéry Montpellier III, Montpellier 2000

Schaeffer J-M: Portraits, singulier pluriel. Mazan/Bibliothèque nationale de France, Paris 1997

Segalen M, N Lapierre, C Attias-Donfut: Le Nouvel esprit de famille. Odile Jacob, Paris 2002

Shorter E: The family in modern society. Sage, London 1970

Simonet-Tenant F: Le Journal intime, Genre littéraire et écriture ordinaire. Nathan, Paris 2001

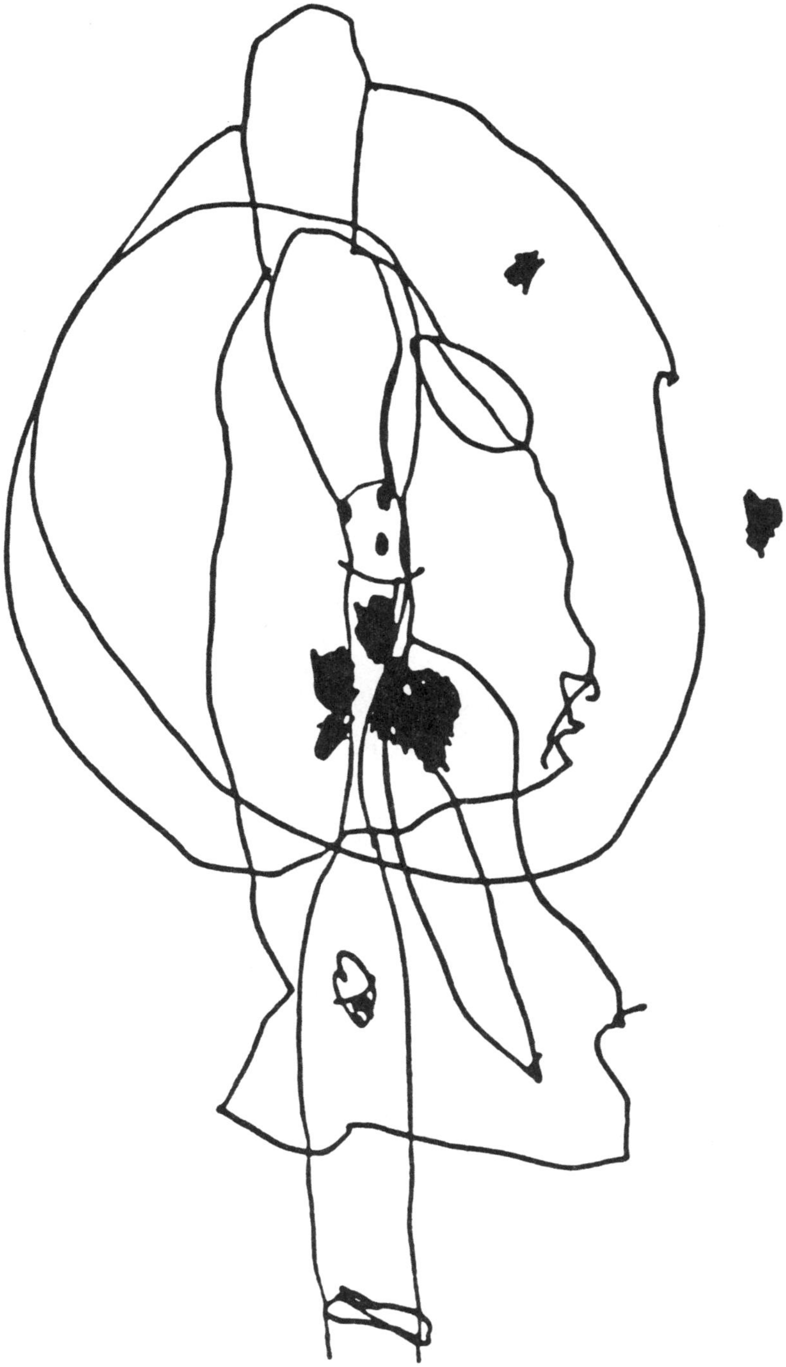

(Stefano, 3 yrs. 2 mos.)
When I was inside my mommy, she knew me.
I saw my mommy through her belly button.

8. The interior experience of maternity

Gina Ferrara Mori; Italian Society of Psychoanalysis, Florence, Italy

An unusual observatory

The choice of this topic is twofold. It stems from my extensive experience in the consulting-room with patients who have become mothers in the course of their treatment and from my many years of observing newborns in their families according to the Esther Bick method.

The decisive moment however, was when I came face to face with a certain work of art which inspired me to dedicate myself to the further exploration and research of what I had accumulated through my own experiences and through observing groups supervised by me and, as I will describe further on, by means of a study and research group I conducted.

The work of art in question is Piero della Francesca's "Madonna del Parto" (The Pregnant Madonna, Figure). In his extraordinary and outstanding pictorial expressiveness he offers us a rich communicative form of the very complex mental activity relating to the interior development process of pregnancy and the dawn of the mother-baby relationship.

Contemplating and interpreting the sublime but at the same time natural representation levels, was for me a kind of in-depth observatory that supplied me with a model and guide to many aspects of the interior experience of maternity, keeping in mind the fact that artists often anticipate many discoveries in their creative works that researchers later make about the human soul.

The fresco has been recently restored and transported to the new exhibition space of the cemetery chapel located in an ex-school of Monterchi. A recent trip allowed me to admire the painting in a new and more appropriate light while my memory filled with (along with personal emotions) the series of counter transferrals which had struck me when working with patients who were pregnant throughout the course of tests. Indeed, I remembered the interviews between observers and future mothers, forerunners to the weekly meetings which aimed to monitor the development of the child its own environment.

We are aware of how, in his visit to Tuscany in 1954, Chagall made a stopover in Monterchi (an ancient village in the high valley of Tiberina near the border of Tuscany and Umbria) after visiting the Arezzo and Sansepolcro frescos, and could not take himself away from the attraction he felt to the Madonna del Parto, situated at the time in the cemetery chapel where the artist's mother was buried (Walter, 1996). The journalist who was accompanying him, after some biographical questions about Piero and knowing that the mother was buried there exclaimed, “Now I understand! It’s the symbol of life that is about to be born from the maternal womb in the place of death, but this is an astounding idea!” There is no way of knowing what went through Chagall’s mind at that moment, but for me the sentiment uttered by a future mother to the observer who had gone to meet her, came to mind, “You know, birth is a change of state, just like death”.

Chagall also devoted himself to the subject of maternity on several occasions during his stay at Paris from 1910 to 1914. Tormented by the nostalgia for his homeland Russia, he painted not Holy Mary, but pregnant peasant women on a background of rural scenes with men and animals. Inside they show an oval shaped image on the abdomen of the baby standing up as if it were possible to see inside the uterus of the mother. The idea probably derives from iconography of the Greek-Orthodox church and Byzantine art. In modern times it is now possible to see the fetus inside the uterus by means of ultrasound which allows the mother to monitor the growth and movements of the fetus during the pregnancy. The desire for the visible internal baby as opposed to the invisible internal one existed before the era of new technology!

There is a story of a cult in honour of Piero’s fresco, that some think continues in secret even today – the pregnant women of Monterchi and surrounding areas make a pilgrimage to the cemetery chapel in the belief of putting themselves under the protection of Piero’s Madonna and asking her help in coping with birth. The belief in the protective role of the Piero’s pregnant Madonna was so strong that still in 1954 the Monterchi women prevented the painting from being transported to Florence to an exhibition, as they did not want to be deprived of her protection for even a short period of time. This cult, which defers to the intense need for a reference figure particularly before the birth, totally disregards the artistic recognition which was attributed to the work.

If we closely and repeatedly observe the Madonna del Parto painting, we are struck by its extraordinary ceremonial fixedness and at the same time by the many signs of human reality and truth similar to those yielded from studies and research on maternity. By depicting the Madonna in her pregnant condition, the artist diminishes the aureole attached to Her, she appears less like “Holy Mary” and more like “Mary”, and makes her seem more “womanly”. In the painting she is standing between two angels who are raising the curtains to reveal her. On the one hand, the curtains highlight the majesty of Mary and on the other, they emphasise the well-known need for protection and refuge linked to the fragility of the particular condition. She is wearing a simple and common dress “well-suited to her pregnant body and as if she could have been any other woman from the village.”

The whole curtain, which in the past also included a large red dome, creates an image of a type of casing and gives an impression of symmetry, solidness and strength, containing in its turn the baby inside. Altogether it gives the effect of the Russian Matryoshka dolls, one inside the next, Mary inside the case and the baby inside Mary.

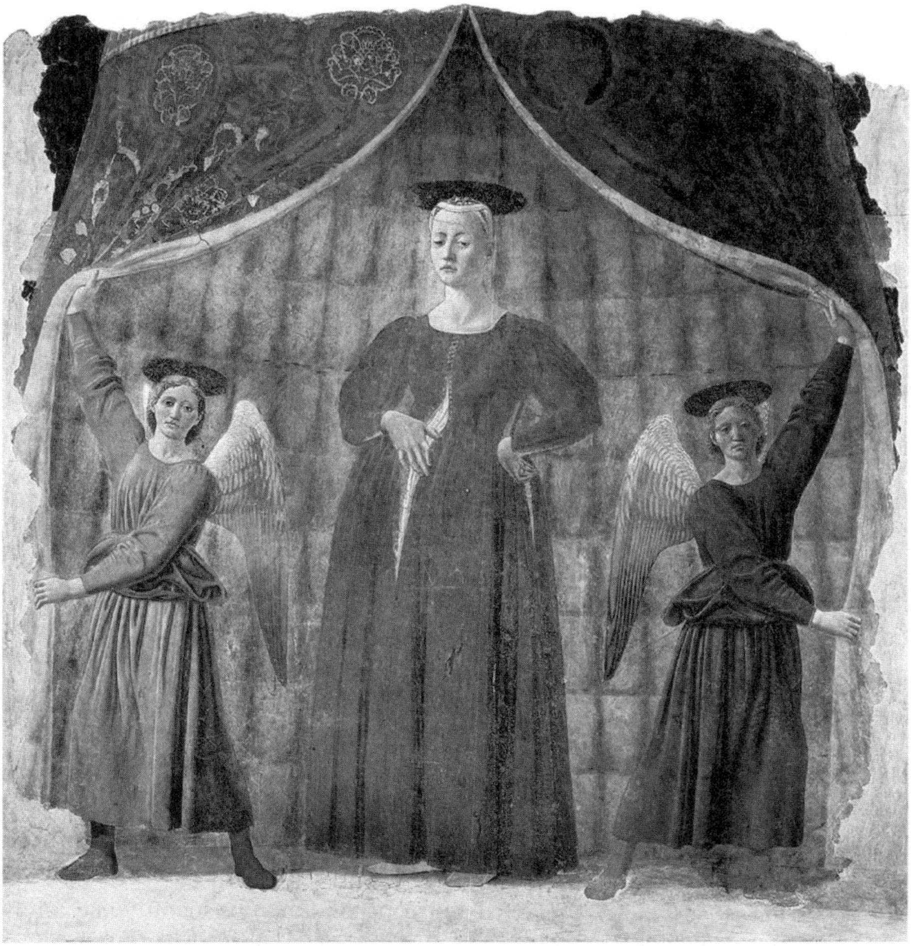

Figure 1. The painting represents the announcement of the coming event: the birth.

Mary's right hand rests on her stomach as if to reassure herself of the baby's presence and to protect him. This is a typical gesture made by pregnant women, the left hand lies on her side with her palm facing outwards. This very much takes away the solemnity of the scene, rendering the figure very realistic and close to the gestures of normal women, which Piero must have observed in the countryside (Piero used this hand position in the Arezzo frescos in the depiction of both the enigmatic young woman from the Flagellazione di Cristo ["The Flagellation"] and the queen of Saba's maid). This depiction of Mary does not show her with a book in her hand like other paintings of Mary at the Annunciation or of the birth, the book signifying another presence – the baby, the Word according to evangelical literature.

Expert observers of future mothers can note the difference of the position of the two hands. The right hand is linked to the concentrated and absorbed expression showing the fullness and intensity of the mother-baby relationship with an attitude of self-admiration. The left alludes to a reality left behind, put aside so that it does not interfere with this communication and privileged fusion which will end in the feared moment of birth. The relationship with the partner, sexuality, commitments and more can be put aside.

Mary's dress opens from the front and does not emphasise the increase in her body size. It shows a white stripe where her right hand is placed, highlighting even more where there is new life and at the same time that it is not easy to have this new being contained inside. The shoulders positioned backwards also seem to indicate the need to support the baby's weight.

Biographies of Piero by Vasari have commented how this image of Mary, very womanly in her pregnant condition, certainly idealized but also very realistic, can be attributed to the artist's attachment to his mother who gave birth to him after the death of his father and lovingly brought him up.

Studies and reflections for an observatory of interior maternity

Pregnancy, which from its beginning is referred to as "maternity", has been described and defined in various ways. It has been the object of multidisciplinary research and studies providing an extremely vast territory of objective and subjective biological experiences and is perceived in many ways from past and present socio-cultural contexts. It is, without a doubt, a major psychosomatic event.

Interior maternity entails the development of the feminine identity and a forming-process of mental representations. It is the place for fantasies, emotions, desires, dreams, and the place where bonds and affections are formed, new relationships made, and it is the home of this fantasized internal baby, soon to become a real external one.

With a group of psychoanalysts and psychotherapists of analytical orientation with a long history of experiences together in the course of studies dedicated to the observation of the newborn in its family environment and to research and study about maternity, we designed an Observatory for understanding this "maternal atmosphere" which develops in the pregnancy period and determines new mental events and transformations in the organisational processes of the individual.

Going back to baby-planning, running through all the stages of the pregnant state, exploring the changes that occur, considering the prenatal status of the infant and maternal management as stages in the development of the child and the mother, have all meant working with a "pre-infant observation" approach, as I defined it on the occasion of the Infant Observation Conference in Florence

(1999), and subsequently at International Conferences on Infant Observation in Krakow (2002) and Florence (2004).

In the initial period of our work we discussed a great deal what methodology to adopt in our exploration of the "interior maternity". We decided to use observation set-up and group discussion according to what we had learned from the work of Esther Bick, choosing to distance ourselves from the vast literature of numerous techniques and research methods, and concentrating instead on the pregnant condition based on questionnaires and structured interviews in different forms, all ways of studying mental representations and/or narrative models.

Reflecting on maternity in today's climate led us to examine the events which have brought about great changes: contraception, medical prevention, abortion laws, artificial insemination techniques, and new social and family pressures. The desire to have a baby or give one up, the desire for a healthy baby, a baby planned for at a stable time, a baby with that particular partner, connote a great freedom of choice rendering maternity a more mature and mindful decision, while we also encounter certain ambiguous sentiments surrounding the mystery of the origins of creative breeding. Behind every new birth and every unborn baby there is a unique story filled with dreams, feelings, unconscious mechanisms, desires, and different realities.

The relative paternal role in the relational dynamics with the future mothers was kept in mind, even if we have not yet been in a position to properly investigate it. We also considered very carefully the idea of exploration methodology which, from the very beginning, leaves the mothers under the biological monitor-control-domain undoubtedly aimed at prevention, preparation, and at the physical well-being of the mother and fetus. It is not certain however, how well this respects the mental life of the future mother. We have our doubts and experiences which bring this into question and have discovered that these kind of interventions can take the mother away from "thinking", from being in contact with her baby still inside her, from feeling the new relationship which is forming, even if this course of treatment is certainly aimed at providing support and reassurance. The pregnant women are definitely placed in a position of infantile regression by this health/prevention system and various types of alliances with or dependencies on the different health workers surrounding them are formed.

The ultrasound is a test which has become routine and is repeated several times during pregnancy. It has a notably important role if we reflect on the amount of information it gives on the life of the fetus and its abilities with repercussions on the fantasies the pregnant women has, transforming the "imaginary" baby into something much more real, an encounter with the real "fetus" already being called a "baby".

The first ultrasound serves as a type of "pregnancy certificate" and guarantees that all is normal. If this is the case and if until that moment the mother had been forming mental representations of herself and the imaginary baby, she now discovers the existence of another independent being and finds herself facing the responsibility of carrying a child, as if already born, inside her. At this point her role is no longer solely that of 'daughter' but also already of 'mother'. Michel Soulé (2000) spoke about the idea of the "abortion of the ghost" in describing the end of the fantasies with the sudden visible and verbal (the words of the ultrasound technician) confirmation of the fetus, now "figurative" and it is uncertain for how long this block lasts. This is certainly the case for some women, but for others it is possible that a re-organisation of the maternal imagination takes place. The first, and in fact subsequent ultrasounds, give the sensation of "worrying extraneousness" (Soulé) which seem to correspond to the Freudian descriptions of "The Uncanny" (1919) and which, if experienced, risks hindering the recommendable amount of imaginary investment in the fetus.

Mainly contributing to this disturbing aspect of the ultrasound procedure is the hesitation in recognising that it is all about a living being. Ultrasound technicians, gynecologists and various staff members involved, already use the word "baby" at this stage in order to humanize it and reduce the sense of extraneousness, bringing the activeness of the fetus to attention, its repetitive or rhythmic movements and the sounds coming from its heartbeats. Of course the other positive aspect of the ultrasound test when carried out in the presence of the future father is that it can also aid the *parentalization* process of the couple.

Before the era of ultrasound tests, the first indication of the activeness of their babies for future mothers was when they were able to feel their movements (around the fourth-fifth month) which are often described in relation to their daily life. They often told their close-ones or let them feel the movements, letting them share the experience and assigning a place to the baby in the family. At one time, these movements had a mysterious communicative significance, they were looked forward to, and attempts were made at deciphering their meaning. They were also observed by external figures, and provoked with physical contact (hands placed on abdomen). The baby became real but also inspired representations and dialogues that were still imaginary because they were "internal".

The amniocentesis procedure, which is currently considered more and more necessary, also has a worrying and anxiety inducing effect as is widely known. One of our colleagues told of one her patient's dreams at the fifth month of her pregnancy: "*I was locked in a room and heard a buzzing sound get louder and louder. I realised it was a helicopter which was circling the house sometimes approaching the window threateningly where I was able to see and hear it more clearly*". Immediately after telling her about this, she went on to say how the previous day she had undergone amniocentesis and hadn't liked it at all. The patient identified with the fetus inside and projected her own anxieties experienced during the test procedure onto it.

Among all the theoretical contributions and research on maternity we have discussed in the course of our study (for example, contributions from Franco Fornari, Massimo Ammaniti, Fausta Ferraro and many others belonging to the vast Italian and international literature on the topic), much interest surrounded the work of Monique Bydlowski (French psychiatrist and psychoanalyst) carried out over many years in a maternity ward. She has published various works including the volume "*Je rêve un enfant*" in which she discusses the interior experience of maternity, along with the culmination of observational, biological, sociocultural, and artistic points of view.

The theory proposed by Bydlowski on "*psychological transparency*", described as "*maternal psychological activity characterized in particular by the decrease in the pregnant woman's normal strength in facing unconscious repressed content with a marked hyperinvestment in her personal affairs and infantile conflicts, accompanied by major fluctuations in mental representations centred on undeniable narcissistic polarization*". "*The state of consciousness seems to become modified and the threshold of permeability in the unconscious and preconscious state is lowered*" (Bydlowski 1991) is much in keeping with our own hypotheses.

Bydlowski notes that the progression of pregnancy can be divided into various stages. Firstly, (in the sense of psychological transparency), the perception of the fetus as a concrete baby due to it being conceived and growing inside the womb, has its corresponding fantastical imagery and should still be considered an "internal object", reactivating deep within the recesses of her mind the baby the mother once was, or believes to have been up to that moment.

Subsequently as she approaches the final month of pregnancy, the fetus, as yet unborn but almost newborn, begins to take on an external status leading the pregnant woman to move away from the idea herself as "the container of the content" but with more of a focus on the future newborn. At this stage the fetus begins to be objectified in the mother's mind.

After birth, all of the mother's attention goes towards her baby which has now become a real external object even though many traces of the previous mental representations still remain. This process does not always happen gradually and does not necessarily coincide with birth. Many women still harbour their dreams of pregnancy after several weeks; they feel like they have lost the internal object while the external baby, driven by the strength of its needs for survival, stimulates her into dialogue (Vallino, 2004).

Other authors have described the various phases of pregnancy, indicating them with respect to corporeal transformations, anxieties, mental representations, fear of labor, and delivery. However, Monique Bydlowski chose to highlight the changing from an "internal object" to an "external object", assigning particular importance because, as already discussed, exploration methodologies and especially the ultrasound test lead to the premature objectification of the future newborn by the mothers, rendered almost newborn in the images and photos.

Esther Bick was not in a position to contemplate the development of these tests which nowadays initiate a dialogue between a (premature?) mother and her baby which, from the first ultrasound, is already perceived as an external object.

The observatory of interior maternity

The structural plan for an Observatory suitable for interpreting and "narrating" the experiences that surround the beginnings of the mother-baby relationship was gradually outlined based on the experiences and competencies of the study and research group on interior maternity.

The locations and real and emotional contexts that allowed the group to deeply explore the experience of pregnancy were vastly diverse, enabling them to "contemplate" and describe:

1. *Preliminary Infant Observation meetings*

The methodology involves a preliminary meeting at the beginning of the observation period, to take place preferably in the final period of pregnancy.

For Esther Bick (1964) the first meeting was important for introducing the observation plan to the future mother, making arrangements, fixing the setting, and making the mother aware and getting her used to the presence of the observer who is non-intrusive but respectful and participates emotionally.

Practical experience demonstrated how important this first encounter between future mother and observer was, as it allowed the sensing of an already emotionally rich 'maternal atmosphere', the immediate and complex transference between the projections of the mother onto the observer and the mother's strong emotional involvement in facing this new experience.

Our research group highlighted how these first encounters include vital moments for the *observation of interior maternity*. It was actually noticed that, from the very beginning, it is possible to observe the state of anxiety felt when birth is imminent and various warning signs in the mother-baby relationship and mother-baby-observer relationship which subsequently set in.

We found a correlation with the research carried out by Peter Fonagy (1992) which highlights the predictions that can be made at this stage about future mother-baby relationships through the study of the maternal mental representations surfacing during the pregnancy. He identified continuity between the maternal style which sets in during the pregnancy and the one carried on after birth. The final phase of pregnancy requires the mother to prepare herself psychologically for the separation from the baby inside her, the typical anxieties surrounding this and the fear of loss.

Donald Winnicott observed and documented the existence of an abnormal *psychological* condition amongst women who had just given birth, a particular condition which, without the involvement of a baby, could be taken for a genuine mental pathology which he refers to as "*primary maternal anxiety*". This condition develops gradually before reaching a sharp sensitivity level during pregnancy, particularly towards the end and after birth (both prenatal and postnatal primary maternal anxiety are referred to, the latter associated with the well-known physiological post-partum depression).

The reality of the anxiety is almost always present at the first encounters and can often be revealed due to the presence of the observer, as if being seen as the concrete representation of the obvious and inevitable fact of the imminent birth (similar to the sudden appearance of the angel at the Annunciation) making the pregnant woman face the reality of the vicinity of birth and interrupting the maternal fantasies and experiences of fusion.

In the preliminary meetings we find ourselves at a point where the interior relationships between mother and future baby have *already begun*. This inspired us to look back and explore the beginnings of the psychological process which brings about the forming of the mother's new identity – from Infant Observation to Pre-Infant Observation.

I cite below a detailed example of *maternal atmosphere and warning signs* in the mother-baby relationship (confirmed at subsequent observations).

At the first encounter, Ms. R., in her thirties, of non-Italian nationality and expecting her first child, was attentive to all the practical and concrete aspects, self-assured, competent and had everything pre-arranged and organized.

Starting from the first statement (". . . my house is small, it's fine for two but maybe not for three") she seemed to have not made any mental space for the baby, she never referred to any fantasies she had about him – we don't know if he was planned for or if she had thought of a name. Even the cot ("wooden rocking cot") is small – a play cot situated in the corner of the couple's large room. The interview is based on the mother's descriptions of how she continued to work and follow a dance course up until the seventh month, only feeling the baby at night, not wanting to "see him" (stressing the importance of the half-light in the delivery room and clinic nursery, "I want the lights dimmed"). She did an accelerated prenatal course in preparing "for the birth". She plans to give birth in the presence of many people; her husband, sister, gynecologist and another obstetrician. The needs and fears surrounding the imminence of birth (due in nine days) seem to be replaced with the organization of an exceptional birth, using her power to create in a narcissistic way, a type of crib where wise men and shepherds are in adoration of Mary giving birth.

The difficulties for this mother in having emotional connections (mental representations) with the future baby are found in the vicissitudes of our observation of mother-baby relationship which continued over two years. Already at the second observation session, the mother tells of how the baby's bottom is red and inflamed, somatically concretizing contact problems. The observer also notes that there is no visual or mental contact with the baby. The mother does not name the baby (as previously alluded to) after the birth. In the first observations she manages to see the baby, which is put to sleep all covered up in its little cot at a safe distance, with difficulty whereas the mother continues to go into – in detail – what the baby "does" and shows the observer photos of the baby and a big album full of photos of the baby's development from zero to three years. At around the fifth month the mother returns to her native country to her mother's house. The baby was hospitalized for persistent atopic dermatitis, kept isolated for a certain period in a sterile room where the mother could see him and give him milk as if they were both in a large incubator. The baby's skin problems are resolved and the mother finds a way to improve contact with the child until she can return to Italy. (Observer Laura Mori)

2. *In the consulting rooms*

In our capacity as psychoanalysts and psychotherapists the pre-infancy period is examined in our consulting-rooms when the patient plans for a baby and then experiences the entire pregnancy and subsequent phases with us. In this context the state of interior maternity is highlighted by means of transference-countertransference movements and expresses itself in ways particular to psychoanalytical methodology.

The presence of clinical facts which induce and/or determine the pregnancy in question are also taken into account along with the displacement of anxieties and defences in many cases. There are changes in the analytical relationship due to the new object which has entered into the patient's life – the fetus playing its own role as transference object, a situation familiar to any analyst who has worked with pregnant women. The psychoanalytical treatment becomes an opportunity for the "active" observation of interior maternity and the mother-baby relationship and at times the patients show a certain level of self-observation in order to speed up the analytical process. The analyst and patient both undoubtedly witness the transformation of the "patient" who is experiencing an "interesting" situation requiring a continuous readjustment of the whole clinical setting. The interpretative as well as control function (non-explicit but on the analyst's mind) are maintained in the treatment room.

Description of a clinical sketch:

One of my young married patients who required treatment for her depression resembling her mother's depression, told me at one of the first sessions of her and her husband's plans to have a baby. After only a few months of analysis did she begin to tell me about the anxieties she had about not being able to have a baby and subsequently about the investigations which had begun to discover the cause of infertility – which turned out not to be attributed to her but to a weak sperm count in her spouse.

Her desire to have a baby became clear throughout the analyses and her need to treat the depression was tied in with wanting to be a sufficiently good mother.

Modern insemination techniques involving her and her husband finally succeed and she becomes pregnant.

Until the 3rd month of pregnancy there are rich fantasies and forming of fears and hopes which climax at the amniocentesis test which indicates that the fetus is a healthy boy. The patient recognises the contribution of the analyses in being able to get in touch with her psychological movement and profound emotions. At around the sixth month the patient at a session tells me that she cannot pay attention to what I am saying. She is thinking about what is happening inside her, about the placenta and the cells of the fetus' organs which are growing and explains that it's not that she's thinking about it scientifically but it is her new role of expressing energy from her mind to her tummy. She speaks of her "displacement". In that moment I realized that I also needed to "move myself" as analyst in order to welcome what was arriving again between us. At this stage in the analysis she vaguely remembered her dreams and appeared to close herself in with the baby silently assuming different positions and moving in a way that made the situation seem "sacred", reminding me of Piero della Francesca's "Madonna del Parto".

The patient contentedly brought the pregnancy to term, the analyses continued and after two years she became pregnant again without external intervention. I had the opportunity to follow her case through the second pregnancy and note that she achieved a balanced maternal role for the second time.

3. *Preparation for maternity*

From our first year of work, we discussed some of our experiences as public health workers and in particular our participation on the *prenatal courses*, which we regarded as important occasions in which to observe interior maternity. The prenatal course is where pregnant women can speak about their subjective experiences. If a warm and intimate maternal atmosphere is successfully created within the group, the women express themselves spontaneously, begin to get in touch with their own body and gradually get closer to the fantastical world linked with their own experience of having been babies with their mothers. They feel the fetus-baby still inside them, not just see it in the ultrasound test.

The courses are generally aimed at women who are in their last months of pregnancy, the period of great changes to the body and extreme physical and emotional tiredness often accompanied by senses of loneliness and isolation. The woman needs a figure of reference and support in this period and tends to favour fellow females. It is important for them to share their maternity experiences with other women, the sentiment of "being one of us", as they say.

The period is accompanied by the sense of loss of their previous state, a type of evolutionary struggle and anxiety of experiencing a transformation of their female identity into a new maternal code. It is necessary for the woman expecting a child to harbour a positive image of maternity and the historical figure of the obstetrician is traditionally characterized as the woman who knows everything, who survives deliveries, who banishes any lurking threat of death.

The women who had given birth described of how they anticipated meeting their baby in their dreams, as though for them it is impossible to imagine the delivery itself – the unknown. They describe: "I dreamt of a baby already grown and nourished, but didn't see his face clearly", "I often dream about a baby who wakes up without crying and who smiles at me when I go to his crib" and "I'm ok now but I had a difficult pregnancy up to the fifth month and I dream of the delivery only from the part where they cut the cord – it's a really nice dream".

Excerpts of two moments from these group atmospheres:

The "baby-mothers" (conducted by Linda Fortini)

In the discussion held at one session (about 15 future mothers), lines of thinking emerge as to the role of the obstetrician at the delivery. Some of the women who had given birth prefer to hand over the management of the delivery, feeling a great need for dependency on a figure of reference. This regression makes them appear like "baby-mothers" ("Here, I am taught what to do and if I didn't know, I'd panic. . .. ")

"The color of the delivery room" (Conducted by: Daniela Martignano)

In this session the simultaneous presence of the obstetrician and psychologist clearly represent two different aspects, like the body and the mind, in one reality (the pregnant individual). The women seem to go from one to another depending on their specific needs. During the session, the topic shifts from the imminent birth to future problems with regard to breast-feeding and then back to the birth again ("we need to go back there"). Anxieties coming from external reality (examinations, preparation for and management of birth) add to internal anxieties and everything seems quite overwhelming, almost like a "mini breakdown", with phases of denial and/or idealization ("Is it possible to choose the color of the delivery room?").

4. *Pre-infant observation*

Our research greatly benefited from the possibility of following the cases of some women right from the beginning of their pregnancies. The most significant moments and changes taking place were discussed in the group which transformed emotionally and intensively to understand the interior maternity of these future mothers.

Below is the brief report of a hairdresser's pregnancy (observer: Luigia Cresti).

This was quite an "atypical" observation case as the young pregnant woman (33 year-old hair-dresser who we will refer to as "Daniela", active and enthusiastic about her job, quite an extrovert and well able to enjoy life, simple but sensitive) was already acquainted with the observer. The observer had known the woman from adolescence to adulthood, albeit not in a professional sense, and had witnessed the gradual definition of her femininity and her sentimental choices and finally the decision to have a baby "with the right man at the right time".

It seems that, up to the second month, D. attributed the role of listener of her interior movements to the client-observer. She tells the observer spontaneously of her pregnancy and immediately describes a dream:

"I was inside a type of big balloon full of water. It wasn't transparent, there were lots of what looked like pumpkin seeds and some peat. I was swimming the breaststroke, without seeing very well in front of me when I caught a glimpse of a little head coming my way – it was a baby girl with chubby face and light-blue eyes and she was looking right at me!

In this dream we notice the normal regressive identification with the fetus-baby, a baby reactivating the same one D. once was and the incipient assumption of the maternal role with the imminent arrival of the intimate meeting with the potential baby. There is an obvious sense of difficulty in "focussing" on this new emotional experience.

The overall course of pregnancy confirms the impression that it signifies an important maturation process for the young woman. Internally, it involves the double identification process with the fetus and her own mother. The series of internal processes dealing with the relationship of her own mother is in the form of a dream in the latter stages of pregnancy" (6th month). "I was dreaming about my mother as she actually is, about 60 years old. I saw her while she was in the throes of labor, she was at home and I offered to accompany her to the bathroom to give birth. Then I saw her with her feet in the bath tub, legs slightly open, but she was telling me to go away and tell my father to come in. Shortly afterwards I saw a baby comes out of the bathroom with a curly head and already walking" (One of her brothers does have, in fact, curly hair).

Here we see fantasies and anxieties of an Oedipal nature towards the mother and her procreative abilities. There is also recognition of the paternal role accompanied by a sense of her own exclusion from the primary scene. This is followed by an unconscious "repairing" anxiety compared to infantile impulses of Oedipal rivalry and perhaps envy to restore fertility to her mother. It seems highly significant in her internal history as a child including the surprising arrival of her little brother.

The observer was able to verify the reorganization process of the young woman's femininity over the course of the months involving her having to renounce aspects of her life, which was not easy – from being an independent, active girl, free to enjoy travelling, dancing, spending time with friends, D. needs to stop working at the 5th month as advised by her gynecologist and then gradually reduce travelling by car, which allowed her to get away for a few weekend holidays until the beginning of the 7th month, after which she is advised to learn how to "keep calm".

In the final months, D. repeatedly expresses the desire to "get some air", reminiscent of claustrophobic anxiety. Her pregnancy is actually quite demanding and there is also a family history of Down's syndrome entailing a *"hidden crisis" of which we detect indirect signs and slightly manic-defensive behaviour. D. smiles, actually laughs a lot, sometimes with an air of excitement, up to the final phases, minimizing her fears surrounding the amniocentesis and birth. (on many occasions the staff points out the possibility of a cesarean delivery). At the 9th month the defence against the anxiety felt towards the birth seems to intensify by means of fantasies and dreams in which D. "by-passes" the birth experience, imagining that her baby has already been born, raised and is walking about. She tells of having dreamt "that she was at the hospital, she knew she had already given birth and she saw the babies walking about. Then she left the hospital with these two little ducks".*

Throughout the course of this pregnancy, the significance of the ultrasound tests and the way of communicating their result was very interesting. The tests seem to have had a significant emotional investment for D. and in fact from the 3rd month they force D. (in a rather traumatic way) to face the idea of an "external object" due to the revelation of the fact that she is expecting twins!

Regarding the "trauma" of discovering about the twins it seems that this was rather quickly and positively emotionally integrated, actually nourishing a "heightened" sense of herself and identification with the idea of being a strong, fertile, mother. The fact that the placentas are distinct contributes to the development of anxieties surrounding expecting twins, and faced with subsequent ultrasound images we see D. constantly making the effort to distinguish between the two fetus (by weight, measurements, position and differing kicks).

It is interesting to note how D. appears disturbed at the vision of the "little pieces" of baby produced by the ultrasound images but as if it inspires a global image of the babies or the perception of embryonic "gestures" which are potentially full of meaning (the fetus scratches its head or seems to open its mouth).

D. develops a rather stable perception relatively early and differentiates the temperament of the two baby girls (one livelier and larger, the other calmer and smaller) showing her mental adaptation to the two babies. At the 8th month, D. shows the observer a homemade piece of furniture, separated into two parts, which she personally made for the two unborn babies. The two distinct spaces are very clearly cut out in the little home for the two babies, each in its own placenta as they were seen in a previous ultrasound. The mother is creating a double space – both physically and mentally for her daughters, still helped and supported by her husband, as known by the observer.

The babies are born by caesarean section, one smaller than the other and the case is followed by the observer for another two years.

Conclusions

In conclusion, I list below some of the main points of our research and experience in the form of "central ideas".

1. Every experience of interior maternity is unique. The uniqueness of every mother-baby relationship has already been highlighted in many IO studies.
2. There is a constant presence of a certain amount of anxiety ("hidden erisis") which fluctuates in the way it emerges and manifests itself in relation to potentially distressing events to do with the development of the pregnancy, with the results of biological monitoring, in particular environmental situations, and most of all, dependant on the transformation of the unconscious mental representations (for example after a dream).
3. There is a need for figures of reference (the mother, obstetrician, gynecologist, partner or observer).
4. The future newborn is precociously objectified, it is perceived as almost already born due to the virtual images from the ultrasound, however still in its internal baby (fetus) state. It has not yet taken its place in the mental space and therefore constitutes a "premature" mother-baby relationship.
5. A complex process of identification of the pregnant woman with her own mother exists.
6. Pre-infant observation and listening to future mothers has a deep transforational function: they change themselves from mothers who feel, see, speak, dream, and suffer to mothers who "think". In IO, the phenomenon of mothers who learn to observe their own baby is often discussed.

The work methodology adopted centred on group discussions, the experiences in various sectors of the observatory (presented here in reduced and limited format), the quantity of theoretical analysis, acquired knowledge and competencies, recording and collection of all the meeting minutes (each group member took their turn to write up the minutes which now form an Archive on interior maternity) are all elements which contributed to constructing a "work in progress" atmosphere in the group over the period of time. Moreover, every group member had a mindset which was very much sensitized to listening, observing and understanding particular psychic processes which accompany the pregnant woman from the baby-planning stages to after the actual maternity experience when the baby has been born.

The Observatory, as well as being a research and study space, became an educational environment with professional figures prepared to develop a new clinical and therapeutic climate for the consultation and treatment of pregnant women when they most need it. I maintain that this helping environment is greatly beneficial to the work of health staff in the maternity sector and can contribute to the prevention of frequent and, at times, tragic post-partum psychiatric disturbances.

The group of co-workers consists of Luigia Cresti Scacciati, psychotherapist psychologist; Linda Root Fortini, psychotherapist psychologist; Isabella Lapi, psychotherapist psychologist; Arianna Luperini, psychoanalyst psychologist; Daniela Martignano, psychologist; Marco Mastella, psychoanalyst neuropsychiatrist pediatrician; Fiorella Monti, psychotherapist psychologist; Laura Mori, psychotherapist psychologist; Gristina Pratesi, psychotherapist psychologist; Gabriella Smorto, psychotherapist psychologist.

References

Ammanniti M: (a cura di) La gravidanza fra fantasia e realtà. Cortina, Milano 1992

Bick E: Notes on infant observation in psychoanalytic training. In: Int. Journ. Psycho-anal. 45 (1964) 558–566

Bydlowski M: Je rêve un enfant. L'experiénce intérieure de la maternité. Odile Jacob, Paris 2000 Bydlowski M: La transparence psychique de la grossesse. In: Etudes freudiennes 32 (1991) 2–9

Ferrara Mori G: (a cura di) L'osservazione dell'interazione madre-bambino nel primo anno di vita: presentazione di una esperienza, riflessioni e testimonianze. In: Quaderni di psicoterapia infantile 4 (1981) 179–200

Ferrara Mori G: Les formes et le niveau du chamgement dans la formation de l'observateur. In Sandri R: (a cura di) L'observation du nourisson selon Esther Bick et ses applications. Césura Lyon Editino, Meyzieu 1994

Ferrara Mori G: Apprendere dall'osservazione. In: Cresti L, Farneti P, Pratesi C et al. (eds): Osservazione e trasformazione. Borla, Roma 2001

Ferraro F, A Nunziante-Cesaro: Lo spazio cavo e il corpo saturato. Franco Angeli, Milano 1985

Fonagy P: La genesi dell'attaccamento: la relazione della donna al feto durante la gravidanza, Trad. it. in Ammanniti M. (a cura di) op. cit.

Fornari F: Il codice vivente. Bollati Boringhieri, Torino 1981

Freud S: Il perturbante, vol. 10. trad. it: OSF 1919

Soulé M: La vita del feto. In: Righetti P, Sette L: (a cura di) Non c'è due senza tre. Bollati Boringhieri, Torino 2000

Vallino D: Essere neonati. Borla, Roma 2004

Walter I: Piero della Francesca – La Madonna del Parto. Franco Cosimo Panini, Trad. it. Modena 1996

Winnicott W: Through Paediatrics to Psycho-Analysis. Tvistock Publications, London 1958

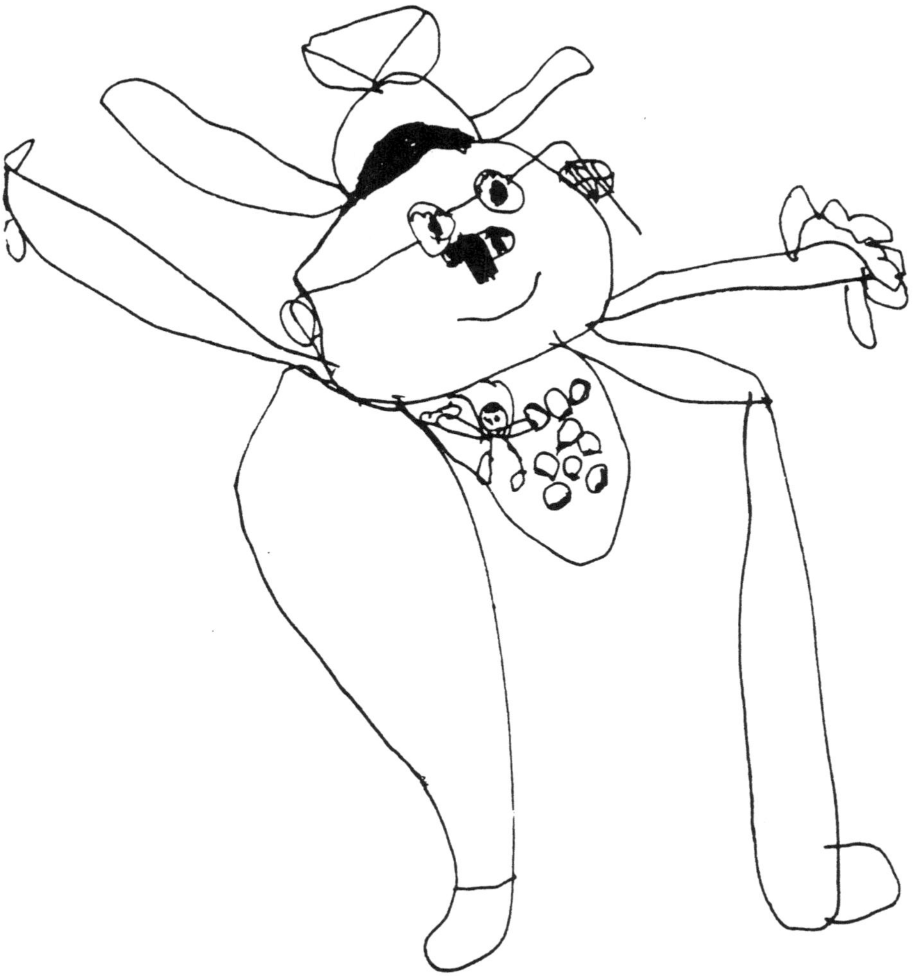

(Federica, 4 yrs. 7 mos.)
I got born again; one time I was born from my mom's tummy, and one time from my dad's tummy.

9. Transition to fatherhood

Adriana Lis; Department of Psychology of Development and Socialisation,University of Padua, Italy
Alessandro Gennaro; Department of Pedagogical and Didactic Psychological Sciences, University of Lecce, Italy
Claudia Mazzeschi; Department of Human and Educational Sciences, University of Perugia, Italy

Within the life cycle, becoming a parent represents a fundamental step involving important changes in the psycho-sociological life of a couple (Zeanah et al., 1990; Abelin, 1971; Bimbi, Castellano, 1990). It also represents a 'marker event' (Levinson, 1987) which has significant repercussions on the development of adult personality.

The birth of a child should be considered within a precise 'context' (understood here as both a socio-psychological network – including the mental relationship, work, social support, and psychological support for the partner – and the socio-cultural context in which the father's role and function are envisaged). Furthermore, even though parenthood is a step which is taken at a particular time, it is nonetheless part of a long process of growth. For this reason many scholars emphasize the significance of this event in terms of 'developmental crisis' or even 'developmental phase'. On the one hand, many scholars underline the growth and the personal development of both parents, on the other, they tend to emphasize how the choice of having a child interacts with various psychodynamic dimensions which refer to: the history of the couple, the family and its intergenerational relations, a revision of the way individuals have experienced maternity and paternity during childhood, the gender differences implied by motherhood and fatherhood respectively, and, in general, the configuration of new identities, which appear to be connected to the sense of the self and to the separation from, and the confrontation with, one's own parent figures (Erikson, 1964; Fonagy, Target, 2001).

As far as the parents are concerned, the need to allow space for a third person, who has the right to occupy a precise place and has a precise role, means developing a complex process which, on a behavioral level, requires reorganizing the couple's schedules and physical spaces and, on a mental level, involves preparing to welcome the baby, by creating an adequate psychological space. In so doing, parents work towards constituting an efficient and well balanced triad, thus avoiding exclusions and the formation of coalitions. In this sense, the function of parents appears simultaneously extremely complex and very delicate. The choice of having a child, which implies important psychological processes in relation to the individual, the couple, and the very notion of generativity –

understood here as the ability to take care of what parents have given birth to together, that is to take care of the other's difference (Mahler et al., 1975; Scabini, Cigoli, 2000) – requires a redefinition of masculine and feminine identity. The birth of a child therefore also implies a change in the way parents relate to each other. On the one hand there is the weakening of 'companionship', that is the pleasure that 'doing things together' can give; on the other, however, there is the intensification of the 'partnership', that is the sense of belonging and supporting each other.

Since the 1980s, researchers and psychologists investigating the function of parents have shifted their attention from a study of the development of maternity to an analysis of the father's function, its development and its influences on the child's development, thus bringing to the fore the importance of this figure which had been neglected for a long time.

One of the first and clear conceptualizations of father involvement is Lamb's work (1987). According to this model, the role of the parent involves three stages: involvement (the parent interacts on a one-to-one basis with the child during activities such as feeding, playing etc); accessibility (the parent is at the child's disposal both physically and psychologically); and responsibility (the parent feels responsible for the child's well-being and his/her care). Although Lamb's work (1987) was the starting point of much research into father involvement, it has also been criticized. For instance, authors such as Hawkins and Palkovitz (1999), Hawkins et al. (2002), Palkovitz (1997) and Daly (2001) maintain that research on fatherhood over the last thirty years, has conceptualized the father's involvement in the child's birth in terms of a specific temporal event in relation to components which are directly observable, thereby sustaining a unidimensional vision of this notion. In contrast, Hawkins and Palkovitz (1999) propose a pluridimensional vision of father participation, which consists of affective and cognitive, as well as behavioral, components which can be directly observed, and which have often been studied in relation to fatherhood.

The development of various positions on father involvement has led contemporary researchers to consider possible ways of conceptualizing and measuring father involvement. In so doing, research contributes to the analysis of this phenomenon, in an attempt to clarify (and, more recently, to extend) existent conceptualizations of fatherhood, increasingly focusing on specific aspects (Day, Lamb, 2004; Doherty et al., 1998; Hawkins, Dollahite, 1997; Lamb, 2004; Palkovitz, 1997; Pleck, Masciardelli, 2004). In particular, Palkovitz (1997) has innovated the concept of father involvement by identifying 15 important categories of parental participation: communication, teaching, control, ability to develop judgments about what is going on, guidance in situations of need, care giving, handling capacity, separation of interests, readiness to help, ability to plan for the future, repartition of the activities, affection, protection, and ability to offer emotional support by advising the child. Research in this field is paying greater and greater attention both to the quality and quantity of the father's participation in his children's lives (Cabrera et al., 2000; Hawkins, Dollahite, 1997). This development is very challenging for researchers, and this is particularly true in relation to the development of reliable criteria of evaluation which could enable an assessment of father participation from a pluridimensional perspective (Day, Daughter, 2004; Hawkins et al., 2002; Marsiglio, Day, Lamb, 2000; Palkovitz, 2002; Parke, 2002; Roggman et al., 2002).

Many researchers have taken up these challenges in the attempt to develop relatively brief and fairly global measures for evaluating father participation, capable of representing the complexity of this pluridimensional construction adequately (Hawkins et al., 2002). It must however be said that occasionally these attempts have lost sight of the complete range of behaviors which reflect the diversity in the way individuals approach their parental role. A fundamental issue related to this problem, concerns the conceptualization of father participation as comprehensive of all the domains which researchers have recently identified or imagined as a unitary construction. This issue is essentially reflected in the identification of father involvement with a unidimensional view of a pluridimensional construction. Indeed, if father participation is unidimensional, it means that participation, as a general construction, is something which should be measured with a single generic variable (for example, we could measure father participation and reach the general conclusion that for those fathers who are less involved it is an extra).

Although various theoretical conceptualizations have been discussed, the surveys on previous research (Russell, Radojevic, 1992; Tiedje, Darling, 1996) have brought to the fore the fact that it is difficult to systematize the data due to the wide range of themes involved, the complexity of the works themselves, and the lack of underlying conceptual models which could integrate the various discoveries in a more wide-ranging perspective. In spite of this, in our opinion, it is possible to emphasize two important perspectives, which remain fundamental even though they present the same limitations highlighted in the surveys mentioned above. The first is a clinical perspective founded on psychoanalysis, which involves the formulation of new models for the interpretation of the father function and the transition to fatherhood. The second is an empiric-psychodynamic approach, which has focused, in particular, on empirical studies of aspects connected to the development of an image of the self, the concept of attachment, and other variables associated with the transition to fatherhood. Clearly we could not avoid referring to a common psychoanalytic background and the implications it might have. These references have emphasized a change in the role of the father (Parke, 1998), who is no longer perceived solely as an authoritative figure, but is conceived of as a more complex one.

The expression 'transition to fatherhood', refers to the lapse of time from the beginning of pregnancy to the first month of the infant's life. During this period, the role of the father, and everything it implies, becomes an 'object of investment' (Farrel, Rosemberg, 1993). This moment of transition must be studied as a specific phase in the development of an individual's personality, during which the individual's level of development until that moment concurs with the specific social network he enters (Hawkins et al., 1993).

The psycho-dynamic clinical approach

Although interest in the 'father' and 'paternity' dates back to the 1980s, there are fewer studies on this subject than on maternity (Chalmers, Meyer, 1996; Barclay, Lupton, 1999). In addition, the literature does not seem to consider the socio-cultural changes which nowadays influence this experience (Draper, 2002). This particular field of research has often been criticized because it seems to be an extension of the research originally conceived as an analysis of the parental experience of mothers (Draper, 2002). The way fathers perceive themselves as fathers and the way in which the socio-cultural context influences contemporary experiences of fatherhood are therefore virtually unknown. Indeed, early research focused on the difficult adaptation of fathers to their new function on a physical (Ferketich, Mercer, 1989; Hyssala et al., 1992; Mason, Elwood, 1995), psychological (Klein, 1991; Mercer et al., 1993), and psychiatric level (Ballard, Davies, 1996; Leathers et al., 1997), thereby offering a sort of 'pathologized' vision of paternity (Lupton, Barclay, 1998), according to which fathers rarely have the opportunity to describe their experience (Sharpe, 1994).

It is precisely in this direction that research has moved in the last few years (Strass, Goldberg, 1999; Catherine et al., 2000; Draper, 2002; Piccinini, 2004; Kugelberg, 2006), by focusing attention on this particular moment of a man's life both within the family and in relation to his own well-being.

Currently, the focus is on the change in the father's role. This change is obviously connected to the transformation of the social representation of the father's function (for example the growing commitments of women in the workplace), the different demographic profile of new families and the increasing debates on children's well being, which are of course related to a proliferation of scholarly works emphasizing the importance of father involvement during the period which precedes birth of the first child (Marsiglio, 1995; Lamb, 2004).

This new broad perspective has led to an increase in the literature on paternity (Cabrera et al., 2000; Day, Lamb, 2004; Tamis-LeMonda, Cabrera, 2002). However, no researcher has offered an exhaustive description of the way boys become parents, and, as yet, no researcher has provided a single theory capable of explaining the complex development which shapes the paternal experience (Cabrera, 2000). For example, if we consider the idea that awareness of the father role and its significance forms during the period which stretches from childhood to the birth of the first child (an idea that is essentially based on the fact that boys become fathers of boys who will, in turn, become fathers in the future), it appears that childhood experience and paternal capability are not directly related. For instance, Hoffert (1999) shows how fathers reveal that they relate to their children more on the example of their fathers than their mothers, even when they admit they had irresponsible fathers.

During pregnancy, the role of the father is defined in terms of the support and help provided in the preparation of an adequate physical and, more importantly, psychological space within the couple, into which the new member will enter. This clearly implies, in the father too, the activation of complex processes of integration and adjustment of identity, which appear intimately connected to the Oedipal phase (Ammaniti et al., 1995). From this perspective, research focusing on changes in the conception of the self, appears particularly interesting. This research has highlighted three different aspects which help the individual's growth: the sense of identity as a parent; the locus of control, and self esteem. These elements reorganize other aspects of the self in order to establish a more coherent sense of the self in various roles, especially in relation to the new role of parent (Strauss, Goldberg, 1999).

These changes, which lead both parents to develop their own parenthood, appear as determinant elements from a psychological perspective, not only in order to categorize the vast range of experiences, but also to interpret future events (Zeanah, Stewart, 1990).

The process of transition to fatherhood, a period which is closely connected to the birth of the first child, is a period of major change and reorganizations, which may occasionally be the cause of drastic personal, conjugal, familial, and social changes. The couple must create a psychological space for their child, and this begins during the last three months of pregnancy, when fetal movements become clear evidence of the baby's presence and encourage parents to fantasize about their child and their new identity as parents (Zeanah et al., 1990). The parents' picture of the child includes phantasmal representations of the child endowed with its own personality and belonging to the mother and father (Stern, 1991). These representations will of course undergo modifications at the child's birth and will influence the quality of the conjugal relationship. In particular, the parents' ability to anticipate their child's mental state is a fundamental process which can lead to the establishment of a secure relationship of attachment with the parents (Fonagy, 1991). In relation to this, Fonagy and co-workers (Fonagy, Steel and Morgan, 1991; Steele, Steele and Fonagy, 1996; Fonagy and Target, 1997), have introduced the notion of 'reflective self', a concept which has become operative through the 'Self Reflect Function Scale' and which refers to the capacity to understand each other's mental states in terms of mental representations.

It is important to remember once again the sequence proposed by May (1982) in relation to the way fathers acknowledge the pregnancy. According to May, fathers are initially suspicious of the pregnancy, and wait for it to be confirmed. They then accept it as a verified fact, and in the end, during a third phase which begins with the third trimester, fathers live the pregnancy as a fundamental stage in their lives, finally defining themselves as fathers.

In relation to father involvement during pregnancy, May (1980) emphasizes that the relationship with the partner can be of different kinds, and identifies three profiles: the observer, fathers who consider the pregnancy as external to their lives and essentially view it as something which falls within their wife's competence (an attitude which leads them to remain at a safe distance from this experience); the instrumental father, who emphasizes his present and future responsibilities towards the child; and the expressive father, who appears emotionally involved in the event and elaborates on the child's life within the couple from the very moment the woman announces she is pregnant.

In spite of these three different levels of emotive involvement, recent research (Piccinini, 2006) indicates that at a low level of emotive involvement, some fathers find it difficult to acknowledge their child as real even during the last three months of pregnancy.

Palkovitz's re-conceptualization of the father's involvement within the couple emphasizes a pluridimensional perspective and also underlines the cognitive and affective functions typical of parenthood, aspects which have not been the focus of, or have not been actually considered by, previous conceptualizations. Other approaches have recently developed from a socio-constructivist (Marsiglio et al., 2000) and social (Amato, 1998) perspective.

Our contribution to this topic

In recent years we have focused on the 'transition to parenthood', in an attempt to broaden the theoretical conceptualization of this period and identify specific methodological tools for an empirical study of these conceptualizations. This aim has been realized thanks to a substantial research on both the pregnancy and the baby's first month of life. The research was carried out on 112 couples at the seventh month of pregnancy, who were contacted again immediately after birth. However, this paper refers only to some aspects of the work carried out, namely those concerning the period of pregnancy. The average age was 24 for women and 28 for men. The socio-economic level, calculated by means of the Four Factor Index elaborated by Hollingshead (1975), indicated a family average of 35.5. In descriptive terms, this suggests that approximately half the parents of both sexes had attended secondary school for at least for a few years. From a professional point of view, more than half of the sample was employed, in professions that ranged from generic workers, to industrial managers earning a good salary. The methodological interest, on the basis of a psychodynamic background, has led to the creation of The Clinical Interview for Parents During Pregnancy (CGG; Lis et al., 2000).

The CGG is a semi-structured interview which aims to study the emotional and affective attitudes of parents during pregnancy, focusing in particular on certain areas such as: the development of pregnancy (sensations, feelings, fears), fetal movements, fantasizing about the baby's physical and mental characteristics.

On the basis of the data offered by the application of the CGG, we have identified the different styles of involvement/detachment which fathers expressed during the interview. These styles conceptually refer to the dimensions highlighted by May (1980) in terms of the father's involvement (observer, expressive, instrumental), and are depicted in terms of scales. Every scale is, in turn, evaluated by the father in relation to the baby, the couple and his own parents (Lis et al., 2000).

The Reflective Self Function of the CGG was also assessed through three sub-scales: the global reflective self function (GRSF), the frequency of low reflective self function (LRSF), the frequency of medium and high reflective self function (HRSF). The father's function was investigated in relation to three main elements: the baby, the couple, and the father's own parents. The value of the Reflective Self Function was assessed on the basis of 5 grades (1, 3, 5, 6, 7 and 9). More precisely, the LRSF was assessed using grades from 1 to 3, while the HRSF by using grades from 5 to 9. The LRSF was interpreted as a sign of low reflective capability, which is explicit but not characterized by a particular sensitivity, whereas the HRSF was interpreted as a sign of a marked reflective ability.

The results obtained through a descriptive analysis of the data (Tables 1 and 2) are given below.

Although parenthood is a fundamental aspect of adult life, there are very few studies on the projected psychological states which the father's role evokes in

Table 1 Standard average values and deviations referring to the fathers' Reflective Self Function.

Level of Reflective Function		Average	SD
GRSF	Infant	0.17	1.24
	Couple	3.16	1.28
	Parents	3.58	1.54
HRSF	Infant	3.27	2.16
	Couple	2.04	1.58
	Parents	1.57	1.44
LRSF	Infant	5.24	0.13
	Couple	2.03	2.40
	Parents	3.25	2.18

Table 2 Standard average values and deviations referring to the style of father involvement/non-involvement evaluated through the CGG.

STYLE		Average	SD
OBSERVER	Infant	3.39	0.14
	Couple	2.24	2.37
	Parents	0.09	2.05
	Total	7.36	5.37
INSTRUMENTAL	Infant	0.18	0.14
	Couple	0.13	2.21
	Parents	0.81	1.26
	Total	7.51	0.42
EXPRESSIVE	Infant	10.31	6.51
	Couple	4.51	3.21
	Parents	0.12	2.39
	Total	17.43	0.21

future fathers (Gerson, 1989). Our results emphasize the complex nature of the Reflective Self Function and father involvement during pregnancy. The fathers who took part in our research were mainly characterized by their expressive involvement, which is followed by their instrumental involvement. In contrast, the 'observer' style seems very limited. Furthermore, we can say that fathers who have an expressive style exemplify this style more when talking about their children than when talking about the couple or their own parents. This aspect seems to fully confirm the available literature on the subject (Abelin, 1971; Gersonv, 1989).

Regarding the level of Reflective Function, as expressed by the fathers we interviewed, they generally show a Low Reflective Function, especially in relation to the child. This aspect, which is also confirmed in existing scholarly works, suggests that fathers are unable to experience this event with an intensity similar to that experienced by mothers: the baby is pictured in more realistic and less imaginative terms, and this probably depends on the fact that the event is experienced differently from a physical point of view (Mebert, 1989; Piccinini, 2006).

References

Abelin E: The role of the father in the separation-individuation process. In: JB Mc-Devitt, CF Settlage (eds): Separation-Individuation: essay in honor of Margaret Mahaler. International Universities Press, New York 1971

Amato PR: Children adjustment to divorce: theories, hypotheses, and empirical support. Journal of marriage and the family 55 (1998) 23–28

Amato P: More than money? Men's contributions to their children's lives. In: A Booth, AC Crouter (eds): Men in Families: When do they get involved? What difference does it make? Erlbaum, Mahwah, NJ, 1998

Amato PR, SJ Rejac: Contact with non resident parents, interpersonal, conflicts and children's behavior. Journal of Family Issues 15 (1994) 191–207

Amato PR, F Rivera: Paternal involvement in and children's behaviour. Journal of Marriage and Family 61 (1999) 375–384

Ammaniti M, C Cancelori, M Pola, R Tambelli: Maternità e gravidanza. Studio delle rappresentazioni genitoriali, Raffaello Cortina, Milano 1995

Andolfi M: Il padre ritrovato. Franco Angeli, Milano 2001

Ballare C, R Davies: Postnatal Depression in fathers. International Review of Psychiatry 8 (1996) 65–71

Barbero Avanzino B: Giovani coppie e immagine paterna. In: Donati P, E Scabini: L'immagine paterna nelle nuove dinamiche paterne, Cortina, Milano 1985

Barclay L, D Lupton: The experiences of new fatherhood: a sociocultural analysis. Journal of Advanced Nursing 29 (1999) 1013–1020

Bimbi F, G Castellano: Madri e Padri, Franco Angeli, Milano 1990

Cabrera NJ, CS Tamis Le-Monda, RH Bradley, S Hoffert, ME Lamb: Fatherhood in twenty-first century. Child Development 71 (2000) 127–136

Cappello C, A Olivieri: La gestazione dei genitori: immagini della gravidanza e del parto del bambino. In Nascere 1 (1991) 6–12

Chalmers B, D Meyer: What men say about pregnancy, birth and parenthood. Journal of Psychosomatic Obstetrics and Gynaecology 17 (1996) 47–52

Daly K: Minding the time in family experience: emerging perspectives and issues. Elsevier Science, Oxford, UK, 2001

Day R, ME Lamb: Conceptualizing and measuring father involvement. Erlbaum, Mahwah, NJ, 2004

Doherty WJ, EF Kouneski, MF Erickson: Responsible fathering: an overview and conceptual framework. Journal of Marriage and the family 60 (1998) 277–292

Draper J: "It's the first scientific evidence": men's experience of pregnancy confirmation – some findings from a longitudinal ethnographic study of transition to fatherhood. Journal of Advanced Nursing 39 (2002) 563–570

Draper J: Men's passage to fatherhood: an analysis of contemporary relevance of transition. Nursing Inquiry 10 (2003) 66–78

Erikson E: I cicli della vita. Continuità e mutamenti. Armando, Roma 1984

Farrel MP, S Rosenberg, HJ Rosenberg: Changing texts of male identity from early to late middle age: on the emergent prominence of fatherhood. In: Demick J, K Burisk, R Di Biase: Parental Development. Erlbaum, Hillsdale, NJ, 1993

Ferketich SL, RT Mercer: Men's health status during pregnancy and early fatherhood. Research in Nursing and Health 12 (1989) 137–148

Fonagy P: Thinking about thinking: some clinical and theoretical considerations in the treatment of a borderline patient. International Journal of Psycho-Analysis 72 (1991) 1–8

Fonagy P, M Target: Attaccamento e funzione riflessiva. Cortina, Milano 2001

Gerson MJ: Tomorrow's father: the anticipation of fatherhood. In: Cath SH, A Gurwitt, L Gunsberg (eds): Fathers and their families. Analitic press, London 1989

Grigio M: Il parto di coppia: il padre. Nascere 3 (1992) 14–18

Gottman JM, LF Katz, C Hooven: Metaemotions. Erlbaum, Hillsdale, NJ, 1997

Hawkins AJ, DC Dollahite: Generative fathering: beyond deficit perspectives. Sage, Thousand Oaks, CA, 1997

Hawkins AJ, SL Christiansen, KP Sargent, EJ Hill: Rethinking father's involvement in child care: a developmental perspective. Journal of Family Issues 14 (1993) 531–549

Hawkins AJ, R Palkovitz: Beyond ticks and clicks: the need for more diverse and broader conceptualizations and measures of father involvement. The Journal Men's Studies 8 (1999) 11–32

Hawkins AJ, KP Bradford, R Palkovitz, SL Christiansen, RD Day, VRA Call: The inventory of father involvement: a pilot study of a new measure of father involvement. The Journal of Men's study 10 (2002) 183–196

Hoffert SL: Report on 1997 data collection for the PSID Child Development Supplement, Retrieved April 1999 from PSID-CDS Web site, 1999

Hollingshead AB: Four Factor Index of social status. Unpublished Manuscript, Yale University 1975

Klein H: Couvade syndrome: male counterpart to psychiatry. International Journal of Psychiatry in Medicine 21 (1991) 882–890

Lamb ME: The role of father in child development. Wiley, New York 2004

Leathers SJ, MA Kelley, JA Richmann: Postpartum depressive symptomatology in new mothers and fathers: parenting, work and support. Journal of Nervous and Mental Disease 185 (1997) 129–139

Lis A, A Zennaro: A semi-structured interview with parents to be used during pregnancy: preliminary data. Infant Mental Health Journal 18 (1997) 306–323

Lis A, A Zennaro, C Mazzeschi, M Pinto: Parental styles in prospective fathers: a research carried out using ma semistructured interview during pregnancy. Infant Mental Health Journal 25 (2) (2004) 149–162

Lupton D, L Barclay: Constructing Fatherhood: Discourses and experience. Sage Publications, London 1998

Marsiglio W, P Amato, R Day, ME Lamb: Scholarship on fatherhood in the 1990s and beyond: past impression, future prospects. Journal of Marriage and the Family 62 (2000) 1173–1191

Mahler MS, F Pine, A Bergman: La nascita psicologica del bambino (trad. it.). Boringhieri, Torino 2000

May KA: A typology of detachment/involvement styles adopted during pregnancy by first time expectant fathers. Western Journal of Nursling Research 2 (1980) 445–453

May KA: Three phases of father involvement in pregnancy. Nursling Research 31 (6) (1982) 337–42

Mercer RT, SL Ferketich, JF DE Joseph: Predictors of partner relationships during pregnancy and infancy. Research in Nursing and Health 16 (1993) 45–56

Palkovitz R: Reconstructing involvement: Expanding conceptualization of man's caring in contemporary families. In: Hawkins AJ, DC Dollahite (eds): Generative fathering: beyond deficit perspectives. Sage, Thousand Oaks, CA, 1997

Palkovitz R: Involved fathering and child development: advancing our understanding of good fathering. In: Tamis-Le Monda C, N Cabrera (eds): Handbook of father involvement: Multidisciplinary perspectives. Erlbaum, Mahwah, NJ, 2002

Parke RD: Fatherhood. Harvard University Press, Cambridge, MA, 1996

Parke RD: Fathers and Families. In: Bornstein M: Handbook of parenting. Erlbaum, Mahwah, NJ, 2002

Pleck JH, B Masciadrelli: Paternal involvement by U.S. residential fathers: Levels, Sources and consequences. In: Lamb ME: The role of father in child development. Wiley, New York 2004

Roggman LA, HE Fitzgerald, RH Bradley, H Raikes: Methodological, measurement, and design issues in studying fathers: an interdisciplinary perspective. In: Tamis-Le Monda C, N Cabrera (eds): Handbook of father involvement: Multidisciplinary perspectives. Erlbaum, Mahwah, NJ, 2002

Russell G, M Radojevic: The changing role of fathers? Current understandings and future directions for research and practice. Infant Mental Health Journal 13(4) (1992) 296–311

Salerno A, AM Di Vita: Genitorialiltà a rischio. Franco Angeli, Milano 2004

Scabini E, V Cigoli: Il famigliare. Legami, Simboli Transizioni. Cortina, Milano 2000

Lee Shapiro J: Il padre in attesa, in Età evolutiva. Gravidanza e Preparazione alla Nascita 95 (1989) 33–37

Sharpe S: Fathers and Daughters. Routledge, London 1994

Stern DN: Maternal Representation: a clinical and subjective phenomenological view. Infant Mental Health Journal 12 (1991) 174–183

Strauss R, WA Goldberg: Self and possible selves during transition to fatherhood. Journal of family psychology 13(2) (1999) 244–259

Tamis-LeMonda C, N Cabrera: Perspectives on father involvement: research and policy. Social Policy Report, Society for Research in Child Development 2002

Yogman MW, D Kindlon, F Earls: Father involvement and cognitive/behavioral outcomes of preterm infants. Journal of the American Academy of Child and Adolescent Psychiatry 343 (1995) 58–66

Zeanah CH, PD Zeanah, L Stewart: Parent's constructions of their infant personalities before and after the birth: a descriptive study. Child Psychiatry and Human Development 20 (1990) 191–206

10. The psychosomatic approach to contraceptive choice

Beth Alder; Napier University, Edinburgh, United Kingdom

The term 'psychosomatic' literally means 'of the mind and body'. Research into the use of contraceptives has tended to concentrate on the somatic rather than the psychological aspects. The use of condoms has been evaluated by those interested in sexual health and sexually transmitted diseases rather than contraceptive choice. It will be argued that to understand influences on contraceptive choice, both psychological and somatic approaches are needed. This paper will address the psychological aspects of contraceptive choice. It also will ask why, in the present state of knowledge, contraception fails, and whether understanding the motivation to overcome infertility can promote our understanding of contraceptive choice (Alder, 2006).

In spite of the development of safe and effective contraceptive methods, unintended pregnancies are common. Effective contraception is relatively inexpensive and available in all European countries but still there are unwanted pregnancies. In England and Wales, the proportion of conceptions terminated by abortion rose from 19.4% in 1991 to nearly 23% in 2002 with the highest percentages in those aged under 20 or over 40. In 2002, the Total Fertility Rate (TFR, sum of age and specific fertility rates expressed per woman, controls for the changing age distribution over time) in England and Wales was 1.65 per woman, which is similar to the rates between 1920 and 1940, before the widespread use and acceptability of contraception (Population Trends 2004, Social Trends 2004, http://www.statistics.gov.uk/).

If women request termination of pregnancy it is usually because of failed contraception, lack of use of contraception, or inappropriate contraception. It might be expected that following a termination request women would be more highly motivated to prevent a subsequent conception. In a study of 100 women in Switzerland, of those attending for termination of pregnancy 69% claimed that they had used contraception in the cycle that had resulted in the pregnancy (Bianchi-Demicheli et al., 2001). Most women (83%) intended to use contraception to prevent another pregnancy. Most women (60%) were using the pill six months later and fewer used condoms. Most women changed their previous method of contraception even though that method would have been recommended (Bianchi-Demicheli et al., 2003).

Sexually active individuals make a choice about which contraceptive method to use. This changes as they get older, or as the relationship develops. In a report based on surveys in 1992, Oddens (1996) suggests that attitudes towards the perceived medical nature of some contraceptive methods (oral contraceptives, sterilization, and IUDs) influence contraceptive choice. Miller and Pasta (1996) carried out a study on the contraceptive choice of 40 couples over a four-year period. They distinguished between method-choice and method-use in decision-making. Method-choice is about continuing with the present method or changing to a new one. Method-use is the actual use of the selected method, e.g. taking the oral contraceptive pill daily or inserting a diaphragm. They found that husbands and wives appeared to have equal influence on method-choice but intentions depended on their own preference.

Although we assume that knowledge about contraception is freely available in Western societies there is some evidence that it is not widespread. Medical students by the very nature of their chosen profession and education might be expected to have a good understanding of sexual health. However a study of medical students in England found that there was poor knowledge of the failure rate of condoms and of abortion rates (Fayers et al., 2003). There was a small effect of increasing knowledge with increasing years of medical training. Gardner (2001), in survey of over 100 nursing school students, found that fear of side effects or health risks were the most frequently cited reasons for stopping pill use, and that the views of health care providers were influential.

Low rates of knowledge in women about the oral contraceptive pill were found by Little et al. (1998). However, by providing an educational leaflet in a randomized controlled trial they were able to increase the knowledge significantly. Knowledge is important in trying to understand contraception choice and many studies have been directed at specific groups such as teenagers. In a study of over a thousand teenagers in Scotland, one third of sexually active girls aged less than 16 years were found to have used emergency contraception (Graham et al., 1996). Scottish teenagers were well informed about the existence of emergency contraception, but many did not know when and how to access it properly. There have been significant changes in patterns of sexual behaviour in the last fifty years and many of these have been attributed to change in contraceptive use. We have seen a rise in sexual activity among young people. The median age for first sexual intercourse in the United Kingdom dropped during the early 1990s and is now stable at around 16 years for both men and women. Even before the age of 15, about 18% of boys and 15% of girls report having had full sexual intercourse, with similar proportions having engaged in oral sex (Tripp, Viner, 2005). These data have clear implications for the risk of pregnancy and for sexual health.

Traditional societies in the West and many societies in other parts of the world assume that for women, bearing children is a natural expression of femininity and that for men, it is a duty to have children. With changes in lifestyle for women and diminished gender inequalities, more couples may choose to remain childless and increasing numbers of couples delay the birth of their first child. The proportion of women who never have children appears to be increasing. It is expected that over a third of women born in 1967 will be childless at the age of 30 (Matheson, Baab, 2002). At the same time there is global concern about the burgeoning worldwide population (Morse, 2000). In some countries there are state policies to regulate fertility and to limit family size. In others, there is concern about the proportionate increase in the ageing population with fewer young people to care for them. In both types of societies, socio-political pressures may centre on the role of women.

In couples of average fertility pregnancies may be unplanned, but not unwanted. In others, who are of lower fertility, there are those who would like to become pregnant, and those that are not concerned about infertility. In their study of nearly 400 couples, Miller and Pasta (1995) found that child-timing intentions followed by child-bearing intentions were the most important factors in predicting attempts to conceive. Women are expected to conform to societies' expectations of the right time to have children and the right number. Using qualitative data, Woollett (1996) describes how women are expected to be free to choose how many children they have, as long as it is not 'no children', not 'only one child', and not 'too many'. They are expected to have children neither when they are 'too young' nor 'too old'. There may be ambivalent attitudes to those who choose to remain childless. Lampman and Dowling-Guyer (1995) gave six scenarios describing couples with different family situations to over 200 undergraduate students. They rated the scenarios on characteristics of the couples and their relationships. The results showed negative ratings towards voluntary childlessness but they were less negative towards involuntary childlessness.

These are the expectations of society and thus may be expected to vary from decade to decade and from culture to culture. Not only do we need a psychosomatic approach to understanding contraceptive choice, we also need a social context. The biopsychosocial model used in health psychology incorporates the biological aspects as well. The model suggests that biological, psychological, and social aspects of a person's life affect health and illness (Schwartz, 1982). Biological factors include genetic inheritance. Individuals differ in their vulnerability to disease, in their physical make up and thus in their potential fertility. Their physical functioning (including sexuality) may be determined by an early experience (e.g. a childhood illness or accident) or later behaviour (e.g. smoking or substance abuse). All these interact with each other and health is a dynamic process. Psychological factors that are familiar to psychologists include cognition, emotion, and motivation. In the context of fertility, cognition might be the desire to have a family life, emotion might be maternal or paternal longings and motivation may calculate the cost benefit of having a child. And all these might account for differences in health behaviour. However, psychological factors influencing health behaviour are, in fact, far more complex and therefore, social cognition models have been developed to understand health behaviour (Conner, Norman, 1996). Social factors include a society which values reproduction, our health behaviour, and our use of health care.

Another way to understand the psychological aspects of contraceptive decision-making is to consider what happens when positive decisions about having children are not fulfilled. Infertility or subfertility has been addressed by advances in reproductive technology but delaying planned pregnancies increases the likelihood of fertility problems. Research studies have found little evidence for psychogenic effects on infertility. Studies that attempt to compare characteristics of patients with apparent organic infertility with those having unexplained infertility are difficult because the extent of unexplained infertility may reflect the sophistication of the infertility investigations (Edelmann, Connolly, 1996). Berg and Wilson (1995) looked at the pattern of distress in 104 couples with primary infertility attending for infertility investigations. Forty per cent of men and 49% of women met the inclusion criteria on the SCL-90-R scale (Derogatis, 1977). In a third of the couples neither were distressed; in 18% the male only was distressed; in 22% the female only was distressed, and in 27% both partners were distressed. Edelmann and Connolly (1996) assessed sex-role type (Bem, 1974) on psychological functioning in a sample of 130 couples presenting for primary infertility but before diagnosis. Masculine men were the least anxious but there were no relationships between anxiety and sex-role type in women. Depressive symptoms may be associated with infertility but the infertility may also be associated with the use of anti-depressant drug therapy (Lapane, et al., 1995).

Overcoming infertility is stressful, possibly painful, time consuming and expensive. Attempts have been made to understand the powerful motivation for parenthood in couples attending for infertility treatment, and this should also promote our understanding of reproductive decisions and contraceptive choice. A simple cost-benefit model has been used but listing of reasons may not reveal the complex motivation of infertile couples. The desire for children can be innate. Coplin et al. (1998) found that the main reason for wanting a child was 'happiness' followed by well-being, motherhood, identity continuity, and social control. The Parenthood Motivation list (Van Balen, Trimbos-Kemper, 1995) showed in a retrospective study few differences between women having in vitro fertilization (IVF) and non-IVF mothers. Langridge et al. (2000) used network analysis to investigate the reasons for parenthood among expectant couples and couples presenting for treatment by IVF or donor insemination (DI). The sample was small (ten expectant couples, ten about to have IVF and 14 presenting for DI) and no recruitment response rate was reported. Similar to the results of other studies, these authors found that the most important reasons were the need to give and receive love and experience the enjoyment of children, and these were strongly interconnected. Pressures from family and friends were not given as reasons.

Clearly contraceptive choice is more complex than assessing acceptability and effectiveness and is bound up with decisions about reproduction. A psychosomatic approach will promote our understanding.

References

Alder B: Contraception. In: Ayers S, A Baum, C McManus, S Newman, K Wallston, J Weinman, R West (eds): Cambridge Handbook of Psychology, Health and Medicine (2nd Edition). Cambridge University Press, Cambridge, UK, 2006

Berg BJ, JF Wilson: Patterns of psychological distress in infertile couples. Journal of Psychosomatic Obstetrics and Gynaecology 16 (1995) 65–78

Bem S: The measurement of psychological androgyny. Journal of Clinical and Consulting Psychology 42 (1974) 155–162

Bianchi-Demicheli F, E Perrin, PG Bianchi, P Dumont, F Lüdicke, A Campana: Contraceptive practice before and after termination of pregnancy: a prospective study. Contraception 67(2) (2003) 107–113

Bianchi-Demicheli F, E Perrin, F Lüdicke, PG Bianchi, D Fert, F Bonvallat, D Chatton, A Campana: Sexuality, partner relations and contraceptive practice after termination of pregnancy. Journal of Psychosomatic Obstetrics and Gynecology 22 (2001) 83–90

Conner M, P Norman (eds): Predicting health behaviour. Open University Press, Buckingham 1996

Coplin H, A De Munter, L Vandemeulebroecke: Parenthood motives in IVF mothers. Journal of Psychosomatic Obstetrics and Gynaecology 19 (1998) 19–27

Derogatis LR: The SCL-90-R Manual: a step in the validation of a new self-report scale. British Journal of Psychiatry 128 (1977) 280–9

Edelmann RJ, KJ Connolly: Sex role and emotional functioning in infertile couples: some further evidence. Journal of Reproductive and Infant Psychology 14 (1996) 113–119

Fayers T, T Crowley, JM Jenkins, DJ Cahill: Medical students awareness of sexual health is poor. International Journal of STD & Aids 14 (2003) 386–389

Gardner JA: Perceptions of the use of oral contraception in female nursing students. Masters in Research thesis, University of Dundee 2001

Graham A, L Green, AF Glasier: Teenagers' knowledge of emergency contraception: questionnaire survey in south east Scotland. BMJ 312 (1996) 1567–1569

Lampman C, S Dowling-Guyer: Attitudes towards voluntary and involuntary childlessness. Basic and Applied Social Psychology 17 (1995) 213–222

Langridge D, K Conolly, P Sheeran: Reasons for wanting a child: a network analytic study. Journal of Reproductive and Infant Psychology 18 (2000) 321–338

Lapane KL, S Zeirler, TM Lasater, M Stein, MM Barbour: Is a history of depressive symptoms associated with an increase of infertility in women? Psychosomatic Medicine 57 (1995) 509–513

Little P, S Griffin, J Kelly, N Dickson, C Sadler: Effect of educational leaflets and questions on knowledge of contraception in women taking the combined contraceptive pill: randomised controlled trial. BMJ 316 (1998) 1948–1952

Matheson J, P Babb (eds): Social Trends, 32. The Stationery Office, London 2002.

Miller WB, D Pasta: Behavioural intentions: which ones predict infertility behaviour in married couples. Journal of Applied Social Psychology 25 (1995) 530–555

Miller WB, D Pasta: The relationship of husbands and wives on the choice and use of contraception, a diaphragm and condoms. Journal of Applied Social Psychology 26 (1996) 1749–1774

Morse CA: Reproduction: a critical analysis. In: Ussher JM (ed): Women's Health Contemporary International Perspectives. BPS Books, Leicester 2000

Oddens BJ: Determinants of contraceptive use: National population-based studies in various West European Countries. Eburon, Netherlands 1996.

Schwartz GE: Testing the biopsychosocial model: the ultimate challenge facing behavioural medicine? Journal of Consulting and Clinical Psychology, 50 (1982) 1040–1053

Tripp J, R Viner: Sexual health, contraception, and teenage pregnancy. BMJ 330 (2005) 590–593

Woollett A: Reproductive decisions. In: Walker A, K Niven (eds): Psychology of Reproduction, Volume 2: Conception, pregnancy and birth. Butterworth/ Heninmann, Oxford 1996

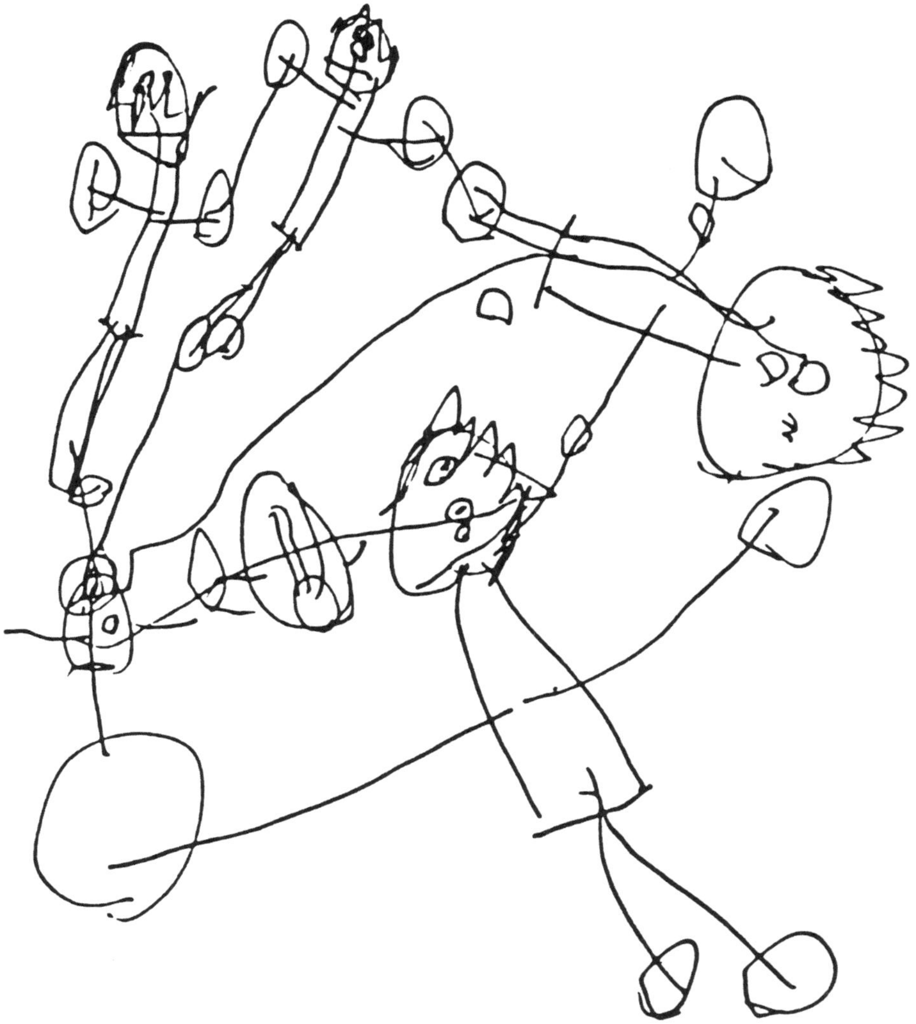

(Giulia, 3 yrs. 8 mos.)
Daddy wanted me because I wasn't there, I wanted Daddy.
Mommy and Daddy wanted me.

11. Counselling for infertility and its treatment

Jacky Boivin; Cardiff University, United Kingdom

Introduction

Counselling for infertility has a long history, and during this time the goals of psychological interventions have changed significantly. From the mid-1940s to the 1970s, most interventions were aimed at dealing with the psychological conflicts that might be blocking pregnancy, whereas from the 1970s to the late 1990s counselling focused more exclusively on the personal, marital and social effects of fertility problems. As we move into the new century, the accessibility of medical intervention for infertility and the numerous treatment options now available to couples means that treatment-related issues are now dominating the counselling.

Counselling to improve pregnancy rates

The first point of entry of psychology into infertility medicine was via psychiatry. The psychosomatic theory was extremely popular in the 1940s and 1950s and it was introduced to obstetrics and gynaecology where it was readily accepted as an explanation for diagnostic mysteries of the time. With "unexplained infertility" diagnosed in nearly 50% of the cases, fertility experts were keen to off-load untreated cases to other specialities while still appearing to have resolved the diagnostic problem. The emergence of psychogenic infertility as a diagnostic category achieved this goal. Whilst infertility was not among the original psychosomatic disorders, Helen Deutsch (1945) wrote extensively on the conflicts that were responsible for reproductive failure in women. Infertility was perceived to be a defensive reaction against pregnancy. If a pregnancy occurred, it would then allow psychological conflicts about motherhood to surface with catastrophic results. Consequently, the "specific" psychic conflicts proposed all involved difficulty assuming the motherhood role: masculine-aggressive personality, feminine-immature personality, hostile dependence on mother, etc. Although Helen Deutsch is frequently cited, many others contributed to the application of such principles to the problems of infertility, for example Benedek (1952) and Sandler (1959) were influential in holding the view of psychogenic infertility best exemplified by Menninger (1943): "Her illness represents a psychic conflict sailing under a gynecological flag".

Ideas of psychogenic infertility were discredited in an early review. Noyes and Chapnick (1964) evaluated 75 studies related to psychogenic infertility and showed that the majority of studies were vague in their assumptions and hypotheses, and clearly biased in favour of finding a psychogenic etiology. Moreover, in most studies psychogenic infertility was diagnosed by the process of exclusion: if no organic pathology was observed, then it was a psychogenic etiology (Sandler, 1959). However, none of the studies provided compelling evidence for the case of psychogenic infertility (Noyes and Chapnick, 1964). In light of the conceptual and methodological flaws identified by the review, Noyes and Chapnick concluded that psychological factors could not be linked in a convincing manner to reproductive failure. Publications of this paper coupled with advances in reproductive surgery reduced the need for psychogenic explanations. For example, Drake et al., (1977) showed that when laparoscopy was introduced, 75% of women with unexplained infertility demonstrated abnormal findings. Although a psychoanalytic approach to understanding fertility problems continues to be an approach (e.g., Christie et al., 1998), it has generally been concluded that longstanding infertility is unlikely to be exclusively caused by psychological stimuli (Wischmann, 2003).

Despite this ultimate demise, the influence of the psychosomatic theory on research and clinical goals is nevertheless immense. First, psychosomatic theories were revised to accommodate multifactorial models of disease etiology, so that researchers in the area of infertility directed their attention to the vulnerability of *all* patients to the physical effects of psychological factors (particularly stress). In the biopsychosocial model, any disease state is thought to have multiple determinants (i.e., biological, environmental, social, and psychological) with extent of individual susceptibility to disease dependent on personal history (e.g., genetic, developmental, and learnt) (Engels, 1977; Lipowski, 1984). In combination with concepts from behavioural medicine and health psychology, much of the research published recently concerns identifying these psychological influences and the trait factors that may moderate their effects.

There is now compelling evidence associating psychological factors with fertility potential. Negative affect (e.g., anxiety, depression) has been associated with longer cycle duration (Hjollund et al., 1999) and reduced conception in healthy women trying to conceive (Sanders & Bruce, 1997). Further evidence for stress effects comes from fertility treatment studies showing that stress indicators are associated with a poorer ovarian functional response to treatment (Lancastle, Boivin, 2005) and reduced fertilization, implantation, and live birth rates, regardless of whether stress is assessed via mood states (Klonoff-Cohen et al., 2001; Sanders, Bruce, 1999; Smeenk et al., 2001) or physiological parameters (e.g., cortisol, Facchinetti et al., 1997; immunological parameters, Gallinelli et al., 2001). These associations remain even after controlling for obvious confounders, for example, life style (e.g., smoking) and health (e.g., weight) factors (Klonoff-Cohen et al., 2001; Sanders, Bruce, 1999). A recent study has estimated via modelling techniques that approximately 13% of the variability in ovarian response to fertility treatment is attributable to variations in psychosocial profile (Lancastle, Boivin, 2005).

Second, psychosomatic perspectives influenced the goals of psychological interventions and this directive persists to this day. Psychological therapy was mainly conceived as a way to address the psychological conflicts that might be blocking pregnancy, and an improved pregnancy rate is still an important goal in many therapies used today (Domar et al., 2000). The link between decreased distress and increased pregnancy rates was initially held on the basis of anecdotal reports lacking validity. For example, reports of couples conceiving after receiving reassurance from the physician (de Watteville, 1957), adoption (Sandler, 1965), holidays (Ayala, 1974), or transfer of the medical burden to medical staff skilled in coping with such situations (Stone and Ward, 1956). Early interventions were mainly recommended for women because male infertility was believed to "lie outside of the psychological domain" (Benedek et al., 1952). The preponderance of women in most clinical evaluations of psychological interventions in infertility (e.g., Boivin, 2003; de Liz, Strauss, 2005) shows that this bias is still in effect, though it is currently known that this may be due to a lack of interest on the part of men (Boivin et al., 1999) rather than a referral bias on the part of medical staff.

Although improved pregnancy rates are a key goal for clinical interventions, a recent review offered only equivocal evidence of the effectiveness of counselling in achieving this goal. In the period 1966–2000, 15 studies evaluated the psychological interventions for infertility and included pregnancy as an outcome variable (Boivin, 2003). In these studies, the variety of interventions which were used could be grouped into either supportive-expressive (e.g., counselling, psychodynamic) or educational (e.g., relaxation or coping training) interventions. Though approaches differed, all proposed that a decrease in psychological distress would be associated with an increase in pregnancy rate. Despite clear indications that therapies reduced negative affect, especially anxiety and depressive symptoms, evidence was not compelling in terms of pregnancy rate. Studies were almost equally divided in terms of the findings, namely, 8 showing no effect of counselling versus 7 providing evidence of an increase in pregnancy rates.

Given such equivocal results, two interpretations were offered for the findings (Boivin, 2003). One possibility was that interventions were effective in producing the kinds of psychological and biological changes necessary to enhance reproductive potential. This explanation would be in line with numerous studies claiming to show that psychological distress can interfere with the biology of reproduction (e.g., Bydlowski, Dayan-Lintzer, 1988). A number of psychobiological mechanisms could account for such effects including effects on gonadal function in both women (Lancastle, Boivin, 2005) and men (Clarke et al., 1999) and negative effects on uterine receptivity and implantation (Boivin, Schmidt,

2005; Rabin et al., 1990). Moreover, such effects would be consistent with a large body of psychological research showing that talking about traumatic events, as would be emphasized in counselling interventions, can have demonstrable effects on physical health (Pennebaker, Susman, 1988).

Alternatively, positive findings may be due to spurious effects introduced by methodological weakness. One factor that would have an obvious effect on pregnancy in these studies is the concomitant use of fertility treatment. Almost all positive effect studies in the Boivin (2003) review sampled patients during treatment so that pregnancies could have been due to medical treatment rather than to psychological interventions. The finding that the pregnancy rate in the studies showing positive effect was similar to that in medically treated patients could support this contention.

Whilst the influence of psychosomatic contributions can still be seen to this day, the last 20–30 years focused more on counselling approaches seeking to improve quality of life of infertility patients through better awareness and management of psychological consequences of infertility.

Counselling to address psychological consequences of infertility

The shift from *cause* to *consequence* in the goals of psychological interventions in infertility is mostly associated with the advocacy movement of the 1970s, in particular the rise of support organizations for infertile people whose goals included increased public awareness of the emotional needs of this population (Menning, 1979). Another potent influence on counselling perspectives of the time was the application of the Kubler-Ross (1969) descriptive framework (of reactions to death and dying) to infertility, whereby the experience of infertility was described as being accompanied by "...a nearly universal syndrome of feelings" that included shock/surprise, denial, isolation, anger, guilt, and grief (Menning, 1979). These contributions re-focused research and clinical work toward understanding and dealing with the psychological consequences of fertility problems rather than their psychological antecedents or cause.

First, a plethora of studies were carried out and aimed at investigating the negative effects of infertility and its treatment on the well-being of individuals and couples. Various methodologies were used including comparisons between infertile and fertile individuals, comparisons across different stages of the medical process and evaluations concerned with the effects of new treatments, to name but a few. The outcomes assessed were also numerous, including mental health, marital and sexual relationships, quality of life, family and social functioning, and so on. By the end of the 1980s, definitive conclusions could be drawn in some areas. For example, psychological functioning was within the normal range, women experienced more intense negative reactions to childlessness than did men, infertility strengthened the marital relationship, and several reviews of this vast literature have since been published (Wright et al., 1989; Greil, 1997). This literature also uncovered risk factors for the development of psychological disturbance following the infertility diagnosis, including gender (woman), parity (childless), pre-existing psychopathology, high need for parenthood, reliance on avoidant coping, and marital conflict (Boivin, 2002). Research with this population lead to an improved understanding of psychological implications associated with medical interventions (e.g., use of donor gametes) and their effect on individual and family life. Such studies revealed, for example, that the cognitive and psychological development of children conceived through donor gametes in heterosexual or lesbian families was similar and in some cases superior to naturally conceived children (Golombok et al., 1996; van Fraussen et al., 2001).

A second major effect of the shift from cause to consequence was that a main aim of counselling during this period became to assist couples, particularly women, to identify, "work through" and thereby resolve the syndrome of feelings that were purported to accompany a diagnosis of infertility. This approach was in keeping with the significant influence of the Kubler-Ross (1969) framework at that time and, the perception that "couples must grieve those losses" (Mahlstedt, 1985). This goal was achieved using diverse theoretical frameworks: ego and self psychology, developmental and crisis, grief and loss, cognitive-behavioural, family systems, and gender-based theories (Hammer-Burns, Covington, 1999). Ningel and Strauss (2002) presented a list of therapeutic goals described in clinical papers concerned with infertility counselling and these could be grouped as those aimed at reduction and management of distress, improvement of marital communication and relations, facilitation of decision-making, and helping people to achieve a "good life" in spite of the infertility.

Recent reviews of infertility counselling interventions would suggest that psychological interventions with this population appear to achieve some of these goals (Boivin, 2003; de Liz, Strauss, 2005). Research has shown that psychological interventions can reduce symptoms of depression, anxiety (Stewart et al., 1992; Wallace, 1984) and infertility-specific distress (Strauss et al., 2002), improve marital and sexual relations (Tuschen-Caffier et al., 1999) and coping (McSweeney et al., 1997) as well as modify negative life style factors (Domar et al., 2000; Clark et al., 1995). Taken together, a review of 25 independent evaluations of clinical interventions in infertility showed strong beneficial effects on the reduction of negative affect and infertility distress, but more minor effects on interpersonal and social relations (Boivin, 2003). The latter findings may be due to the fact that changes in longstanding behaviour may be more difficult to produce or evaluate using short-term interventions and follow-up periods that mark the psychological interventions used in this population.

The lack of spectacular effects for counselling, coupled with emerging evidence that couples were not using the offered psychological services (Boivin et al., 1999) prompted clinicians and researchers to take a more critical approach to the psychological services being offered. In other words, more research is now directed to understanding the 'who, what, and when' of effective interventions: who benefits, from what intervention, and when. The need for such reflection has become more pressing as evidence-based principles are introduced into psychological fields (Chambless, Hollon, 1998). The increased utilization of medical treatment has also an appreciable impact on the type of psychological services required (and requested) by infertility patients and lead to another change of focus in counselling that emphasizes medical decision-making and coping with medical intervention.

Current and future directions in psychological interventions for infertile couples

In Europe, 2.1% of children are now born using assisted reproductive technologies (ART) and more than 300,000 ART cycles are performed every year (Nyboe Andersen et al., 2005). Although success rates for individual cycles is 20%, cumulative pregnancy rates show that more than half of the couples embarking on ART treatment can expect to eventually conceive (Stolwijk et al., 2000). The utilization rate of ART increases every year, with a cumulative increase of 40% since 1997 (Nyboe Andersen et al., 2005). The treatment options available expanded significantly since the introduction of in vitro fertilization (IVF) and related technologies, so that effective treatments are now available for problems considered irresolvable in the early days of infertility medicine, for example, male infertility (i.e., ICSI) or advanced female age (i.e., oocyte donation and ovarian preservation). However, these treatments have relatively low success rates and numerous factors, including psychological variables (Lancastle, Boivin, 2005) influence whether they will be initiated or successful. The increased number of treatment options, the significant investment that couples make in pursuing treatment, and the impact of psychological factors on implementing and success suggest that treatment-related issues frequently dominate counselling for infertility.

Three treatment influences on counselling have emerged. First, it is apparent that psychological factors determine initiation and continuation of treatment. This view is based on two recent findings that have implications for what counsellors do in fertility clinics. First, it has become obvious that a relatively small proportion of people pursue medical treatment (about 40%) even though parenthood is a significant life goal for most (Greil, McQuillan, 2004). Ambivalence about parenthood, a reluctance to acknowledge the existence of an infertility problem and negative attitudes toward medical technology all seem to contribute to treatment initiation. Second, it is obvious that people discontinue treatment prematurely and that for a significant proportion this is due to psychological factors (Smeenk et al., 2004). Therefore, individuals are increasingly seeking counselling to help in decision-making regarding the continuation or termination of treatment (Boivin et al., 2005).

Decision-making interventions in health contexts are becoming more and more important. Historically, decision-making was considered to be solely the domain of the treating medical team. However, the changing attitudes within health contexts, increased education of patients generally and through self-directed research (i.e., internet, Epstein et al., 2002) points to the fact that patients increasingly want to share in the decision-making process. A growing body of research shows that interventions aimed at increasing active patient involvement and shared decision-making (e.g., through the use of Decision Aids) ensures that people feel better informed about how their health conditions are going to be treated or managed, with the result that things would work out better (O'Connor et al., 1999). Informed patients feel better about the decision process. Their decisions are more likely to match up with their preferences, values, and concerns. These patients are more likely to comply with the required treatment regimens, and they often end up rating their medical experience after treatment as better than those who play a more passive role in decision-making.

A second effect of the significant investment in treatment has been the need to address factors that may compromise the success of medical interventions. Research on treatment success showed that life style factors (e.g., smoking, alcohol use, weight, and stress) are important in determining whether people achieve a pregnancy naturally or in treatment (Klonoff-Cohen et al., 2005). These findings indicate that infertility counsellors need to focus on interventions that help people address these problematic life areas. Health psychology offers an impressive array of interventions designed to decrease health risk behaviours (e.g., smoking, obesity) and increase health-promoting behaviours (e.g., exercise). However, only a few researchers have thus far focused their interventions on modification of maladaptive behaviours to improve quality of life and pregnancy rates (Domar et al., 2000; Clark et al., 1995). For example, the Mind Body program, a cognitive-behavioural intervention, does not only aim to reduce anxiety and depression, but also to minimize the negative effects of life style factors (e.g., obesity, poor nutrition) through additional sessions focused exclusively on exercise and diet education (Domar et al., 1990). It is clear that such interventions will increasingly facilitate success rates, as well as improve quality of life for infertile patients.

A third consequence of the considerable amount of time spent in treatment is the increased emphasis during counselling on identifying and implementing effective coping strategies to manage the rigours of treatment. The relationship between coping and adjustment to infertility is more or less consistent with the general literature on coping. First, emotion-focused types of strategies, for example, disregarding negative treatment information like low success rates, avoiding pregnant women, or fantasizing about life with children are associated with more distress in terms of depression, negative psychological symptoms and marital distress (Morrow et al., 1995). Second, problem-oriented strategies are associated with less distress on these measures. For example, obtaining information about infertility, seeking advice, or dealing with the problem directly is associated with better adjustment after treatment (Litt et al., 1992). Social support has been associated with better adjustment to infertility generally and during treatment (Boivin, Takefman, 1996). Finally, individuals who cope by re-appraising infertility in terms of its benefits, for example, strengthening the marital relationship or seeing the problem as a challenge rather than a threat, report better adjustment than couples coping in other ways (Lancastle, Boivin, 2005). Developing ways to help women cope with the strains of fertility diagnosis and treatment is an important consideration and aspect of counselling these patients.

Conclusions

Infertility counselling has a long history, influenced by both medicine and psychology. Evaluations of counselling in this field show promising results but it is apparent that interventions delivered to the patients need to keep pace with changes in the demography of parenting as well as new emerging technologies, as these determine the needs of individuals and couples trying to achieve a pregnancy. Traditional approaches focused exclusively on distress reduction for the purposes of pregnancy are still warranted, but more needs to be done to improve quality of life during the long period in treatment.

References

Ayala G: Sterility. Holidays. Fertility. Gynecologie 25 (2) (1974) 211–212

Benedek T: Infertility as a psychosomatic defense. Fertility and Sterility 3 (1952) 527

Boivin J: Who is likely to need counselling. In: Boivin J, H Kentenich (eds): Guidelines for Counselling in Infertility. ESHRE Monographs, Oxford University Press, Oxford 2002

Boivin J: A review of psychosocial interventions in infertility. Social Science and Medicine 57 (12) (2003) 2325–2341

Boivin J, J Takefman: Stress reactions across an IVF cycle in pregnant and non-pregnant women using daily monitoring prospective data. Fertility and Sterility 64 (1995) 802–811

Boivin J, Schmidt L: Infertility-related stress in men and women predicts treatment outcome 1 year later. Fertility and Sterility 83 (2005) 1745–1751

Boivin J, L Scanlan, SM Walker: Why are infertile couples not using psychosocial counselling? Human Reproduction 14 (1999) 1384–1391

Boivin J, J Takefman, A Braverman: Giving bad news: "It's time to stop". In: Macklon N (ed): IVF in medically complicated patient: A guide to management. Taylor & Francis, London 2005

Bydlowski M, M Dayan-Lintzer: A psycho-medical approach to infertility: 'suffering from sterility'. Journal of Psychosomatic Obstetrics and Gynaecology 9 (1998) 139–151

Chambless DL, SD Hollon: Defining Empirically Supported Therapies. Journal of Consulting and Clinical Psychology 66 (1) (1998) 7–18

Christie GL: Some socio-cultural and psychological aspects of infertility. Human Reproduction 13 (1) (1998) 232–241

Clarke R, SC Klock, J Geoghegan, E Travassos: The relationship between psychological stress and semen quality among in vitro fertilization patients. Human Reproduction, 14 (1999) 753–758

Clark AM, W Ledger, C Galletley, L Tomlinson, F Blaney, X Wang, RJ Norman: Weight loss results in significant improvement in pregnancy and ovulation rates in anovulatory obese women. Human Reproduction 10 (1995) 2705–2712

De Liz TM, B Strauss: Differential efficacy of group and individual/couple psychotherapy with infertile patients. Human Reproduction 20 (2005) 1324–1332

De Watteville H: Psychologic factors in the treatment in the treatment of sterility. Fertility and Sterility 8 (1957) 12

Daniels KR, K Taylor: Secrecy and openness in donor insemination. Politics and the Life Sciences 12 (2) (1993) 155–170

Domar AD, M Seibel, H Benson: The mind/body program for infertility: A new behavioral treatment approach for women with infertility. Fertility and Sterility 53 (1990) 246–249

Domar AD, D Clapp, EA Slawsby, J Dusek, B Kessel, M Freizinger: Impact of group psychological interventions on pregnancy rates in infertile women. Fertility and Sterility 73 (2000) 805–811; Development 79 (2000) 439–449

Drake T, D Tredway, G Buchanan, N Takaki, T Daane: Unexplained infertility: A reappraisal. Obstetrics & Gynecology 50 (6) (1977) 644–646

Deutsch H: The Psychology of Women, Volume II, Chapter: Motherhood. Grune, New York 1945

Engels GL: The need for a new medical model: A challenge for biomedicine. Science, 196 (4286) (1977) 129–196

Epstein YM, HS Rosenberg, T Venet Grant, N Hemenway: Use of the Internet as the only outlet for talking about infertility. Fertility and Sterility 78 (3) 2002) 507–514

Facchinetti F, ML Matteo, GP Artini, A Volpe, AR Genazzani: An increased vulnerability to stress is associated with a poor outcome of in vitro fertilisation-embryo transfer treatment. Fertility and Sterility 67 (1997) 309–314

Gallinelli A, R Roncaglia, ML Matteo, I Ciaccio, A Volpe, F Facchinetti: Immunological changes and stress are associated with different implantation rates in patients undergoing in vitro fertilisation-embryo transfer. Fertility and Sterility 76 (1) (2001) 85–91

Golombok S, A Brewaeys, R Cook, MT Giavazzi, D Guerra, A Mantovani, E van Hall, PG Crosiggnani, S Dexeus: The European study of assisted reproduction families: Family functioning and child development. Human Reproduction 11 (10) (1996) 2324–2331

Greil LA: Infertility and psychological distress: A critical review of the literature. Social Science & Medicine 45 (11) (1997) 1679–1704

Greil LA, J McQuillan: Help-Seeking Patterns among U.S. Women. Journal of Reproductive and Infant Psychology 22 (4) (2004) 305–319

Hammer-Burns L, SN Covington: Infertility Counselling: A comprehensive handbook for clinicians. Parthenon, New York 1999

Hjollund NH et al.: Distress and reduced fertility: A follow-up study of first-pregnancy planners. Fertility and Sterility 72 (1) (1999) 47–53

Klonoff-Cohen H: Female and male lifestyle habits and IVF: what is known and unknown. Human Reproduction Update 11 (2) (2005) 180–204

Klonoff-Cohen H, E Chu, L Natarajan, W Sieber: A prospective study of stress among women undergoing in vitro fertilization and gamete intrafallopian transfer. Fertility Sterility 76 (4) (2001) 675–687

Kubler-Ross E: On death and dying. Macmillan, New York 1969

Lancastle D, J Boivin: Dispositional optimism, trait anxiety, and coping: Unique or shared effects on biological response to fertility treatment? Health Psychology 24 (2005) 171–178

Lipowski ZJ: What does the word "Psychosomatic" really mean? A historical and semantic inquiry. Psychosomatic Medicine 46 (2) (1984) 153–171

Mahlstedt P: The psychological component of infertility. Fertility and Sterility 43 (3) (1985) 335–346

McQueeney D, A Stanton, S Sigmon: Efficacy of emotion-focused and problem-focused group therapies for women with fertility problems. Journal of Behavioural Medicine 20 (1997) 313–331

Menning BE: Counselling infertile couples. Contemporary Obstetrics and Gynecology 13 (1979 101–108

Menninger K: Sterility. Bulletin of the Menninger Clinic 7 (1943) 7

Ningel K, B Strauss: Psychological diagnosis, counselling and psychotherapy in fertility medicine. In: Strauss B (ed): Involuntary Childlessness: Psychological assessment, counselling and therapy. Hogrefe and Huber, Seattle 2002

Noyes RW, EM Chapnick: Literature on psychology and infertility: A critical analysis. Fertility and Sterility 15 (1964) 543–558

Nyboe Andersen A, L Gianaroli, R Felberbaum, J de Mouzon, KG Nygren: Assisted reproductive technology in Europe, 2001: Results generated from European registers by ESHRE. Human Reproduction 20 (5) (2005) 1158–1176

O'Connor AM, V Fiset, C DeGrasse, ID Graham, W Evans, D Stacey et al.: Decision aids for patients considering health care options: Evidence of efficacy and policy implications. Journal of the National Cancer Institute, Monograph 25 (1999) 67–80

Pennebaker JW, JR Susman: Disclosure of traumas and psychosomatic processes. Social Science and Medicine 26 (1988) 327–332

Rabin DS, EO Johnson, DD Brandon, C Liapi, GP Chrousos: Glucorticoids inhibit estradiol-mediated uterine growth: Possible role of the uterine estradiol receptor. Biology of Reproduction 42 (1990) 74–80

Sanders K, N Bruce: Psychosocial stress and treatment outcome following assisted reproductive technology. Human Reproduction 14 (6) (1999) 1656–1662

Sandler B: Emotional stress and infertility. British Journal of Clinical Practice 13 (1959) 328–330

Smeenk JMJ, CM Verhaak, A Eugster, A van Minnen, GA Zielhuis, DDM Braat: The effect of anxiety and depression on the outcome of in-vitro fertilization. Human Reproduction 16 (2001) 1420–23

Smeenk JMJ, CM Verhaak, AM Stolwijk, JAM Kremer, DDM Braat: Reasons for dropout in an in vitro fertilization/intracytoplasmic sperm injection program. Fertility and Sterility 81 (2) (2004) 262–268

Stewart DE, KM Boydell, K McCarthy, S Swerdlyk, C Redmond, W Cohrs: A prospective study of the effectiveness of brief professionally-led support groups for infertility patients. International Journal of Psychiatry in Medicine 22 (1992) 173–182

Stolwijk AM, AMM Wetzels, DDM Braat: Cumulative probability of achieving an ongoing pregnancy after in vitro fertilisation and intracytoplasmic sperm injection according to woman's age, subfertility diagnosis and primary or secondary infertility. Human Reproduction 15 (2000) 203–209

Stone A, ME Ward: Factors responsible for pregnancy in 500 cases of infertility. Fertility and Sterility 7 (1956) 1–14

Strauss B, U Hepp et al.: Focal counselling for women and couples with an unfulfilled desire for a child: A three-step model. In: Strauss B (ed): Involuntary Childlessness: Psychological assessment, counselling and psychotherapy. Hogrefe and Huber, Seattle 2002

Tuschen-Caffier B, I Florin, W Krause, M Pook: Cognitive-behavioural therapy for idiopathic infertile couples. Psychotherapy and Psychosomatics 68 (1999) 15–21

Vanfraussen K, I Ponjaert-Kristofferson, A Brewaeys: An attempt to reconstruct children's donor concept: A comparison between children's and lesbian parents' attitudes towards donor anonymity. Human Reproduction 16 (9) (2001) 2019–2025

Wallace LM: Psychological preparation as a method of reducing the stress of surgery. Journal of Human Stress 10 (1984) 62–77

Wright J, M Allard, A Lecours, S Sabourin: Psychosocial distress and infertility: A review of controlled research. International Journal of Fertility 34 (1989) 126–142

Wischmann TH: Psychogenic infertility – Myths and facts. Journal of Assisted Reproduction and Genetics 20 (12) (2003) 485–494

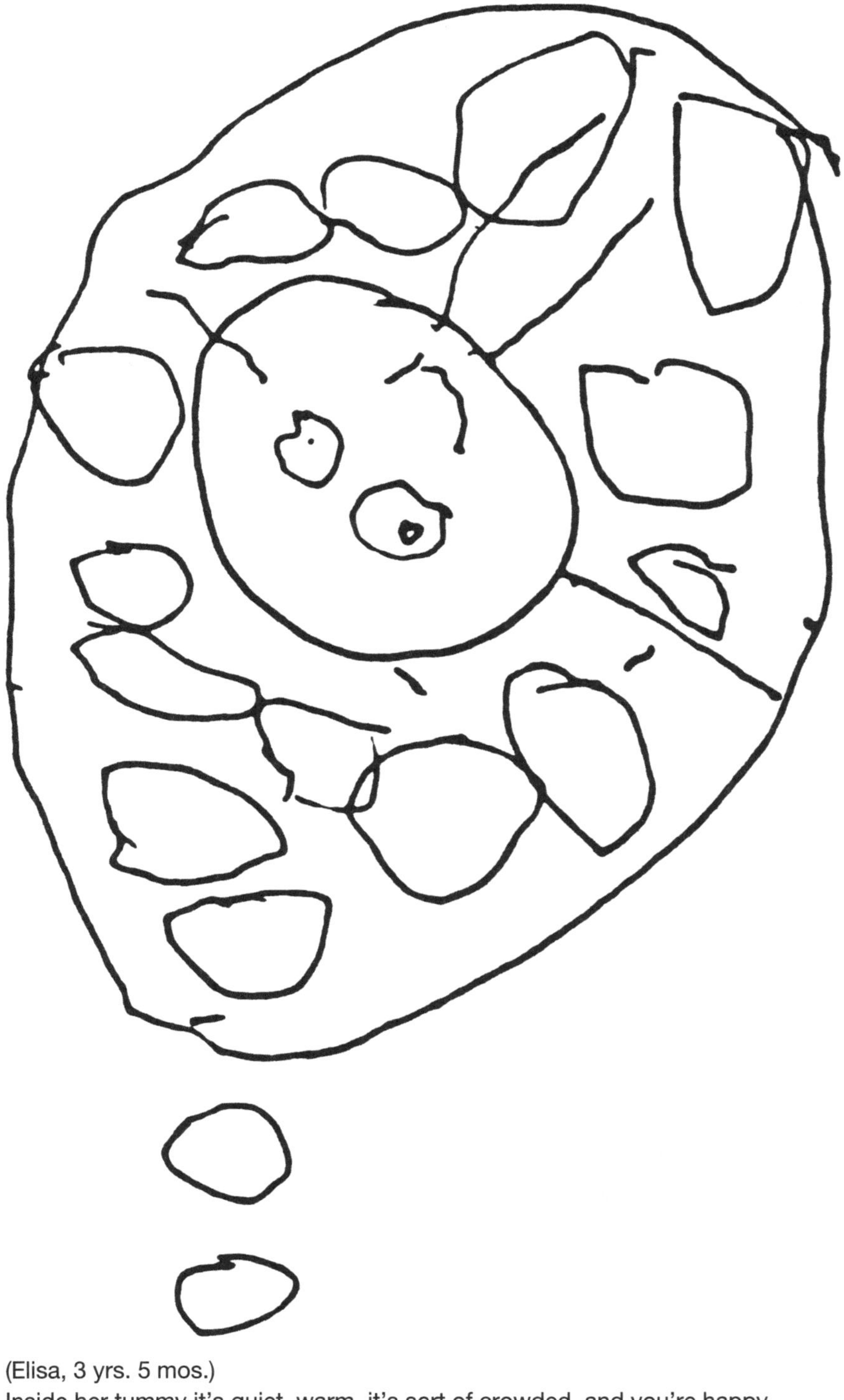

(Elisa, 3 yrs. 5 mos.)
Inside her tummy it’s quiet, warm, it’s sort of crowded, and you’re happy.
It was cold and I was squashed.

12. The maternal and paternal experience between sterility and procreation

Piergiuseppina Fagandini; Department of Motherhood and Infancy, S. Maria Nuova Hospital, Reggio Emilia, Italy
Fiorella Monti; Faculty of Psychology, University of Bologna, Italy
Francesca Agostini; Department of Psychology, University of Bologna, Italy
Ramona Fava; Modena, Italy
Giovanni Battista La Sala; Department of Obstetrics and Gynaecology, S. Maria Nuova Hospital, Reggio Emilia, Italy

"Knowledge enlightens ignorance,
without ever enlightening mystery."
Renè Magritte

The extraordinary progress in medical and biological technology is changing how we are born, live, and die, and causes us to reconsider what are self, a mother, a father, and a family. Biotechnology encourages us to reconsider our notions of what is possible and what affects the very heart of our most primitive and omnipotent fantasies.

This "revolution of thought", which has been triggered by biotechnology, has already come to pass in other historical epochs: "*Our very own sense of 'being' and society could change just as it did when the spirit of the early Renaissance period ran through medieval Europe over seven hundred years ago*" (Rifkin, 1998).

If we move through space and time, we come across the age-old custom of celebrating the anniversary of conception rather than birth, as it happens for instance in China. In this way, birth is intended not as coming into the world but rather the moment in which parental desire and thought generate life. It is one way of enhancing the internal world in a physical sense (the body of the mother who is carrying the fetus contains the unborn child and prepares for the birth) and in a psychic sense (the process of mental gestation, fantasies and dreams which accompany the pregnancy). Thinking about distant time and space which have already been experienced, and about what has already happened, may help suspend our mental categories in order to explore these new realms whilst respecting the mystery of life which accompanies us in our work every day.

"Mystery lies within existence itself, in the duality between the "I" and the "You" in which it is generated, between the subject and the object in which it is known, between the body and mind in which it is represented, between soma and psyche which gives it meaning, between the energy and substance with which it takes shape, between waking and sleeping in which one dreams" (De Toffoli, 2003).

The facts, in as far as we are able to understand them, entangle themselves with our imagination. Biotechnology is complex, but the psychological experiences of its application are just as complex. The epistemology that we are referring to assumes that both body and psyche are categories of the conscience, as concepts through which we get to know a single reality which is unknowable for us; we accept the hypothesis that the ontogenetic development of the psyche and the whole organism are parallel and concurrent once the fetus is formed in relation to the body and psyche of the mother, and in a different way, to that of the father.

Current techniques, including biotechnology, may not be an attack on nature but rather a human contribution to it, if, as Francis Bacon points out, *ars est homo additus naturae*. What seems important to us is that man manages to "think" this continuous overlapping of nature and technology, and thus assimilate its elaboration and deep meaning. This means embracing the continual transformation implicit in every phase between nature and civilization, which can be achieved by working on the social imagination and the symbolic elements implied therein. The postmodern condition excludes neither naturalness nor artificiality, but it requires their transcendence through a different symbolic and relational perspective.

At present, we are witnessing an invasion of the biological dimension in many aspects of our existence, thus restricting the scope of our imagination concerning questions about life and existence. Nonetheless, it is limited to an unknown, unspecific margin representing that which makes the experience of being human specifically unique and unrepeatable. In this way, psychoanalysis can help re-evaluate this field, redefine the identity of those subjects involved in various experiences, by not avoiding the "unnerving" element within the new generative power, and it can assist in finding the instruments to render this conceivable. A reorganization of meanings may help introduce a dimension of grieving and working through loss instead of denying the limitation and retreating behind omnipotence.

In the hope of achieving a confrontation between bioethics and psychoanalysis, Preta (1999) suggests that the experience of "disturbed" feelings, which more than ever characterize the current historical moment, should neither be underestimated nor overestimated. Rather, it should be rendered thinkable, thus preventing "*reality from overshadowing and silencing the mind*".

The subjective experience of fertility and sterility

> *That which is written most amongst all writings the prince of writings so difficult to read beyond its uniform exterior, is the body.*
> Pierre Legendre

Procreation recalls the mystery of birth, the enigma of sex and desire, affective, existential and cultural bonds. Every parental couple, every pregnancy is from the very beginning highly complex, and involves unique and "special" feelings. "Families" have always managed these feelings within various cultures in a sufficiently effective way by going beyond them, and bringing up the child. For centuries, the process of coming into the world was not an event that it was possible to arrange but instead was a natural occurrence, unpredictable, uncontrollable; the fact that it was endured *"determined a certain estrangement and precariousness, from which followed an unburdening of both expectations and feeling of guilt; elements that both currently occupy an enormous space, something which has also been caused by the most complex socio-cultural transformations"* (Bettheleim, 1987).

The World Health Organization (WHO) currently estimates that the proportion of sterile couples in the industrial countries of the Western world is around 20% (Cecotti, 2004) and this figure is constantly increasing. Social factors and cultural values influence fertility; in today's "westernized" society, with its extremely low reproduction rates, there is an increasing demand for sterility treatment. This contradiction can be explained in part by the value attributed to self-determination and reproductive planning. Free and conscious procreation, whilst representing a milestone in social development which cannot be given up, would appear to lend support to the omnipotent expectation, unconscious but socially recognized, that the control action can be reversed, in a kind of mechanism which can negate the influence of desire and subjectivity, both central to the relationship between the sexes.

The instinctive impulse to procreate is surrounded by a cultural framework which interacts with individual intentions. The value of a child has undergone an important change, its "weight" has gradually become concentrated in the affective content of emotive capital, more and more often the result of choice and not chance: the outcome of a decision made by the couple. Yet, if expecting a child emphasizes the elements of decision, sterility may highlight the irrational, unconscious aspect of the desire for paternity and maternity.

The parents who bring forth a life are carriers of representations, scenarios which are for the most part conscious, significant impressions originating in their history, and in a cross-generational manner, that of their ancestors. In this way, pregnancy can be understood as the manifestation of the joint desire of the two partners. The male and female desires for a child are characterized by their differing natures. If it is true that for both we can recognize the essential vehicle of the desire to become parents in the nostalgia for the relationship with the pre-oedipal mother, it is in the woman's body, in the "cavity", that this fusion thrust exists. (Nunziante Cesàro, 2000). For the man, the symbolic aspect of generational transmission would appear to satisfy the generative desire for the most part: rediscovering his own image in a kind of narcissistic duplication and comforting his mortal self-recognition. For the woman, the awareness of her own generative potential conditions female psychology so deeply as to make it one of the determining elements, even when the maternal function is not actually realized.

The willingness expressed, however, does not always coincide with the underlying desire and "the couple is the preferred place in which to express the ambivalence of the desire" (Lemaire, 1979). The partners, even when they agree on procreation, do so partly from mutually estranged positions, if it was not for the gift they exchange, the baby, who "comes" in answer to an order of desires and fantasies of which we know very little. If we reflect on the meanings which a child may represent for the couple, there are three children within the parents' desire (Fraiberg, 1999): the *child of the mind,* the ghost of childhood heritage and subconscious, the *child of the heart*, the affective project which at times may also involve the families of origin, and the *real child* who does not coincide with the one expected by the surrounding world. A mental space is needed where the real child can be placed and this is the transforming function of the desire.

The experience of desire manifests itself in the waiting dimension, where the possibly unfulfilled desire itself is also placed; at times the absolute imperative of procreation may greatly exceed the desire to have a child and need may prevail over desire. Desire is a creative and transforming act which "principally concerns thought and the affective world" (Cecotti, 2004), whilst need represents an indelible moment "related to reality, experienced as an inseparable part of self-fulfillment" (Passarelli, 2002). The birth of a child does not lead to our origins as could be thought, but instead leads us to the real world as it is unknown: a living person seen as a stranger, this is always the real trauma of birth, even the so-called "normal" birth.

Conception, which has always been a private event, is "exposed" in medically assisted procreation (MAP), subjected to an external, scientific, eye which facilitates it, renders it possible and witnesses its achievement: the "primary scene" changes. The exclusion of genital sexuality from procreation, or an intrusion by external elements, as occurs in MAP, may tend to diminish the responsibility of the creative act, turning technicians and/or one or both of the members of the couple into omnipotent ghosts: the paradox of the technical excess is the risk of colluding with the realms of magic.

Reproductive medicine provides techniques to try and realize that which the domain of the will asks for, but, in giving an entirely somatic answer to a subjective problem, risks creating a divide between the physiological and psychic aspects of procreation. A suppression of the symptom through MAP makes the matter of infertility less important, whilst not eliminating it. Paradoxically, the widespread notion that the body and subjectivity are inseparable supports the waiting approach, which, if the body becomes fertile, the subject will also do so; therefore the miracle of reconciliation between having and being is expected from biological maternity and paternity, that is having the child and being father/mother/parent (Fiumanò, 2000).

Being fully aware of this complex issue which affects our daily work, we believe it is necessary to consider the phenomenon of sterility in the light of a "psycho-physical interaction", in which neither the psychic events nor those of the body are foremost, but are reciprocally influenced by each other: "the body speaks by means of symptoms . . . the body is the scenario that the mind chooses as its representation" (Nunziante Cesàro, 2002) and the biological processes "are mirrored by those activities which are subconscious fantasies in the mind " (Cecotti, 2004).

Learning from experience: research

"One arrives on earth, one arrives in time, it is up to us to become part of history"
Sant'Agostino

Even before the 40/2004 law came into effect (Law no. 40, February 19, 2004, "Rules governing medically assisted procreation" represents the first legal provision concerning assisted reproduction techniques in Italy), The Centre for Reproductive Medicine of the S. Maria Nuova Hospital in Reggio Emilia carried out neither embryo freezing nor heterologous fertilization. The research studies which we are to look at here, therefore concern children conceived using MAP with in vitro fertilization techniques on oocytes and the transfer of embryos obtained in vitro to the uterus (IVF) or intracytoplasmic sperm injection (ICSI) within a parental couple.

We began reflecting on these issues of our work in 1998 "from the baby in arms", with a follow-up on infants conceived with MAP; then, by way of a seemingly "backward" route, with two other research projects (2003 and 2006), we followed the children in the first two years of life, the birth, the pregnancy back as far as the conception, again only on couples who "manage" to become parents.

The first project (Fagandini, et al., 1998) analyzed the psycho-physical development of the children conceived through MAP in the first five years of their lives, whilst the second (La Sala et al., 2003) investigated the psycho-affective relationships between the parents and the children conceived through ICSI at 1 and 2 years from birth. We are currently completing a research project which aims to gather parents' representations of the "imagined child" during pregnancy and of themselves as mothers and fathers, and the parents' representations and fantasies in the first few months following the birth of their child. We have therefore passed from the "result" of MAP, i.e. the "baby in arms", to the relationships between parents and child, and finally the fantasies and desire which precede the child and accompany its growth. It is an attempt, albeit highly complex and still experimental, to "keep together" parents and child, physical and psychic experiences, real and imaginary experiences, the external and internal world in the research project, in an experience such as that of conception, pregnancy and childbirth where the "internal" and "external" worlds continually overlap. The parents themselves showed us the "backward route", this "return to our origins", from the very first project.

1998 "Special children and parents?"

The 1998 research project confirmed for our sample what had already been reported in literature (Braverman et al., 1998; Cook et al., 1997; Golombok et al., 1998) on children conceived through MAP, that development is on the whole normal and that there is generally a good aptitude in parents when carrying out their role. As a parallel, most international research projects show that the experience of parenthood, both individually for fathers and mothers, as well as for the couple having gone through the experience of infertility and MAP, seems more delicate. (Colpin et al. 1998; Cook et al., 1998; Gibson et al., 1996).

The children in the research project, with Italian parents and aged between 1 and 5, showed psychophysical development similar to that of the children in the control group. For the same age, weight, similarity, MAP does not in itself differentiate in auxological growth and psychomotor and intellectual development of children conceived with these techniques from "naturally" conceived children. Children conceived with MAP are therefore not "*special children*", but in spite of this reassuring fact, their parents feel like "*special parents*".

The second part of the questionnaire, which is specifically aimed at both parents, analyzes maternal and paternal experiences. The main diversity would appear to be between being a father and being a mother, rather than being a MAP parent or a "natural" parent. But one of the questions strongly differentiates between the two parental groups: "Have you spoken with your child about their birth?" This question really marks the watershed between the two groups of parents. 78% of MAP mothers answered NO versus 38% of mothers from the control group; 83% of MAP fathers replied NO versus 64% of fathers from the control group.

For the second question, which asked "In what way?", we observed that 92% of MAP parents interpreted the word "birth" as "conception", whereas all those parents in the control group used the word "birth" to mean "pregnancy and childbirth".

The way an individual and couple processes conception achieved through MAP techniques represents a problem, even after many years, to the extent that not speaking about the conception seems to stop the parents speaking to the children about their true expectancy and birth. This differing interpretation of the question and the differing chain associated with it introduced us to the topic of the *secret*, of the *unsaid,* of *infertility grief still present.*

2003 "Children conceived with ICSI and their parents"

The 2003 research project represents one of the first investigations conducted in Italy into characteristics of the parent-child relationship in families which have conceived offspring with the assistance of medical techniques also for the therapy of male sterility (ICSI). For ICSI, in particular, there are few long-term studies which reliably illustrate how the psycho-affective development of children conceived using this technique for male sterility proceeds. Bowen's work (1999) suggests the possibility of slight delays in the psychomotor development for these children at the age of 1 year. Our study repeats the same level test (Bayley, 1993), but completes the investigation by observing the parent-child relationship using the Care-Index (Crittenden, 2003) to single out the behavioral indexes in the context of the inner family relationship and using a clinical interview and questionnaires for mother and father in order to observe the parents' experiences in greater detail.

The children, (aged 1 or 2) in the experimental group were conceived using ICSI at our center. The experimental group includes 50 children conceived using ICSI between February 1998 and June 2000, in families resident in Central-Northern Italy. The control group comprised 51 children. For the level test (Bayley), evaluating the overall results, no significantly different indexes of development between the two groups of children emerged as far as cognitive and motor development were concerned. There was no differentiation in the results on the mental scale and motor scale in the two groups either for 1 and 2 year-old children. Only one significant difference emerged concerning behavioral development for the 1 year-old children whereby children in the experimental group have a significantly lower average in "motor quality" for the behavioral scale ($p = 0.04$), that is, they appear to present greater "emotive fragility" in behavioral development compared to 1 year-old children in the control group. At the age of 2 this difference disappears and the two groups are the same in all scales of development (mental, motor, behavioral).

The only difference observed at the age of 1 seems to concern the parent-child relationship rather than the characteristics of the children themselves. In order to investigate this hypothesis, we analyzed the results of the Care-Index which indicate significant differences between the parents from the experimental group and those from the control group. The results of the Care-Index indicate that at the age of 1 year, ICSI mothers are less "sensitive" than other mothers (p = 0.041) and more "controlling" (p = 0.013), whilst the children do not appear to be less cooperative. At the age of 2 years, there are no longer any significant differences. ICSI fathers appear to be less "sensitive" (p = 0.007) compared to fathers from the control group and more "controlling-intrusive" (p = 0.008). The children are significantly less cooperative. Just as the significant differences in the Bayley test on the children's development disappear at the age of 2 yars, so do the differences in the parent-child relationship for the Care-Index at the same age.

According to this study, there are thus no differences in the cognitive and motor development between ICSI-conceived children and naturally conceived ones. Interestingly, the only difference concerns behavioral development, which varies between 1 and 2 year-old children and concerns differences in the parent-child relationship rather than characteristics in the children themselves. It would appear that the differences in the parent-child relationship, triggered by the lack of re-elaboration in parents in the MAP sterility-conception process, can reflect on the child during the first year as far as behavioral development is concerned. Our hypothesis is that this particular relationship has a protective function; the parents' behavior would appear to protect the children, limiting contact with the parents' concerns and painful experiences. At the age of 2 years significant differences in the tests no longer exist in any of the children's developmental areas, nor in the parent-child relationship.

During the first year of the ICSI child's life, the parents maintain greater emotive "control", which allows the children to develop adequately in both mental and motor aspects, but affects their behavioral development. The "healthy" development of the child would appear to promote a more sensitive behavior in the parents and therefore a better parent-child interaction, as well as an improved development in the child in the second year.

Parents can be in greater emotive harmony with their children once they have grown up and become more autonomous: In the second year, parents seem to have overcome the difficult transition which exists between fantasizing about the desired child and thinking about the real child, creating a mental space in which the relationship with their "own" baby can develop, their own child.

It would seem that the transforming function of the attachment process, which needs time and "protection" to complete itself, is thus confirmed. The transforming process for ICSI parents and their children seems to be more prolonged and complex compared to that of parents of naturally conceived children, but that at the end of the second year it is certainly possible. The choice of a sample with two different ages (1 and 2 years old) compared to the Australian study (which only investigated 1 year-old children) and the use of the Care-Index as well as the Bayley test seems to enable us to underline this process.

Despite unresolved personal grief in infertility, ICSI parents activate personal resources and those within the couple and their children, the real children, work in harmony with their parents' resources and use them to grow up "normally".

The hypothesis which has emerged from interviews conducted and statistically significant results in the questionnaires, is that "ICSI" parents are not special parents, but they are special in the way they see themselves in the parental role, "they feel" special.

The narcissistic wound which results from the experience of sterility also features in this study. We obtained the same results for the question "Have you spoken to your child about his/her birth?" as those in the 1998 study: the group of ICSI parents interpreted birth = conception (through MAP). The parents in the control group interpreted birth = birth (pregnancy/childbirth). The ICSI parents, even the ICSI mothers, and even 2 years after birth of their child, still focus on the conception, and do not consider pregnancy and childbirth in their true procreative function. Instead, pregnancy and childbirth are experienced as potential dangers for the "*gift*" child. It would therefore seem that, even 2 years after the birth of the real child, the grief associated with sterility has not yet been sufficiently overcome. Birth of the real child appears unable to completely "repair" the narcissistic wound. The ICSI parents seem more tried, more vulnerable when compared to themselves as individuals and as a couple, but at the same time these aspects do not appear to affect the relationship with their real child, their child's development and their real parental functions, at least not after the age of two.

The greater complexity of MAP parents' emotions, in particular for the fathers, (ICSI directly concerns male sterility), appears to give them a greater depth of understanding and awareness about the parental relationship. These reflections led us to conduct our final research project, and we "went back" to the pregnancy to take the "physiological" route from pregnancy to childbirth, to the first three months of the child's life.

2006 "Maternal and paternal representations in MAP"

The main objective of the 2006 research study was to explore some of the psychological aspects which primarily characterize the transition to parenthood in a comparison between MAP and "natural" procreation. We have referred to the possible presence of psychopathological signs (symptoms of depression and/or anxiety), and the qualitative characteristics of maternal and paternal representations, regarding the child, the Self, their partner, their own parents, which develop in the course of the pregnancy.

For this purpose a longitudinal research plan was conceived, which observed MAP parental couples from the 7th-8th month of pregnancy until the 3rd month after childbirth. The research study is currently ongoing, and the partial results are therefore presented, relating to the first two meetings with the parental couples. The sample, from the part of the study presented here, comprises 70 individuals, 38 women and 32 men, subdivided into an experimental group and a control group.

The experimental group consists of 35 subjects, 18 women and 17 men, thus 17 couples and 1 mother who has taken part in the study individually. The study concerns subjects who have undergone MAP (IVF-ICSI) at our center and represent couples expecting their first child. The control group comprises 35 subjects, 20 women and 15 men; in terms of parental couples, the group comprised of 15 mother-father couples and 5 women who have taken part in the study individually. The couples, who are expecting their first child and have no procreation problems, were contacted on the ward or during prenatal courses in the Obstetrics and Gynecology Division at the same hospital.

As far as the selection of the sample was concerned, it was decided that only Italian nationality will be included, in order to limit the influence of socio-cultural factors on parental representations and the manifestation of psychological symptoms. The control group and experimental group do not differ regarding the following socio-demographic characteristics: place of origin (mainly from the North of Italy), middle class, civil status (mainly married), one third of the sample took part in prenatal courses. However, they differ in age, which is higher in the MAP group (control group 33.23 years old, experimental group 37.77, $p < 0.0005$). If a comparison is made between the control and the experimental group, separating mothers and fathers, the socio-demographic characteristics again do not differ, whilst age does (women: control group 31.95 vs. experimental group 36.05 years old, $p = 0.005$; men: control group 34.93 vs. experimental group 39.58 years old, $p = 0.01$).

Concerning the procedure, the psychologists involved in the study contacted the couples at the hospital clinics in the 20th–24th week of pregnancy when they presented the project and supplied the consent forms. In the 30th–32nd gestational week, each psychologist called at the homes of the parents-to-be, supplying them with a questionnaire on anxiety (ASQ-IPAT) and another on depression (EPDS), conducting an interview on parental representations during pregnancy, IRMAG (maternal representations) and Ra.Pa.G. (paternal representations). Between the 3rd and 5th day after birth, each psychologist once again met the couple at the hospital and asked them to complete additional EPDS and ASQ-IPAT questionnaires.

During the 3rd month after birth, a final visit was made to the parents' homes, and the same questionnaires were completed and an interview on maternal and paternal representations after the birth (IRMAN and Ra.Pa.N respectively) was conducted. This meeting has not been included in this study, as it has not yet been carried out for some of the couples, both MAP and non-MAP couples.

In the 30th–32nd week of gestation, both partners had a *semi-structured* interview, designed to collate information on socio-demographic and cultural aspects (nationality, age, education, occupation, etc.), EPDS, ASQ-IPAT and an interview on representations. The *Edinburgh Postnatal Depression Scale* (EPDS), (Cox et al. 1987), is a self-evaluation questionnaire in widespread use at international level, purposely created as a "*screening*" tool to identify symptoms of postnatal depression (PND, Postnatal Depression). The *ASQ-Ipat Anxiety Scale*, by Krug et al. (1976), is a tool designed to obtain general clinical information on anxiety, latent/hidden anxiety and manifest anxiety in a rapid, objective and standardized way.

The interview on maternal representations during pregnancy (IRMAG, Ammaniti et al., 1995) and the one on paternal representations during pregnancy (Ra.Pa.G, DiVita et al., 2002) are generally conducted between the 28th and 32nd week of gestation because in this phase the presence of the baby has had time to establish itself within the "maternal psychic space, and has not yet been invaded by pervasive anxieties connected to the imminent birth" (Ammaniti et al., 1995).

During the interview, five lists of adjectives are compiled, creating a structured description of the representations dependent on an evaluation of the meaning attributed to 5 concepts or people by the woman/man: the baby, her/himself, their own partner, her/himself as mother/father, their own mother/father. The unusual thing about the lists is the fact that they are designed around a model of "semantic differential which enables the affective meaning of some concepts to be measured, by means of a qualification process. The semantic differential is usually presented to the subjects in the form of a diagram with steps, each one made up of a pair of adjectives with opposite meanings" (Ammaniti et al., 1995). The first three lists of adjectives, concerning the individual characteristics of the baby, the woman and the partner, comprise the same pairs of adjectives, 17 to be precise. "The adjectives used in the first three lists basically refer to aspects of personal behavior, interpersonal manner, and affective orientation" (Ammaniti et al., 1995). The other two lists, which concern the maternal and paternal characteristics in themselves and their own mother/father, are also made up of 17 pairs of adjectives and are the same and comparable. In these two lists the adjectives refer to the affective area, personal behavior, parental role, and parental sensitivity. In this way it is possible to establish to which extent the expectant mother and her partner wish to approach the maternal and paternal model that they experienced in the relationship with their own parents, or whether they differ from this, and in contrast, start to build their own "parental approach" to be put to the test with their own child in time. In the present study, only data regarding the semantic differential for IRMAG and Ra.Pa.G has been presented.

In order to establish possible differences between the MAP and non-MAP groups, the data obtained through the EPDS (using Fisher's exact test and the linear-log analysis) and the ASQ-IPAT (using ANOVA) was compared. The data obtained from the semantic differential on parental representations was worked out using the mixed ANOVA model.

Results

Depressive symptoms

Pre-natal depressive symptoms, identified using the EPDS questionnaire (cut-off 8/9), are present in 24.2% of the MAP group and 5.7% of subjects in the control group ($p = 0.03$), (Figure 1).

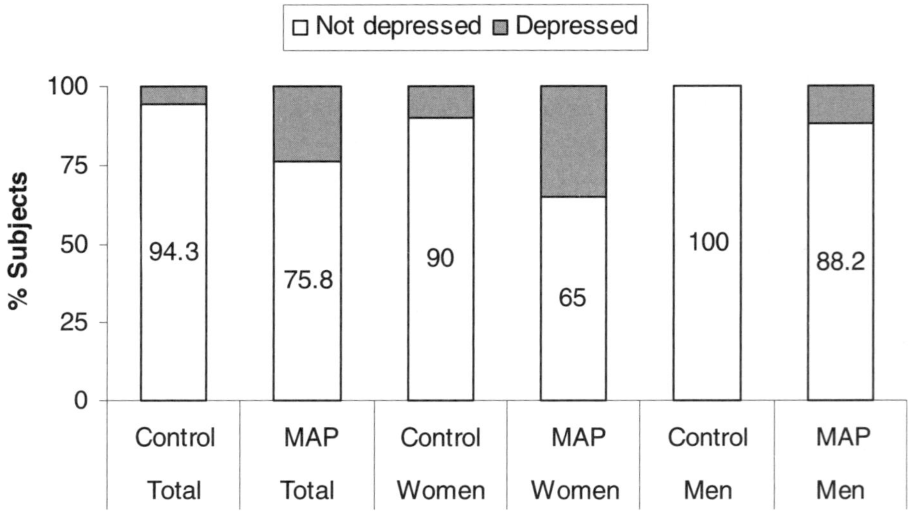

Figure 1. Percentage of subjects with ante-natal depressive symptoms.

A comparison between the MAP and control group, carried out separately for women and men, shows differences which, although perhaps not significant, may be relevant:

1. In the comparison between women, the proportion of depressed MAP women (35.5%) is higher than that of depressed women in the control group (10%);
2. In the comparison between men, 11.8% of the MAP group is depressed, whilst in the control group nobody is reported as being depressed (we would point out that in the MAP group fathers with sterility problems have been included, the couples where the fathers are reported as depressed are couples who have used ICSI).

After birth, depressive symptoms are reported as 20% in the MAP group, and 17.1% in the control group (Figure 2).

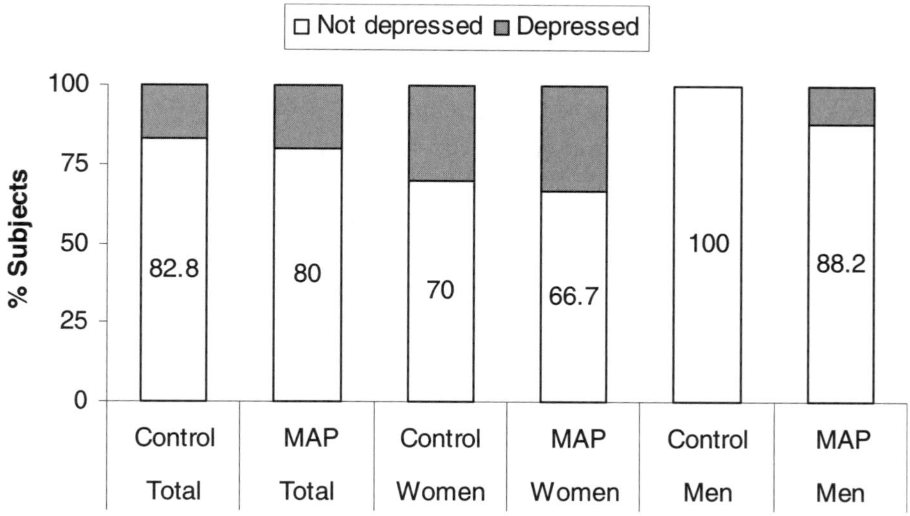

Figure 2. Percentages of subjects with post-natal depressive symptoms.

The comparison between women in the two groups showed a similar proportion of depressed MAP women (33.3%) and depressed women in the control group (30%), whilst in the comparison between men in the two groups, it is still 11.8% in the MAP group as opposed to 0% in the control group.

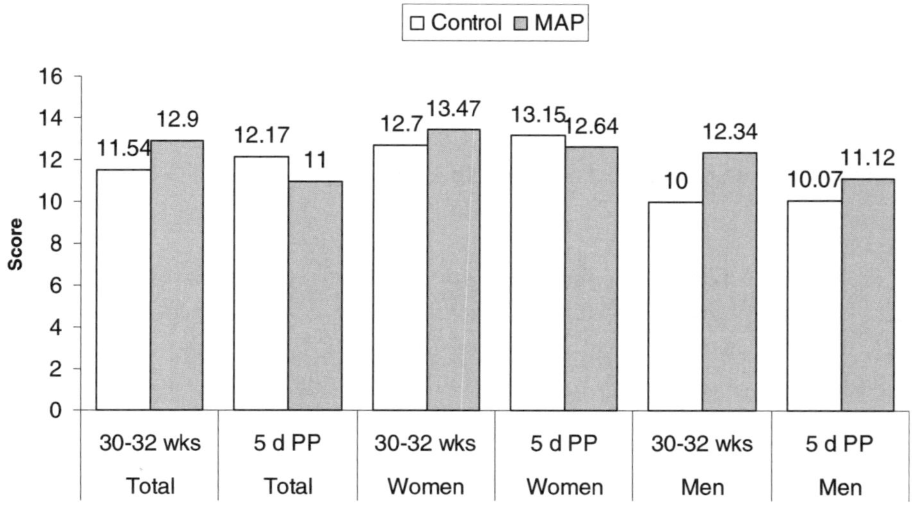

Figure 3. Scores for latent anxiety before and after the birth.

Anxiety

Three scores taken from the ASQ-IPAT test were considered. The first one is a score A, which indicates subconscious, hidden anxiety (Figure 3).

For the first ante-partum meeting, the A scores do not significantly differ when compared to the MAP variable, the parental gender variable and the MAP and parental gender interaction. The same can be observed in a separate comparison for males and females. For the post-partum (PP) meeting, no significant differences emerge in the A scores distinguishing between the MAP and non-MAP groups, between mothers and fathers, taking into account the MAP and parental gender interaction. Considering men and women separately, no significant differences emerge in either case.

The second score which was considered was the B score, i.e. conscious, manifest anxiety (Figure 4).

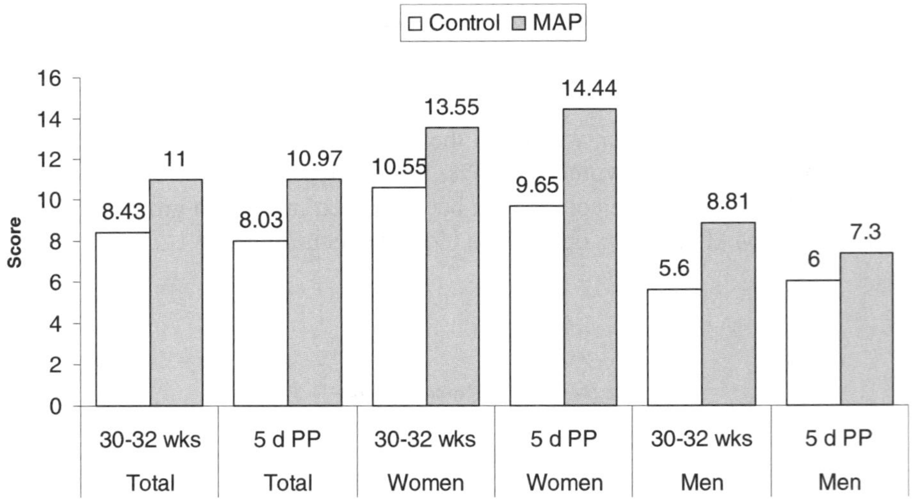

Figure 4. Scores for manifest anxiety before and after the birth.

In the 30th–32nd week, the MAP group reached a significantly higher score than the control group ($p = 0.02$). If the groups are compared according to gender, the MAP women show a score of 13.05, and those in the control group a score of 10.55 ($p = 0.05$), whilst men in the MAP group show a score of 8.81 as compared to 5.60 in the control group ($p = 0.04$). At the meeting after the birth, the B score differs significantly between the MAP group and the control group ($p = 0.02$). The MAP women show 14.44, whilst those in the control group 9.65 ($p = 0.05$), men in the MAP group 7.30 as opposed to 6.0 in the control group (not significant).

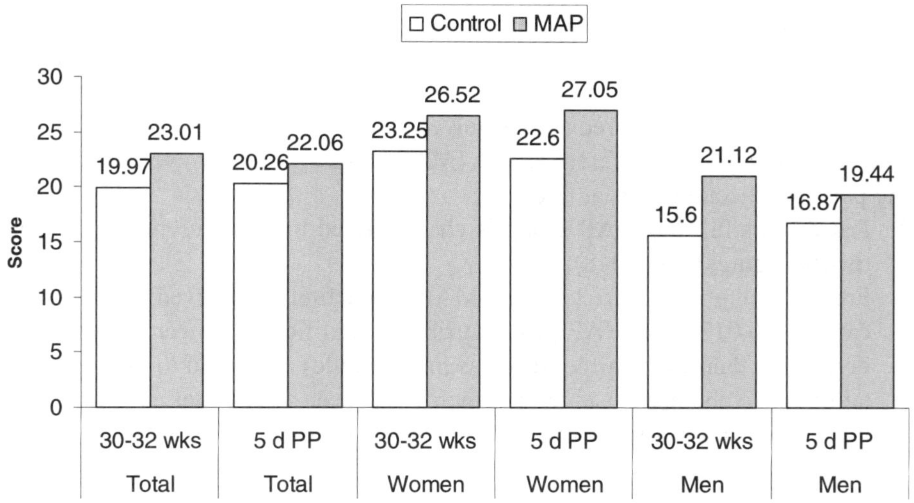

Figure 5. Scores for global anxiety before and after the birth.

The third score considered was the one representing the total level of anxiety (the sum of A and B) scores, (Figure 5).

Before the birth, the MAP group achieves a significantly higher score compared to that of the control group (23.91 vs. 19.97, $p = 0.04$), whilst after the birth, the total A + B score does not differ significantly when compared to the MAP variable. Considering women and men separately, no significant differences emerge either before or after the birth.

Maternal and paternal representations during pregnancy

The results relating to the 5 lists of adjectives establish representations concerning the child, the Self and his/her own partner, all characterized by the same pairs of adjectives (e.g. passive/active, excited/calm), and those concerning the self as mother/father and her/his own mother/father, described by the same pairs of adjectives (e.g. non-affectionate/affectionate, insecure/confident). In the present study, only significant data which is of interest for the purposes of the study has been considered, in order to avoid too many unnecessary details.

Individual characteristics of the child, Self and the partner

The statistical analyses carried out have revealed that, for 7 of the 17 pairs of adjectives, there is a significant difference between the scores of the three figures (child, the Self, partner), irrespective of whether they come from the control or the MAP group. This would appear to presume that such representations are similar in both types of couples. The parents, both MAP and non-MAP, tend to view their own child as more sociable, more forward, cleaner, happier, more intelligent, livelier, compared to themselves and their partner.

Concerning the two different groups (MAP and control), however, the following pairs of adjectives appear to differ:

1. Fearful/trustful: the MAP group is characterized by a representation of less trustful figures ($p = 0.048$);
2. Fragile/strong: the figure type and MAP interaction is observed to be significant ($p = 0.012$): the MAP group attributes significantly lower values when describing their own partner (seen as more fragile) compared to the representation made about themselves and their child, seen as stronger, as opposed to the control group which attributes similar values to the three figures.

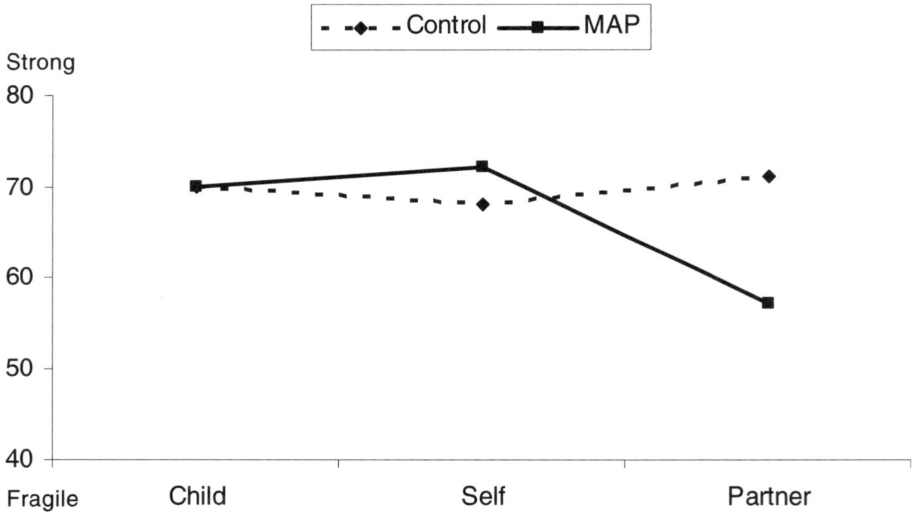

Figure 6. Comparison between representations "fragile/strong" from control and MAP groups.

Considering the parental gender factor, besides the MAP factor, some ANOVA questionnaires were carried out, which established that 8 of the 17 pairs of adjectives (e.g. passive/active, difficult/easy, detached/affectionate, remissive/resolute) differ significantly between mothers and fathers: the women, irrespective of the type of figure and group (MAP or control), tend to have a more positive representation than the men. Moreover, taking the mother and father groups separately, several results worth noting have emerged.

As far as the women are concerned, the following differences are of interest:

1. Shy/forward ($p = 0.029$): the women in the MAP group tend to view their child and their partner as less forward than the women in the control group do, whilst they view themselves as more forward;
2. Fearful/trustful ($p = 0.030$): the representations made by the women in the MAP group concerning the child, self and the partner are characterized by a higher degree of fear.

Regarding men, the differences related to the following pairs of adjectives are worth noting:
1. Excited/calm: the figure type and MAP interaction is observed to be significant ($p = 0.04$): whilst men in both groups view the child in a similar way, halfway between excited and calm, the same men differ in the way they view their partner, who is seen as much calmer by the MAP men;
2. Shy/forward: the figure type and MAP interaction is observed to be significant ($p = 0.03$): men in both groups view their child as quite forward, whereas they differ in the way they view their partner, who is seen as much more forward by the MAP men;
3. Remissive/resolute: the figure type and MAP interaction is observed to be significant ($p = 0.016$): the child is view as much more resolute by the MAP men, whilst both groups see the partner as quite resolute;
4. Not lively/lively ($p = 0.04$): the representations made by men in the MAP group concerning the figures are characterized by greater liveliness compared to those made by men in the control group;
5. Fragile/strong: the figure type and MAP interaction is observed to be significant ($p = 0.04$): men in both groups view themselves in a similar way to the child (quite strong), whilst men in the MAP group see their partner as much more fragile.

Maternal/paternal characteristics for self and own mother/father

The results from the ANOVA questionnaires show that, out of the 17 pairs of adjectives, 9 pairs differ with regard to the figure type, irrespective of the group type, thus showing some similarities in the representations made by the control group and the MAP group. The parents from both groups tend to view themselves as significantly more positive parents compared to the way they view their own families: they see themselves as more affectionate, more helpful, more flexible, protective, patient, playful, cheerful and active than their own parents.

Regarding the comparison between the MAP group and the control group, the differences which emerge from the following pairs of adjectives are of interest:
1. Inflexible/flexible ($p = 0.005$): the representation made by the MAP group is much more flexible compared to that of the control group;

2. Non-accepting/accepting: the MAP group is characterized by the representation of Self as a parent and the one of their own parents as more accepting ($p = 0.046$);
3. Insecure/confident: the figure type and MAP interaction is observed to be significant ($p = 0.047$): in the description of Self the two groups are the same (quite confident), whilst in respect of their own parents, the MAP group describes them as much less confident than the parents in the control group;
4. Controlling/letting go: the figure type and MAP interaction is observed to be significant ($p = 0.029$): whilst the two groups report a similar description concerning their own parents (relatively controlling), in the representation of the maternal/paternal characteristics in themselves, the MAP group describes itself as much more controlling in comparison with the control group;
5. Anxious/calm: the figure type and MAP interaction is observed to be significant ($p = 0.008$): the two groups attribute roughly the same degree of calmness in their representation of their own parents, but the MAP group pictures itself as a visibly more anxious parents than the control group.

Taking the parental gender factor into account, ANOVA tests were also conducted in this case, in which 14 of the 17 pairs of adjectives differ greatly, so far as the women have a more positive representation than the men, irrespective of figure type and group. Separate ANOVA were also conducted for the men and women. In the comparison between the women in the MAP group and those in the control group, significant differences emerged regarding the following pairs of adjectives:

1. Inflexible/flexible ($p = 0.01$): the women in the MAP group describe their own maternal characteristics and those of their own mothers as more flexible when compared to the control group;
2. Impatience/patience ($p = 0.04$): the women in the MAP group represent themselves and their own mothers as much more patient when compared to the control group;
3. Controlling/letting go: the figure type and MAP interaction is observed to be significant ($p = 0.05$): the women in the MAP group judge themselves as much more controlling when compared to the women in the control group, whilst both describe their own mothers as quite controlling;
4. Anxiety/calmness: the figure type and MAP interaction is observed to be significant ($p = 0.029$): the women in the MAP group represent themselves as much more anxious parents then those in the control group;
5. Not giving in/generous ($p = 0.05$): the women in the MAP group describe themselves and their own mothers as more generous.

No significant differences connected to the pairs of adjectives emerge, however, in a comparison between men in the MAP group with those in the control group.

Discussion of the results

In terms of socio-demographical characteristics, the two samples are homogeneous, except for the age factor, which is higher in the MAP group and probably linked to the complex route leading to the decision and planning for assisted parenthood. Concerning signs of psychopathological risk, it is worth noting that the number of parents with symptoms of depression is higher in the MAP group, in particular prior to birth, with no distinction between women and men. In this regard, bearing in mind the fact that this is a small sample, it is possible to observe that at a descriptive level, men are only included in the group of depressed MAP parents, whereas only women in the control group are reported to be depressed, and to a decidedly lower degree.

In the MAP group, depressive symptoms prior to the birth could be linked to an amplification of genetic anxieties which, despite being part of every planned pregnancy, may inhibit the work of the psychic maternity in situations where infertility is present, due to their intensity. Immediately after birth the two samples are the same in terms of the presence of depressive signs, which are connected to the maternity blues: the surrounding environment (hospital and family) and the newborn baby will enhance the resilience of the MAP parents concerning their more complex and often traumatic transition to parenthood.

With regard to hidden anxiety, the two groups show no difference, even when the gender of the parent is taken into account, both before and after birth, whereas interesting results emerge for the manifest anxiety and global anxiety. This could be attributed to the test itself, which may be seen as intrusive in a moment of "psychic and transparent vulnerability", such as during pregnancy, and therefore may not facilitate representative access to contents that are in part subconscious. As far as manifest anxiety is concerned, the MAP group shows a generally higher score compared to the control group. In a separate examination of men and women in the MAP group, we can observe that both groups achieve a higher score compared to men and women in the control group. This can also be observed in the 30th–32nd week and is also maintained after birth. In the MAP group manifest anxiety therefore tends to be more intense and it could be presumed that just as genetic anxieties are more pervasive, so parental anxieties have a greater influence on the representation of the self as parents dependent on techniques and the representation of the child as precious and vulnerable. The level of global anxiety is higher in the MAP before birth, but not afterwards, as if for all parents the birth represented a positive outcome of their project.

Concerning the representations, in particular the first three categories: child, the Self, and partner, it appears that the two groups do not differ significantly, but rather attribute similar scores to the representations of the child, themselves and their partner.

In both groups the higher score is attributed to the child, represented as much more sociable, more forward, cleaner, more cheerful, more intelligent and livelier compared to the Self and the partner. Only with regard to the adjective tidy do mothers and fathers describe themselves as tidier than the child and the partner. For both parents in the MAP group and those in the control group, the child is an object of love, libidinal investment, which is naturally idealized as it represents the goal of our own desire and a need to be confirmed in terms of the integrity and the ability of the internal and external world: *being* parents and *having* a child. It would therefore seem that depression and anxiety, which are much higher for MAP parents in this phase of the pregnancy, do not involve fantasies about the child which will be born.

It is important to point out another "common aspect": the gender variable affects the intensity of the representations; in fact women in both groups achieve a higher score than men, in most cases. The mothers, irrespective of the group, allow their fantasies to emerge more as well as a much more accentuated investment regarding the child.

The representations concerning the partner in the two groups only differ in the aspects about trust, which are lower in the MAP group, and fragility aspects, which are higher in the MAP group; the MAP couple has had to tolerate traumatic experiences and feelings of inadequacy regarding their own and reciprocal expectations and appears to be painfully aware of this.

Considering the representations of the Self as a parent and of their own parents, however, we can observe another common aspect: the two groups are similar in the scores on the self image as a parent, which is perceived more positively than that of their own parent, as more affectionate, helpful, protective, patient, playful, satisfied, cheerful and active.

To imagine oneself emotively and knowingly, being and becoming a "better" parent than one's own, may be a way of creating a model of parenthood that can be passed down in an ever more positive way, and therefore a task which is carried on towards higher goals, so that one's own childlike side may also be protected and sheltered.

Differences between the two groups can be observed in the representation of Self as father and mother; in the MAP group both parents view themselves, on the one hand, as more flexible and more accepting, but on the other, as more anxious and controlling compared to the control group. These parents have certainly had to accept and go through a more inaccessible route, physically but above all psychologically, and they find themselves having to anxiously "watch over" their objective.

This representation of the Self as parents who "control" points us to the results of the 2003 research study, in which the MAP parents were in fact more controlling on the Care-Index, in the first year of their child's life, compared to parents in the control group. We observed that the gender variable is once again a determining factor. It has emerged that the MAP mothers, in particular, describe themselves as more flexible, more patient, more generous and at the same time as more anxious and controlling compared to mothers in the control group. For the MAP fathers, there are some significant differences, which are less important. Pregnancy for MAP mothers, in a medically assisted and often unstable environment, appears to demand a much more complex psychological process than that of the mothers who conceived "naturally".

Conclusions

The MAP experience involves, even if in an amplified way, fears, doubts, anxiety and a natural feeling of inadequacy which is present in any planned parenthood. Getting to know the "parental representations" and the parents' depressive and anxious experience when conceiving with MAP, helps us move away from the prejudice of presumed "omnipotence" of these couples. The results of the test and interviews with the MAP parents help us to understand how suffering caused by the narcissistic wound of sterility, and the subsequent exhausting and painful experience of MAP, may represent a more complex route, but also a deeper one when working towards parenthood.

We know from previous studies that the psycho-physical development of children conceived using MAP is not different from that of children conceived "naturally". The differences in the experiences and the various defense mechanisms which accompany the waiting and the parental experience of MAP parents would therefore seem to be functional for the "protection" of the child's development starting with pregnancy.

Putting this into practice means more questioning the clinical routes in order to offer more effective solutions, setting aside failures and, above all, allowing the couple to internally "take back" responsibility and actively participate in the process.

It is important to limit the fantasies of omnipotence in patients and primarily those of physicians, in a situation in which sliding back in this direction is implicit. This assertion would seem to apply to many problems in perinatal medicine; the risk is that the parents, physicians and the child itself, may become obsessed with the techniques used, which as a result, could condition the parents' relationship and the child.

The facilities in the health service surrounding MAP should be carefully assessed and conceived paying particular attention to the transition to parenthood and to the follow-up of the child; the emotive experience of pregnancy may become an opportunity to work through the narcissistic wound of sterility both for mothers and fathers. We have observed that achieving conception and the birth of the same child do not in themselves "automatically" repair the grieving caused by MAP.

The risk in medically assisting procreation may become a warning for physicians, so that they should encourage the idea that progression of events following "conception" must be accepted as far as possible as a physiological experience, in order not to risk halting the process of internal elaboration relating to procreation.

It is just as important to promote an interdisciplinary and integrated culture amongst physicians of birth and parenthood which focuses on and encompasses, whilst not confusing the internal emotive aspects, alongside the physical ones. We believe that our role as technicians in the field of MAP, involves "supporting" the desire for parenthood, dealing with all the physical and psychic risks of MAP, but at the same time we believe it is vital to promote the idea of the "normal complexity" of the birth and conception and return this to the parents. Even in MAP, the parents and their children, not the technicians or the techniques, are and should be the main players of the parental experience: *"put the subject (child, mother, father) back in their own story"* (Ansermet, 1999).

In the *silence of the senses* it is the body that speaks of discomfort, experiences of anguish and suffering, in its silent yet explicit language. The medical answer risks dealing even more with the body, sure of finding a subconscious willingness to accept it, to put aside the mental dimension in an apparently reassuring way. It is instead necessary to *"refresh the value of the verbal function, encouraging affable medicine, that is one which does not forget the fundamental necessity of the word that is genuinely spoken and listened to, to avoid both defensive protections of tradition, as well as a rash euphoria for unreflective technology"* (Francesconi, 2005).

References

Ammaniti M, C Candelori, M Pola, R Tambelli: Maternità e Gravidanza. Cortina, Milano 1995

Ansermet F: Clinique de l'origine, l'Enfant entre la médicine et la psychanalyse. (Psyché), Payot, Lausanne 1999

Bayley N: Bayley scales of Infant development, second edition. The Psychological Corporation. Harcourt Brace, San Antonio 1993

Bettelheim B: Un genitore quasi perfetto. Feltrinelli, Milano 1987

Bion W: Apprendere dall'esperienza. Armando, Roma 1972

Bindt C, K Ohlsen, M Berger: Parenthood and child development after reproduction medicine treatment. Psychosomatic follow-up of 46 parents after assisted reproduction. Fortschr Med 114 (27) (1996) 337–40

Bowen JR, FL Gibson, GI Leslie, DM Saunders: Medical and developmental outcome at 1 year for children conceived by intracytoplasmic sperm injection. Lancet 351 (1998) 1529–34

Braverman AM, AS Boxer, SL Corson, C Coutifaris, A Hendrix: Characteristics and attitudes of parents of children born with the use of assisted reproductive technology. Fertility and Sterility 70 (5) (1998) 860–5

Cecotti M: Procreazione Medicalmente Assistita. Aspetti psicologici della sterilità, della genitorialità e della filiazione. Armando, Roma 2004

Colpin H, A De Munter, L Vandemeulebroecke: Parenthood motives in IVF-mothers. Journal of Psychosomatic Obstetrics and Gynaecology 19 (1) (1998) 19–27

Cook R, S Bradley, S Golombok: A preliminary study of parental stress and child behaviour in families with twins conceived by in-vitro fertilization. Human Reproduction 13 (11) (1998) 3244–6

Cook R, I Vatev, Z Michova, S Golombok: The European study of assisted reproduction families: a comparison of family functioning and child development between Eastern and Western Europe. Journal of Psychosomatic Obstetrics and Gynaecology 18 (3) (1997) 203–12

Crittenden PM: CARE-Index. In: Lambruschi F (ed): Psicoterapia cognitiva dell'età evolutiva. Bollati Boringhieri, Torino 2003

De Toffoli C: Il lavoro somato-psichico della coppia materno-fetale: come "ciò" diviene "tu". Richard e Piggle 11 (3) (2003) 271–284

Di Vita AM, F Giannone: (a cura di) La famiglia che nasce. Angeli, Milano 2002

Eugster A, AJ Vingerhoets: Psychological aspects of in vitro fertilization: a review. Social Science & Medicine 48 (5) (1999) 575–89

Fagandini P et al.: Bambini e Genitori Speciali? Atti Convegno Internazionale 30–31 Ottobre 1998, Percorsi/Carocci, Roma 1999

Fiumanò M et al.: L'immacolata fecondazione. La Tartaruga, Milano 1996

Fiumanò M: A ognuna il suo bambino. Nuova Pratiche Editrice Il Saggiatore, Milano 2000

Fraiberg S, E Adelson, V Shapiro: I fantasmi nella stanza dei bambini in Il sostegno allo sviluppo, Raffaello Cortina, Milano 1999

Francesconi M: L'infertilità: limite o divieto? Richard e Piggle 13 (1) (2005) 58–72

Gibson FL, JA Ungerer, GI Leslie, DM Saunders, CC Tennant: Development, behaviour and temperament: a prospective study of infants conceived through in-vitro fertilization. Human Reproduction 13 (6) (1998) 1727–32

Gibson FL, JA Ungerer, CC Tennant, DM Saunders: Parental adjustement and attitudes to parenting after in vitro fertilization. Fertility and Sterility 73 (2000) 565–574

Golombok S, A Brewaeys, R Cook, MT Giavazzi, D Guerra, A Mantovani; E van Hall, PG Crosignani, S Dexeus: The European study of assisted reproduction families: family functioning and child development. Human Reproduction 11 (10) (1996) 2324–31

La Sala GB et al.: Developmental outcomes at one and two years of children conceived by intracytoplasmic sperm injection. International Journal of Fertility 49 (3) (2004) 113–119

Lemaire JG: Vita e morte della coppia. Cittadella, Assisi 1979

Nunziante Cesàro A: (a cura di) Il bambino che viene dal freddo. Angeli, Milano 2000

Nunziante Cesàro A: Psicoanalisi e Bioetica nella PMA. In: Riccardi E, F Monti, C Passarelli, L Lombardini: (a cura di) Procreazione medicalmente assistita. Incontro di professionalità diverse tra i sintomi del corpo e i desideri della mente, Casalecchio di Reno. Grafiche MM, Bologna 2002

Passarelli C: Genitorialità non biologica e PMA. In: Riccardi E, F Monti, C Passarelli, L Lombardini: (a cura di) Procreazione medicalmente assistita. Incontro di professionalità diverse tra i sintomi del corpo e i desideri della mente, Casalecchio di Reno. Grafiche MM, Bologna 2002

Preta L: L'esperienza del "perturbante" nell'impatto con le biotecnologie. In: Preta L: (a cura di) Nuove geometrie della mente. Laterza, Milano 1999

Rifkin J: The Biothec Century: Harnessing the Gene and Remaking the World. Tarcher/Putnam New York 1998

Soulé M, J Noel: Après l'échec des procréations médicalement assistées. Neuropsychiatrie de L'Enfance e de l'adolescence 38 (1990) 669–72

13. Integrative functions of the brain and origins of fetal psychism: Some theoretical and clinical reflections

Mauro Mancia; Professor Emeritus of Neurophysiology, University of Milan; Training analyst of the Italian Psychoanalytical Society, Italy

Introduction

Neurophysiological and psychoanalytical research referring to prenatal and perinatal life support the hypothesis according to which there is no differentiation at the beginning of life between somatic and psychic functions. Ultrasonographic evidence now enables us to hypothesize a developing process which is managed by early 'organizers' of the motor, respiratory, vegetative, sensory, and integrative functions, which are related to fetal cycles of rest and activity, which are precursors of restful and active sleep, the latter of which anticipates, in turn, the baby's REM phase (Mancia, 1981).

The study of this aspect pertains to neurophysiology, but these functions form an apparatus through which the fetus relates to the mother and the uterine environment. Clearly, this is extremely relevant to the branch of psychoanalysis which studies early relations to objects, their dynamics, and the emotional and cognitive consequences they have.

Ontogenetic constants

I would like now to analyze the ontogenetic constants which, in the human fetus, can be considered as a sign of its development. These constants refer to (a) motor and sensory functions, and (b) the integrative functions of the central nervous system (CNS). By observing these functions, I have tried to suggest some hypotheses on prenatal life, in an attempt to establish the relevance these functions may have for the development of the fetal mind and the consequences they might have on the primary relations of the newborn. Finally, I have tried to connect early traumatic experiences (which might be experienced by the fetus during the last few weeks of pregnancy), and the development of a mental and/or psychosomatic pain, which can find a plausible cause in these traumatic experiences.

1. Motor and sensory functions

The seminal work by Michael Corner (1978), which dates back to almost thirty years ago, has demonstrated that even in less developed animals fetal movements begin at a very early stage, and from the very beginning of the development of the CNS, they are characterized by a constant rhythm. These movements represent the mechanism of a developing biological clock whose workings, at least in the human fetus, is extremely complex (De Vries et al., 1985).

From the very early stages of pregnancy, we can register, in the fetus, generalized and partial movements, hiccups, clonic spasms, as well as breathing and swallowing movements, which become very noticeable during weeks 12 and 13 (Joseph, 2000; Piontelli, 2006). These movements belong to those *primary motor patterns* (PMP) that Milani-Comparetti (1981) described 25 years ago, and they coincide with behavioral modules which are genetically defined and which can become functionally significant in relation to fetal development of sensorimotor and other brain functions.

Early fetal movements express a *reflex activity* stimulated by a variety of stimuli (Cohen et al., 1988; Steriade, McCarley, 1990; Cowie et al., 1994; Blessing 1997) and a rhythmic activity of *automatic* origin. Joseph (2000) has demonstrated that the development of the brain mainly concerns the encephalic trunk from the bulb and then progressively upwards, to the pons, the mesencephalon, the hypothalamus, the limbic and striated systems, and finally, to the cerebral cortex. The cerebral trunk contains the neurons which, from a phylogenetic point of view, can be considered most ancient (Vertes 1990; Joseph 1996). It is these neurons which control the various vegetative (essential for fetal survival) and sensorimotor functions. They also participate in (a) the synaptogenic functions of other cerebral structures; (b) the integrative functions which enable the organizations of rest/activity cycles (the *basic rest-activity cycles* which were first described by Kleitman (1967)) and (c) the production of alternate *clusters* which concern, on the one hand generalized and partial movements and, on the other, breathing movements (Piontelli, 2006).

During the *later stages of pregnancy*, the fetal movements and its posture assume more integrated and complex features, and are so specific as to offer some indication of what the baby's behavior will be like that in the future (Piontelli, 1992). These movements might not be simply reflex or automatic movements ascribable to the trunk, but they might involve other prosencephalic structures (which develop only later) and the neocortex itself.

Approximately during the 30th week of pregnancy, the body movements decrease and we can observe some rest periods, which can be ascribed to an increase in the *inhibition* exercised by the cerebral trunk on the motor function. In addition, breathing movements decrease as well when the fetus comes closer to term.

Corresponding to the reduction of the fetal general and breathing movements, is an increase in eye movements. These begin to achieve a certain organization from the 28th–30th weeks, and develop according to a path which seems to run contrary to that followed by the movements of the body, in so far as, while the former increase, the latter decrease. The late appearance of eye movements can be ascribed to the fact that the mesencephalon completes its development rather late. These movements are also important for the fetal integrative functions, the rest/activity cycle (which anticipates restful and active sleep) and finally the baby's REM sleep, which is anticipated by the active phases of fetal sleep.

Fetal *sensoriality* represents an important part of its development. The mother sends the fetus rhythmic and randomized stimuli which are produced by her respiratory, cardiovascular and gastro-enteric systems. Through the maternal 'container', the fetus can be reached even by external stimuli. But the most important stimulus which reaches the fetus through the mother (and which will assume a fundamental importance also for postnatal communication), is her voice, with its *specific quality, tone, volume, and musicality*. Indeed, it is the mother's voice that constitutes an essential relational element which conveys love and emotions. Furthermore, it represents a sort of continuity in the discontinuity created by the fetal passage from the intrauterine to the external environment.

A fundamental aspect of this sensorimotor interaction between mother and fetus is represented by the *regularity and rhythmicity* which characterize fetal *containment functions*. As its response to tactile, kinaesthetic, thermal, auditory, and gustatory stimuli well demonstrate (Koupernick, Arfouilloux 1970) (as well as its sensitivity to pain and light), the fetus begins to be affected by such stimuli from the 20th–24th week of pregnancy.

Later in pregnancy, fetal sensoriality becomes the basis of those episodes characterized by a sensory content, which the fetus can now experience and which participate in the organization of more complex cortical functions. It is precisely from these functions that some proto-representations concerning fetal sensorimotor experiences can develop. Through the somatosensory areas, data reach the amygdala, which can then transmit to them an emotional quality. Emotions are therefore the first experiences which the fetus may have and memorize.

2. Integrative functions

Fetal integrative functions appear in their complete form when the brain stem is almost completely developed, approximately during the 28th week, and when the cerebral cortex is sufficiently developed, so that it can interact with subcortical structures and enable the elaboration of sensory content. This occurs from the 36th to the 38th week of pregnancy, a period during which the brain reacts to various stimuli (in particular the mother's voice) with both reflex movements of the body and the head, and with an increase of the heart rate (Joseph, 2000).

During the 36th week, the tonotopic organization of the cochlea reaches maturity and the fetus is able to discriminate between different frequencies of sounds (also in relation to the mother's voice and her language), assigning them an emotional meaning on the basis of the intense and mutual connections with the amygdala.

This is the moment when the trunk and its reticular structures can constitute the anatomo-functional basis of an *experienced integration* (intégrations experiencielles) which, back in 1954, Alfred Fessard (Fessard, 1954) suggested to be the cause of the formation of a basic consciousness generally identified with awareness. But this is also the moment when the cerebral cortex, which developed also thanks to the synaptogenic stimuli coming from the brain stem, becomes the place where the sensory experiences (for example acoustic and somoesthesic) can enable the fetus to develop a form of *consciousness with sensory content* (Burgess, Tawia 1996), which could then be able to create some *proto-representations*.

These experiences can be stored in the corresponding cortical associative areas, in order to constitute a *first form of memory*. This memory cannot be but *implicit*, due to the maturity of the amygdala and the immaturity of the hippocampus, which is necessary for the late organization of the explicit or declarative memory (Joseph 1996; Siegel 1999). This first form of memory can be the site of an *unconscious proto-function* of the mind, on top of which other sensory, affective, and emotive experiences, characteristic of a baby's life, will be organized in layers. It is in this memory that the prenatal experiences of a traumatic nature, which can determine the baby's mental development after birth, are collected.

During the final stages of pregnancy, between the 36th and the 38th week, heart rate, body and eye movements, metabolic and hemodynamic response to stimuli, can be grouped into episodes which are linked to the fetal phases of rest and activity (Timor-Tritch et al., 1976; Romanini, Rizzo, 1995). These cyclic phases, which are present from the very beginning of pregnancy, turn into states of wakefulness and sleep towards the end of pregnancy, with phases similar to REM (Romanini, Rizzo, 1995; Nijhuis et al., 1982) and phases similar to non-REM comparable to those of adults (Emde, Koenig 1969; Emde, Metcalf, 1970). Various researches on premature infants who were born between the 6th and the 8th month of pregnancy have confirmed the presence of a continuous state of sleep that appeared atypical and that presented similar characteristics to the active one, which could thus be considered a precursor of REM sleep (Petre-Quadens, 1967).

It is possible that the fetus, in a similar way to the newborn, immediately enters the REM phases without going through non-REM ones. This can be explained by referring to the fact that the systems of the thalamocortical synchronization typical of non-REM phases, develop later, and always after birth. This might also be the reason why the baby can enter a REM phase also with its eyes wide open, while it is feeding (*eating REM; sucking REM*) and even when it is crying (*fussing REM*) (Spitz, 1962).

In order to validate the data referring to human fetuses, we can look at the experience of animals such as calves and lambs, whose gestational period is comparable to that of humans. In these cases, as Ruckebush (1972) and Ruckebush et al. (1977) have demonstrated, during the 8th month of pregnancy, periods of wakefulness alternate with periods of resting, active, intermediate or transitional sleep, which, from a qualitative point of view, is similar to that observed in adult ruminants. In these animals, the phases of sleep can occupy 85–90% of gestation time and are dominated by active phases. This demonstrates that the biological desynchronizing mechanisms of sleep similar to REM develop ontogenetically before the synchronizing ones.

It is interesting to observe here that the active phase of sleep, which predicts the baby's REM sleep, can become the biological container of important physiological and psychological hereditary functions. For example, Valatx (1977) and Cespuglio et al. (1975) have demonstrated that during this phase there is an hereditary transmission of physiological characteristics concerning REM sleep, such as its duration, its rhythm, the characteristics of the PGO waves, and the eye movements. In addition, Jouvet (1962) hypothesized that during the REM phase of sleep, recurrent and periodic genetic organizations might take place. The fetal active sleep, which anticipates REM sleep, could therefore represent the ideal biological framework for the transmission of the parents' genetic code, in particular those elements which characterize its early mental experiences not only on a physiological but also on a psychological level. Perhaps, it is precisely this genetic code of which Bion, as well as many of us, think, when talking about the baby's equipment, an apparatus that determines its response to its environment and reality.

3. Relevance of the observations on prenatal life for psychoanalytic theory and clinic

The large quantity of active sleep in the fetus, which anticipates the REM sleep of full-term babies, has led us to think that during this phase significant developmental transformations of the synaptic functions might occur, to which might correspond increasingly developed psychic ones (those functions which will eventually enable the baby to face its primary relationships). At this point, we cannot avoid the issue of when the fetus begins to perceive, memorize and transform into proto-representations, those experiences which are characterized by sensory content.

In my opinion, the maturation of the cerebral cortex is essential in order to allow for the elaboration of sensory information and permit these processes to affect the amygdala, which confers an emotional quality to the sensory experience. Furthermore, this sensory quality will act on the synapses and their plasticity, thereby creating a condition for possible memorization.

Joseph (1996) states that from a very early stage (after 12 weeks), the fetus is capable of complex behavior that entails a very small participation on the part of the prosencephalon and the cerebral cortex while being mediated by the activities of the brain stem. This is confirmed by recent sonographic observations, which demonstrate an integrative function of the brain stem, facilitated by the development of the inhibitory interneurons (Piontelli, 2006).

Subsequently, the cerebral cortex assumes an increasing importance and becomes essential for the sensory experiences of the fetus to be able to produce a proto-representational activity (albeit rudimentary), which places it in the most suitable condition to enter extra-uterine reality. It is this proto-representational function which, in full-term fetuses, facilitates the development of a sense of the Self connected to fetal body functions: a proto-Self, or better, a *neurobiological Self*, which works as a modulator of homeostasis, and which is capable of creating an awareness of its own somatic limits, thereby enabling the fetus to distinguish, at birth, its own Self from 'the other' Self (that is, the Self of others).

Several authors (Piontelli, 2006; Bergeret et al., 2006) now claim that research into prenatal life is extremely important in order to enhance the psychoanalytical theory of the mind. As I will try to demonstrate below, it can also be very helpful in the psychoanalytical clinic.

The "psychological DNA"

Today, the discovery of the implicit memory (Mancia, 2003–2006), which does not need the configurations of the explicit memory in order to attain a form of structure, enables us to suggest that mental life might begin a long way back in ontogenetic time which has its roots in an early and essentially emotive (implicit) memory. We think that this memory might begin with the development of the cerebral cortex (around the 30th week of pregnancy); in particular, we think it might coincide with the development of the amygdala, which develops long before the hippocampus. This memory posits itself within a circuit which, besides the amygdala, involves the basal ganglia, the cerebellum, and the temporo-occipital-parietal cortical areas of the right hemisphere. We know that this hemisphere controls emotions (Gainotti, 2006; Phelps, 2004) and establishes mutual connections with the amygdala. Taking this line of thought further, we can say that the implicit basic memory which stores the first sensory and motor experiences of the fetus could constitute a primitive sketch of an *unconscious function of the mind which does not undergo repression*, and cannot be remembered.

At birth, other relational experiences (the mother's voice, her language and the care she provides for the baby's body), together with the emotions and affections they carry, will be able to organize themselves in layers on top of the basic structures of the implicit memory which was shaped during fetal life, and thus contribute to the formation of an unrepressed *unconscious nucleus of the Self which does not undergo repression*, and which will condition the newborn's primary relationship, its learning processes, and the development of its explicit memory, as well as its affective, emotional and cognitive life.

Using a metaphor borrowed from genetics, we could say that this memory is the subject's "psychological DNA". Its main characteristic is that it developed during the prenatal and perinatal period, which is a pre-symbolic and pre-linguistic period that by definition is incapable of being remembered. This memory will determine the individual's emotions, his/her affections and his/her thoughts during his/her whole life. During analysis, it will manifest itself in dreams and in the transference.

The theoretical-clinical presupposition which we can draw from the above considerations is that structural situations of a psychopathological nature such as psychoses, borderline states and depressive syndromes, have their salient etiology in the earliest (prenatal) traumatic events which involve the infant's development.

The question that contemporary psychoanalysis asks is the following: what is the relationship between the affective and emotional traumas experienced by the fetus and the development of the subject's character and personality, including the psychopathology we can observe in adults? The question is also justified by Freud's work, according to which there is greater continuity between intrauterine life and early infancy than what the trauma of birth might lead us to think.

The clinical experience emphasizes the reality and the importance of early traumas which occurred during the prenatal period. They are often difficult to interpret, and throughout time, they have been (and often still are) met with mistrust, both by patients and analysts themselves, and they are confronted with skepticism by the psychoanalytical community. In these cases, the fetal ability to memorize its early experiences (beginning with the mother's biological rhythms, which act as a container for the fetus itself), are not taken into serious consideration. Similarly, there is a tendency to ignore the fundamentally affective significance of the intonation of the mother's voice, the first source of 'tonal' and musical stimuli outside the self. It is these stimuli which help fetal containment and favor the establishment of an affective and emotional continuity during the passage from the interior of the uterus to the exterior; as such, they stimulate the fetal early fantasies (or proto-fantasies).

The perception of the mother's voice, in fact, involves the constitution of an object which the fetus can endow with affection early enough, through its sense of hearing. The fetus can memorize the affection and the fantasies conveyed by the mother's voice (De Casper, Fifer, 1980) and these can become the first emotional objects stored in the fetal implicit memory, the first one which actually works at the very beginning of life, thanks to the early development of the amygdala (Joseph, 1996; 12, LeDoux, 1996, 2000; Siegel, 1999).

Early memorized prenatal traumas can be reactivated by traumatic situations experienced later in life, to such an extent that they can emerge in transference and dreams. Dreams in particular can confer a form of figurability to those prenatal experiences that cannot be represented. An element which can play a fundamental role in this process, is sensory trans-modality (Stern, 1987), that is, a procedure which enables the fetus to integrate various sensory experiences well before sight develops. The late development of sight prevents the fetus from creating visual representations. We should therefore assume that primary fantasies (or proto-fantasies) have at their root some "neural configuration" created by sensory experience. These fantasies seem to coincide with the 'original ghosts' described by Bergeret (2004), which he defines as a "souvenir non-souvenir", a literary way of talking about an implicit memory whose memory will never be able to surface.

Bergeret et al. (2006) think that projective identification itself originates from traumas experienced during fetal life. They link this traumatism to three fantasies or proto-fantasies: 1) the imaginary and rival baby inside the mother's womb; 2) the father's penis which enters and shakes the mother's womb and, indirectly, the fetus itself; 3) the meconium which fills the mother's womb.

An important aspect entailed by this idea of the French authors, and which we can now link to the discovery of the implicit memory operating from a very early age, concerns the possibility we currently have to extend the Freudian notion of *Nachträglichkeit* (*après coup*, in French). This notion, in fact, implies that the concept of *Nachträglichkeit*, which Freud links exclusively to the repressed content, could in fact be extended to the early and prenatal emotional content, which was stored in the implicit memory and which therefore did not undergo repression.

Furthermore, from Kandel's work we can develop the idea that prenatal stimuli (in a similar fashion to postnatal ones), might be able to act on genes and condition their expression. It is precisely this protein expression which, from an early stage, is able to regulate the development of the synapses and their plasticity, thereby steadily modifying fundamental cerebral circuits. We are now able to put forward the hypothesis that archaic, prenatal (as well as neonatal) experiences of an affective nature leave behind indelible marks which, in a similar way to family secrets, continue to disturb the subject's affective and relational life even during adulthood. In consideration of the extension of the *Nachträglichkeit* concept, we can now create a sort of metaphorical bridge between the present disorder activated by the transference, and the early experiences described above, regarding them as the traumatic causes of the disorder itself.

Mr. B

A brief section of the analysis of Mr. B illustrates the clinical aspects of this theoretical discussion. Mr. B comes under analysis 4 times a week. The therapy was required because of some character difficulties, a sort of physical and mental heaviness, a marked awkwardness when trying to relate to women, incapacity to part company, and his recurrent concern about his sexual potency.

I will describe only a brief phase of this case history, namely the period when my patient began to report a sudden loss of sight from one eye, which specialists diagnosed as an initial and progressive form of retrobulbar optic neuritis. This disorder appeared in a period characterized by insistent self-punishing fantasies in which Mr. B seemed to be the victim of a cruel and irreducible part of himself which threatened him from the inside and which made him aggressive and often violent with people at work and his occasional sexual partners. Mr. B was heavy, adhesive and rigid, also from a physical point of view. My counter-transfer in that period was characterized by a sort of discomfort triggered by his exasperate requests, aimed at the containment of his aggressive and violent parts (which he projected onto me), and the continuous masturbatory moves which he would usually make at the moment of parting company. Furthermore, I felt incapable of helping him and very often I would feel bored because of his repetitiveness, monotony, and heaviness. I thus began to reflect on these counter-transferal feelings and think that they were the answer to his transference, which was very adhesive and defensive in relation to any distance I might try to establish between the two of us. As a consequence of the anxiety he seemed to have felt in a restricted uterine space, Mr. B made me feel enclosed in a restricted mental space. Furthermore he seemed to be resentful for some traumas that I thought he might have experienced during that period of his development. This elaboration of his transference was confirmed a little later, when very significant dreams made their appearance. Neither of us had any difficulty in recognizing that these dreams could be considered symbolic representations of traumatic experiences connected to his fetal life.

In the first of these dreams, Mr. B *is in the garden of a countryside priest (associated with a man who likes women), and he creates for himself a sort of hideout amongst a thorn bush full of thorns. He conceals himself inside the hideout, as if he were a very young child who can look out from within without being seen.* Mr. B associates this dream with the memory of a gamekeeper who used to work on one of his parents' estates, who told him about some dangerous snakes which lived in the woods, and also to some tale about his mother, who was rumored to have played, in her childhood, sexual games in the very wood of Mr. B's hideout.

I suggest that in the analytic garden of a priest/father/analyst who loves women, some voyeuristic fantasies capable of exciting him are activated. I said that his concealing himself inside his hideout creates the image of a fetus that retreats into a womb full of thorns from where he can exercise his voyeurism, but where he feels threatened by a paternal snake/penis which can penetrate inside the mother's vagina and hit his voyeuristic eye.

Mr. B meets my interpretation with silence, and gives the impression that he was emotionally involved, to such an extent that in that precise transference moment he identifies with the child/fetus of the dream, whose suffering eye was threatened.

During the following sitting, he reports another dream: *in a thick bush in his countryside he wants to crouch and withdraw, just like a very small baby. He hides behind the bush but he is very worried that a horse galloping by might hit him on the head with its hoof.* He associates the film *Gandhi*, where the horses appear to stop in front of the crowd, but become very dangerous when they meet an individual, alone, on the ground. He then remembers his countryside, where a man had fallen on the ground and was hit on the head by a horse's hoof. After a short silence, he brings up a fantasy: that of Polyphemus and the cave where Ulysses and his companions blind the giant by piercing his eye with a burning pole.

I am positively impressed by this dream and by his associations. I therefore try to associate it to the previous one, by showing the patient the continuity of his dream work, which again seems to point to Mr. B's identification with a small fetus withdrawing inside a maternal uterus/container, which is very dangerous since the paternal hoof/penis is able to enter rhythmically the interior of the mother's body/garden and hit the fetus on the head. I also tell him that the fantasy about Ulysses, who blinds Polyphemus with a pole, can represent a metaphor of the trauma of a pole/penis which hits and destroys his voyeuristic eye.

I feel that Mr. B is very close and impressed by my hypothesis. He remains silent, as if in a state of intense reflection and emotional involvement.

The following week, Mr. B reports another dream, which I hear as an elaboration and a continuation of the preceding ones, despite its different form. In the dream, *Mr. B with his fiancé is paying a visit to a friend who is seriously ill. He lies down on a bed, which, however, becomes a bath, and he lowers himself into it.* After narrating his dream, he remembers how, as a child, bath time made him fear that he might die. It was always during his bath time that Mr. B, left on his own by his mother, used to have masturbatory fantasies. He also remembers how, as a child, he was always confused with his mother who, in her turn, found it difficult to let him go. He then says that he is afraid his eye disorder might be progressive and lead to blindness and death, and then he concludes by saying: "I feel as if I was in a uterine cavity and I feel pain in my eyes. I've spoken to my mother about this, but she doesn't seem too worried".

I tell him that in his dream, the analyst's couch becomes a lethal bath, full of amniotic liquid/meconium in which, in a similar way to what used to happen during his childhood, he could not be left on his own by his mother/analyst. Indeed, if that were to happen, he would run the risk of dying or of being obsessed by masturbatory fantasies. I also tell him that the fact that he considers his mother not particularly worried, could indicate his faith in the therapeutic and reparatory possibilities of our elaborations during analysis.

The work on these dreams has occupied us, with various alternations, for several months. One day, during a period in which his acting out was much less and the vision of his sore eye seemed definitely improved, Mr. B described *a dream in which he is still in his countryside, but in an entirely remade car. The car-body repairer has reconstructed the body of the car and he feels satisfied. Then he gets on his bike, sets out for a big mound and then enters a big house full of maze-like corridors, from which he gets out in the open air. From the roof, he can see a hilly landscape full of light, which feels very different from the oppressive and deadly atmosphere of the house interior.*

Mr. B associates his dream with the fact that his eyesight has improved, that his worries have decreased and that he is astonished by the fact that during analysis he is able to transform his mental pain into physical agony. We both acknowledge that in the dream the situation has changed, in so far as he is now able to get out of the lethal house, which stands for the intrauterine regressive period. Similarly, his dream makes it clear that he is now able to get out of the nightmare of a deadly confusion with his interior mother, in order to see the light and the vitality of the landscape, as if he was born a second time.

After this dream, Mr. B tells me that the specialists who had been monitoring him throughout this period, told him that his eyesight and the optic disk itself had resumed their normality. They could not explain satisfactorily the regression of this disorder which, in their opinion was probably caused by a temporary vascular disorder.

As analysts, I think we are authorized to put forward the following hypothesis: the dangerous lesion of this patient's eye was a serious psychosomatic experience which became apparent during analysis and which was repaired through a process of mentalization and emotional elaboration, even in the absence of memory, thanks to the work on his transference and his dreams. This has permitted a metaphorical bridge to be built between the actuality of transference (relational heaviness and ocular pain) and the prenatal psychic trauma, and has allowed his unconscious emotional history stored in the implicit memory to be reconstructed.

References

Bergeret J: Les "souvenirs/non-souvenirs". Colloque du Vinatier, Lyon, 27 novembre 2004

Bergeret J, M Soulé et al.: Anthologie du foetus. Abords Pluridisciplinaires. Dunod, Paris 2006

Blessing WW: The lower brainstem and bodily homeostasis. Oxford University Press, New York 1997

Burgess JA, SA Tawia: When did you first begin to feel it? – Locating the beginning of human consciousness. Bioethics 10 (1996) 1–26

Cespuglio R, R Musolino, G Debilly, M Jouvet, JL Valatx: Organisation différente des mouvements oculaires rapides du sommeil paradoxal chez deux souches de souris. Comptes rendus de l'Académie des sciences, Paris 280 (1975) 2681–4

Cohen AH, S Rossignol, S Gillner (eds): Neural control of rhythmic movements in vertebrates. Wiley, New York 1988

Corner MA: Sleep and the beginning of behavior in the animal kingdom. Studies of ultradian motility cycles in early life. Progress in Neurobiology 8 (1978) 279

Cowie RJ, MK Smith, DL Robinson: Subcortical contributions to head movements in Macques. Journal of Neurophysiology 72 (1994) 2665–2885

De Casper AJ, WP Fifer: Of Human Bonding: Newborns Prefer their Mothers' Voices. Science 208 (1980) 1174–6

De Vries JP, GHA Visser, HFR Prechtl: The emergence of fetal behaviour. II. Quantitative aspects. Early Human Development 12 (1985) 99–120

Emde RN, KL Koenig: Neonatal smiling and rapid eye movement states. American Academy of Child Psychiatry 8 (1969) 57–67

Emde RN, DR Metcalf: An electroencephalographic study of behavior and rapid eye movement states in the human newborn. Journal of Nervous and Mental Disease 150 (1970) 376–86

Fessard A: Mechanisms of nervous integration and conscious experience. In: Delafresnaye JF, editor. Brain mechanisms and consciousness. Ch C Thomas, Springfield 1954

Gainotti G: Unconscious Emotional Memories and the Right Hemisphere. In: Mancia M (ed): Psychoanalysis & Neuroscience. Springer, Milano 2006

Joseph R: Fetal Brain Behavior and Cognitive Development. Developmental Review 20 (2000) 81–98

Joseph R: The brainstem, midbrain, DA, 5HT, NE, cranial nerves, and cerebellum. In: Joseph R (ed): Neuropsychiatry, neuropsychology, clinical neuroscience. William and Wilkins, Baltimore 1996

Jouvet M: Recherches sur les structures nerveuses et les mécanismes responsables des différentes phases du sommeil physiologique. Arch Ital Biol 100 (1962) 125–206

Kleitman N: Phylogenetic, ontogenetic and environmental determinants in the evolution of sleep-wakefulness cycles. Res Publ Ass Nerv Ment Dis. 45 (1967) 30–38

Koupernick C, JC Arfouilloux: Neurobiologie et neurologie du développement. In: Gratiot-Alphandery H, R Zazzo (eds): Traité de Psychologie de l'Enfant, 2. PUF, Paris 1970

LeDoux JE: Emotion Circuits in the Brain. Annual Review of Neuroscience 23 (2000) 155–84

LeDoux JE: The Emotional Brain. Simon and Schuster, New York 1996

Mancia M: On the Beginning of Mental Life in the Fetus. International Journal of Psychoanalysis 62 (1981) 351–357

Mancia M: Dream actors in the theatre of memory: their role in the psychoanalytic process. International Journal of Psychoanalysis 84 (2003) 945–952

Mancia M: Implicit memory and early unrepressed unconscious: Their role in the therapeutic process (How the neurosciences can contribute to psychoanalysis). International Journal of Psychoanalysis 87 (2006) 83–103

Mancia M: Implicit memory and unrepressed unconscious: how they surface in the transference and in the dream. In: Mancia M (ed): Psychoanalysis & Neuroscience. Springer, Milano 2006

Mancia M. Sentire le parole. Archivi sonori della memoria implicita e musicalità del transfert. Bollati Boringhieri, Torino 2004

Mancia M: Feeling the Words. Resonant Archives of the Implicit Memory and Musicality of the Transference. Hove, Routledge (in press)

Milani-Comparetti A: The Neurophysiologic and Clinical Implications of Studies on Fetal Motor Behavior. Seminars in Perinatology 5 (1981) 183–89

Nijhuis JG, HFR Prechtl, CB Martin, RSGM Bots: Are there behavioral states in the human fetus? Early Human Development 6 (1982) 177–95

Petre-Quadens O: Ontogenesis of paradoxical sleep in the human newborn. Journal of the Neurological Sciences 4 (1967) 153–7

Phelps EA. Human emotion and memory: interactions of the amygdala and hippocampal complex. Current Opinion in Neurobiology 14 (2004) 198–202

Piontelli A: From Foetus to Child. An Observational and Psychoanalytic Study. Tavistock-Routledge, London 1992

Piontelli A: On the Onset of Human Fetal Behavior. In: Mancia M (ed): Psychoanalysis & Neuroscience. Springer, Milano 2006

Romanini C, G Rizzo: Fetal behaviour in normal and compromised fetuses. An overview. Early Human Development 43 (1995) 117–31

Ruckebush Y, M Gaujoux, B Eghbali: Sleep cycle and kinesis in the fetal lamb. Electroencephalography and Clinical Neurophysiology 42 (1977) 226–37

Ruckebush Y: Development of sleep and wakefulness in the fetal lamb. Electroencephalography and Clinical Neurophysiology 32 (1972) 119–28

Siegel SJ: The developing mind: Toward a neurobiology of interpersonal experience. Guilford, New York 1999

Spitz RA: Il primo anno di vita del bambino. Giunti Barbera, Firenze 1962

Steriade M, W McCarley: Brainstem control of wakefulness and sleep. Plenum, New York 1990

Stern D: Il mondo interpersonale del bambino. Bollati Boringhieri, Torino 1987

Timor-Tritch et al.: Classification of Human Fetal Movement. Am J Obstet Gynaecol 6 (1976) 70–7

Valatx JL: Sleep behaviour: genetic regulation. In: Development du cerveau chez le fetus et le jeune enfant: aspect normaux et pathologiques. Josiah Macy Foundation, New York 1977

Vertes RP: Fundamentals of brainstem anatomy: A behavioral perspective. In: Klemm WR, RP Vertes (eds): Brainstem mechanisms of behavior. Wiley, New York 1990

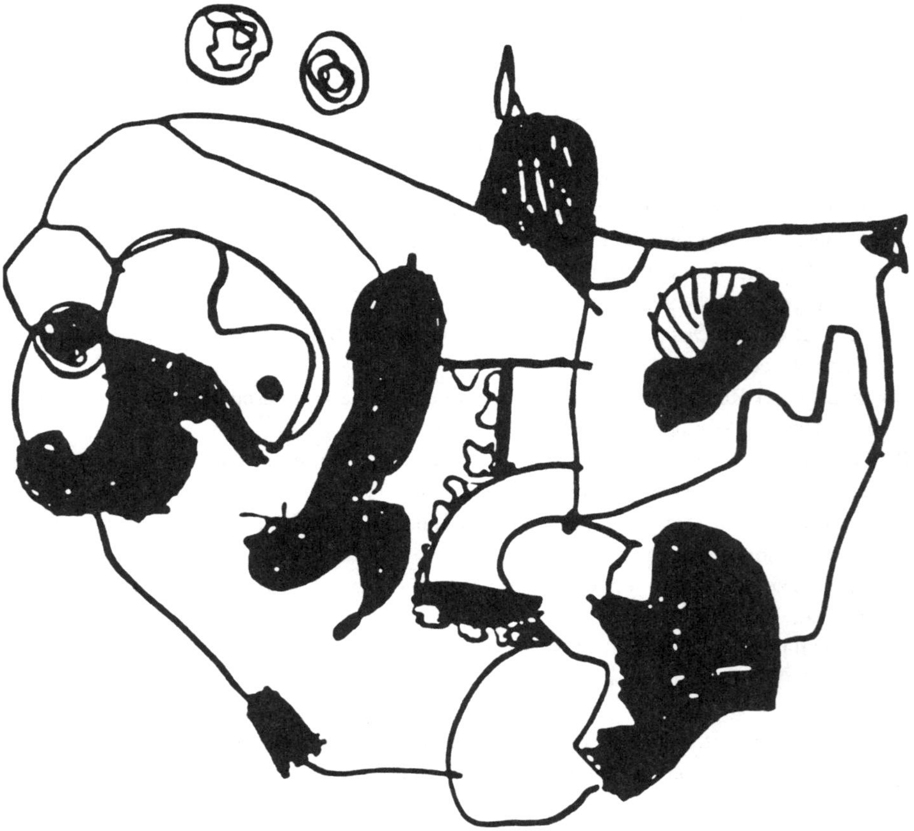

(Elisa, 3 yrs. 5 mos.)
I've never seen a baby being born and I don't know who decides about being born: the mother or the babies. I don't know, I don't remember anything.

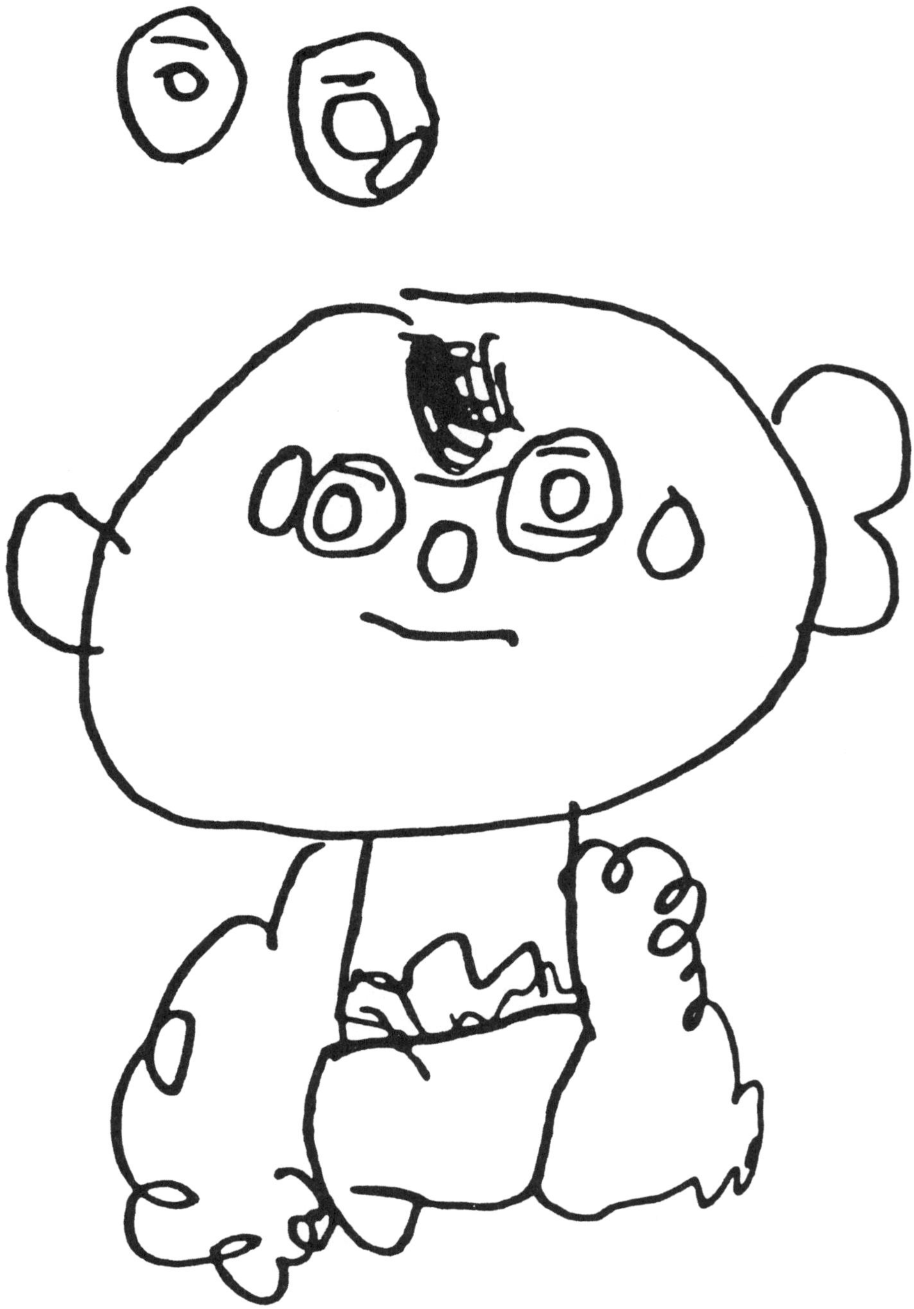

(Serena, 3 yrs. 7 mos.)
When I was born, everybody wanted to touch me – I was so pretty!
I had beautiful eyes, a beautiful mouth, and beautiful hands.

14. Death and birth

François Ansermet; European School of Psychoanalysis
University of Lausanne, Switzerland

Can one be dead before being born? Along with the problems posed by death in the uterus, the question of death before birth presents itself today in a new light following progress in prenatal diagnosis and predictive medicine, with their influence on the therapeutic interruption of pregnancy.

Death during birth is a classic clinical question, whether it is infant or maternal mortality (which will not be discussed in this paper), both of which constitute major public health indicators. This does not stop the possible occurrence of death during birth from touching an (impossible to think of) link between the end and the beginning of life, sometimes even before birth.

Death and birth unite two inexpressible situations. Death is inexpressible, as Freud put it: "The fact is that our own death is inexpressible . . . no one, at the end of the day, believes in his own death or, what recalls it: in the subconscious, each of us is persuaded of his own immortality." The same is true for our origins (Ansermet, 1999). The questions of infants, assiduous researchers, who often leave their immediate circle at a loss are proof of this. Like the little boy who, after his parents had given all the possible explanations they could following the death of his grandfather, continued to interrogate them: "Yes, but once I am dead and buried, when my body is in the ground and my soul in heaven, where will *I* be?" Or that other child, whose pregnant mother had just tried to divulge the secret of her maternity, of the role of the father and mother, of love, of the little seed. . ., who replied in a more than pertinent fashion: "Yes, I understand, but before being in your tummy, where was I?" (Balmary, 1993).

Death at birth – and with good reason, above all, death before birth – adds to the inexpressibility of death and of our origins. And the advances in prenatal medicine as well as the resulting change in the status of the fetus, absolutely force us to face the inexpressibility of life and death before birth.

Change in the status of the fetus

Ultrasound, with the image it unveils, gives a concrete existence to the fetus as a child to be (Muller-Nix et al., 2000) and sometimes, during the exam, one no longer speaks of the fetus but of the baby. An echographer told me that she only used the term fetus when some malformation was unequivocally revealed. Even if it is via a virtual image, the infant takes on a material existence through ultrasound. The dimensions of its body, already resembling those of a baby, become real. Its position is singled out, it is seen in movement: sucking, yawning, stretching, rubbing its feet against each other; in short, it takes on the solid reality of a child being already there. In case of dath, it is the loss of a dear being which one has felt living inside, whose ultrasound image had already been put into the photo album.

Predictive prenatal medicine thus faces impossible choices in the case of detecting pathology. Sometimes a certainty is determined, but more often a probability, a risk, is quantified. It is something which does not stop subjects from living the probability as a certainty. Every decision of therapeutic interruption of pregnancy implies a 'sending into crisis' of the inevitable ambivalence which accompanies bringing a child into the world, most often kept inhibited.

The birth of ambivalence

Every birth is, in fact, accompanied by certain ambivalence: in the face of bearing the child, the transformation from two as a couple to three as a family, the transition of the woman to a mother and the man to a father. This ambivalence can be accompanied by all sorts of indirect manifestations, through a tendency to depression, unexpected behaviour, or attacks of anxiety. The sexual origin is difficult to imagine, more often than not supressed. The standpoint of the change in generations leaves one perplexed. Sometimes, it is put on the child, unconsciously. Killing of a child (Leclaire, 1975) is a major spectre, central, and strongly inhibited, which gambles with all births. Nonetheless, our culture participates in staging it in all its multiple forms, among mythical tales and tragedies, from the exposition of Oedipus to the massacre of the innocents, without considering the cases of those tales for children where this theme is often prevalent. This is also what epidemiological findings reveal: according to Marks (1996), the risk of murdering a child less than one year old is way above that of an older child, and the risk of infanticide by one of the parents is considered as maximal during the first 24–48 hours of life.

The loss of a child during pregnancy is particularly difficult to consider. It plunges those who live it into torments of perplexity: Have they lost a child? Have they lost a part of themselves? Were they already parents? Has nothing happened? Did the lost fetus already have the status of a child or is it only about a narcissistic loss? This question is central and difficult. As Freud shows (1969) it is absolutely necessary to recognize the true nature of the parents' tender love towards the child, which is that of a resuscitation of their own narcissism. A desire for immortality, which reality destroys, comes to find refuge in the child. Thus the loss of a child before birth is also a narcissistic loss for those who are expecting it.

The trauma of perinatal death

The loss of a child before or at the moment of birth is a relatively frequent situation, extremely painful, still too misunderstood, and insufficiently considered. This is true for the time it occurs and for its long-term effects: too often it is downgraded to a simple fact in anamnesis during psychotherapy, ignoring its effects on the couple and the siblings already born or yet to come, who can find themselves confused in their role as surrogate children.

The reaction to a perinatal death is to be understood from clinical studies on trauma. Everything suddenly stops (Soubieux et al., 2005). All that was being invested swings in a brutal fashion, in an instant plunging into a state of stupor, of loss of equilibrium, of confusion. A reality which one was not prepared for – even if reduced to the essence of an ambivalent conflict – forces its way in. The unthinkable and the unspeakable break into a scene which was prepared to welcome life. The pain remains the sole link with the missing baby even if never born. That pain, paradoxically, protects from torment; it is a defence mechanism to be respected, the only outcome in the acute moment of the child's disappearance. As Pontalis (1977) wrote: "There where there is the pain, it's the absent, lost object which is present". This psychological pain, acute, is paired with a physical pain. The integrity of the body, ready for the child, is struck, amputated of a part of itself, everything about it being marked by an absence which is only too real, lived directly by the mother and indirectly by the father.

But death is not only the loss of a vested object. As Lacan shows (2004), the loss of the object unveils in the same stroke the imminence of an inexpressible object, which came to mask the vested object. Hence the anxiety is not linked to the little baby but to the arising of an inassimilable reality, up to that point veiled, covered over by the vested object. It follows that it is not only to the depression, but to the anxiety – and to the trauma – that we must refer in order to understand the effect of a loss. Death, the effects it provokes, would thus to be understood departing first from an excess of 'presence', the too great proximity of an inexpressible object, forward to the vested objects of reality, and nearer to an impulsive reality. The death of the child realizes a baring of the impulse which underlies the investment, hence the traumatic break-in and the torment implicated by perinatal death.

It is possible to suspect this from the text by Kafka (1980) – *Le souci du père de famille* – which features a strange object, named Obradek, a bobbin of twisted thread, which tumbles down the stairs, crosses the house from top to bottom. Obradek provokes the perplexity of those who are there. They know that this object precedes them and will survive them. It is perhaps thus that the pain linked to mourning is to be understood. Anxiety, a signal of confrontation with reality, arises. We are dealing with a state of distress, *Hilflosigkeit* (Freud, 1926). Lacan (1986), regarding the state of distress, distinguishes *abwarten* from

Erwartung. *Erwartung* means the expectation of something. What designates *abwarten* is a widespread expectation, without any anticipation of that which is expected. This is what is involved in the loss which death implies: "the experience of absolute disarray, at which level anxiety is already a protection, no longer *abwarten* but *Erwartung*" (Lacan, 1986). A state of distress, in series with any intervention from others, occurs. It is this type of distress which the confrontation with extreme situations provokes, like that of perinatal death, where death coincides with birth, projecting into a distress "where man in this relationship with himself which is his own death [. . .] expects help from no one" (Lacan, 1986).

Perinatal mourning

That traumatic introduction of a real impulse is not the property of perinatal death, even if it manifests it more than any other loss. It is a lesson which that particular situation brings in a general manner to the clinical treatment of mourning and coping with death in psychotherapy.

Mourning and the travail of mourning are first of all dealing with that 'break-in', which returns to the person himself, as suggested by Freud (1976) when he examined the relationship between mourning and melancholy and the phenomenon of the pain of mourning. The travail of mourning consists in re-involving in a different way the investment bared by the loss of the object. In fact, it is about travail of substitution. As Lacan (1986) indicated, mourning consumes "for a second time the loss of the loved object provoked by the accident of destiny". This travail is complex. It consists of restoring the link with the veritable object of the relationship, the object masked by that which was lost. Every object is, effectively, in a certain manner a replacement of a fundamental object, the cause of a desire. The cause of a desire is distinct from its end. The object which causes the desire is other than that which is targeted in the investment (Miller, 2005). As we have seen, it is that dichotomy which the clinical treatment of mourning brutally reveals, more so when it is about a child that one was unable to know, provoking the resurgence of the object in question in the desire, on the side of the potentially vested object.

In the case of perinatal death, the fetus is a particular object, an object which is not yet a non-object, vested with potentiality, in the narcissistic valences. It is thus that the fetus can be seen as a melancholic object. Along with the fetus, a part of oneself is lost. It coincides with the shadow of the object and it is the "I" which is amputated. It is the immortality of the "I" that is involved in the narcissistic expectation of the parents which is checkmated. It is thus an instantaneous melancholic process, based on a narcissistic identification with the object, which will be transformed into mourning later on. It is about a non-accomplishment of a part of oneself, lost before knowing it, a strange situation where something still unidentified is brutally lost, leading to a fundamental distress.

The process of mourning and burial

Such a particular situation obliges us to reflect on the process of mourning in association with the proposed 'process of burial'. The process of mourning in the situation of a perinatal death is primarily a means of dealing with the involved distress. In front of the inexpressibility of death, an action imposes itself. This action deals with the anxiety. Sometimes this is the initiation of a transition to action in the subject him/herself, an eruption that can go as far as self-destruction and suicide. This is why it is necessary to pass through an action which must be accepted by others, to allow a symbolic and imaginary dealing with the reality which the loss implicated by death reveals, even more so when it occurs before birth.

The travail of mourning thus involves what could be called travail of burial: burial of the inexpressible object, so that this can be symbolically re-involved and pre-sanctified as absent. The travail of burial thus consists in restoring the link to that inexpressible object which covers the vested object. It is about burying the inexpressible object, so that a substitute can be created. At the end, one does not mourn, one only replaces, substitutes, finds objects suitable to mask the inexpressible object, existing already before the object. Life obliges us to pass from substitute to substitute, to deal with the inexpressible reality of death, which passes through new objects, but also by a process of idealization, of eternalization of what has been lost. That idealization being perhaps alienating, as mentioned regarding the child called 'surrogate', where the dead child can hurt those who follow him. This phenomenon can be still more significant when death took place before birth. Nothing comes to form a barrier against idealization. Hence the importance of burial, of the travail of burial, should be acknowledged.

The role of the teams of obstetricians and liaison psychiatrists is, in this framework, fundamental. The legal norms are today still changing, blurred, not always known, and in any case behind the advances in medicine. Is it necessary to show the dead fetus, to present it in a non-frightening fashion, after preparation, in a coffin, to show some photos, give it a first name, declare it to the registry office, and to organize some funeral rites. Usually it is after 22 weeks of gestation (and birth weight greater than 500 g) that these practices are introduced, different if the fetus is born alive or stillborn. But it is, above all, necessary to take into account the subjectivity of the parents, of their manner of living the prenatal death. At certain times, it is only after a while that they wish to see the photos taken, give a first name, go back to visit the burial place (certain cemeteries reserve specific places), and make it their own.

Impossible questions

Following the progress in perinatal medicine we are in a domain of full-blown perturbation. We really do not know when to secure the beginning of life. Is it already at the stage of the unfertilized egg, the zygote, the embryo, the fetus, starting at how many weeks? How and when to define the beginning of life?

This question presents itself even more readily now, when perinatal medicine is flooded by situations where the limit between death and birth is blurred. The extreme situations may be related to medically assisted procreation, where the status of neither dead nor alive defines cryopreserved embryos. With this type of biotechnology, there is also the limit that can be lost, through the possible use of the zygote or embryo in therapeutic cloning.

We could refer in this regard to the possibilities opened by pre-implantation diagnosis, with the selection of a zygote unaffected by a known genetic disease for implantation. When the choice is made, an unthinkable status is given to the eliminated zygotes. Even more so, the selection of zygotes by this sort of technique may end as a baby conceived to allow the treatment of a child already born but affected by an incurable disease and requiring specific transplants. Similarly, numerical reduction of embryos from a multiple pregnancy following assisted procreation, confronts the gynecologists with questions related to the extent of their action and the choices they make.

The list of new questions presented by prenatal medicine is almost infinite. The examples mentioned are here to show the cardinal points involved in the fact of being able to intervene in reality without anticipating the subjective results which may ensue. The point to which these new technologies take those who undergo them, just as those who apply them, are surely the frontiers of what is today considered thinkable. The result is puzzling for everyone and often taken well beyond the particular context in which these questions were originally asked.

References

Ansermet F: Clinique de l'origine, l'Enfant entre la médicine et la psychanalyse. (Psyché), Payot, Lausanne 1999

Balmary M: La divine origine. Dieu n'a pas créé l'homme. Grasset, Paris 1993

Freud S: Pour introduire le narcissisme (1914). In: La vie sexuelle. PUF, Paris 1969

Freud S: Considérations actuelles sur la guerre et sur la mort. In: Essais de psychanalyse. Petite bibliothèque Payot, Paris 2001

Freud S: Inhibition, symptôme et angoisse (1926). PUF, Paris 1973

Freud S: Deuil et mélancolie. In: Métapsychologie. Gallimard, Paris 1976

Kafka F: Œuvres complètes, t. II. Gallimard, La Pléiade, Paris 1980

Lacan J: L'angoisse (1962–63), Le Séminaire, Livre X. Seuil, Paris 2004

Lacan J: L'éthique de la psychanalyse (1959–1960), Le Séminaire, Livre VII. Seuil, Paris 1986

Leclaire S: On tue un enfant. Seuil, Paris 1975
Marks MN: Characteristics and causes of infanticide in Britain. International Review of Psychiatry 8 (1996) 99–106
Muller-Nix C, C Maillard, P Holfeld, F Ansermet: Le statut de la mort prénatale: conséquences cliniques et thérapeutiques. Psychothérapies 20 (2) (2000) 87–93
Pontalis, JB: Entre le rêve et la douleur. Gallimard, Paris 1977
Miller, J-A: Introduction à la lecture du Séminaire l'Angoisse de Jacques LACAN. La Cause Freudienne 59 (2005) 67–103
Soubieux M-J, M Soule: La psychiatrie fœtale. PUF, Paris 2005

15. Prenatal counseling

Johannes Bitzer; Department for Social Medicine, Clinic of Obstetrics, University of Basel, Switzerland

Introduction

For the largest part of human evolution, embryonic and fetal existence has been hidden away in the maternal womb and the development of the child to be has been the subject of fantasies, hopes, fears, and rituals. With the implementation of ultrasound, cytogenetics, and molecular biology, medicine has intruded into this formerly "dark continent" and replaced speculation with knowledge, subjective images with objective ones, hopes and fears with new diagnostic categories. For the first time in human history, physicians shared their insight of intrauterine life with the future mothers and thus become companions during the process of embryonic and fetal development. What was formerly a possible internal dialogue between the pregnant woman and her child to be is now a "trilogue" between mother, physician and embryo/fetus. The new technologies have thus opened up new opportunities for knowledge which carry with them new options and possible decisions for pregnant women. It is the task of the obstetrician to help women to achieve the best use of this new knowledge and to support them in their decision-making according to their personal values and objectives. This means that obstetricians have to take up the role and responsibility of counsellors.

Specific characteristics of prenatal counselling

Obstetricians take responsibility for two persons – the mother and the embryo/fetus. The embryo/fetus cannot be included into the communication. The mother acts as a representative. The obstetrician communicates with the mother and indirectly with the fetus through the relationship between the pregnant woman and her child to be. This relationship is very variable and dependent on socio-cultural and personal values and emotions. Thus, prenatal medicine means communication regarding the values of the pregnant woman and her relationship with the child to be.

Prenatal investigations provide information about the developing child. The developing child is overloaded with intensive emotions and is reflected in the imagination of the mother to be. Prenatal investigations have an influence on this subjective image and may modify it profoundly. Prenatal medicine, therefore, means communication about patients' imagination and emotion.

Some investigations are based on rather complicated statistical theorems and methods, which provide complex information about probabilities. Some of this information may be ambivalent, cause insecurity and anxiety, and disturb the prenatal mother-child relationship. Prenatal medicine means, therefore, communication regarding numbers and statistics in a way which is understandable for pregnant women.

Such diagnostic procedures as CVS and amniocentesis entail a low, but real, loss rate for the pregnancy. "Therapeutic" interventions comprise, among other things, also the termination of pregnancy, which involves fetocide. Both situations are unique in medicine. Prenatal medicine is, therefore, also communication about ethics.

Communicative and counselling skills for obstetricians

Obstetricians in this specific setting should learn to apply basic principles of patient-centred communication with elements of non-directive counselling, patient education, and shared decision-making.

These elements are integrated into a process which comprises the following "steps":

- Clarification of the patient's objectives and the obstetrician's mandate
- Providing individualized information and education about prenatal investigations
- Shared decision-making regarding tests and investigations
- Breaking (bad, ambivalent) news
- Caring for patients with an affected child

Clarification of the patient's objectives and the obstetrician's mandate

This can be done by:

a) Directly asking the patient:
   E.g.; *Do you already have some information about pregnancy care and prenatal medicine? What are your wishes and concerns regarding pregnancy care…?*

b) Giving basic information about routine care and then asking about individual concerns:
   E.g.: *In our routine care we see pregnant women every four weeks. The check-ups serve two purposes, one to assure that you are in good health and are not suffering from any related complications, and the other is to follow and assure the normal development of the child. Do you have special concerns or wishes…?*

Providing individualized information and education about prenatal investigations:

The general principles are:
- Structure the information
- Give information in small units
- Announce important pieces of information
- Encourage questions
- Ensure feedback

This can be memorized as the Elicit-Provide-Elicit Sequence
- Elicit: patients pre-existing knowledge and questions
- Provide: give information in small units and short sentences.
- Elicit: patient's understanding and evaluation of the information. "What does this information mean to you".

The complexity of the information about tests and prenatal investigations demands a clear explanation of the statistical information and the use of images and visualizations. Important issues in talking about numbers are:
- Give absolute frequencies and not relative probabilities
- Use always the same basic unit
- Explain not only risks but also chances
- Put the numbers into an everyday perspective

A basic instrument is the table with 1000 small symbolic figures, which serves as a basic unit. With this table the different probabilities can be visualized. E.g.: *The probability of the child having Down syndrome is 4 in 1000. (4 red figures are drawn on the 1000 figure table). This means at the same time that in 996 pregnancies of women of your age children do not have this disease.*

Shared decision-making

Shared decision-making means that physicians provide information based on evidence and that patients contribute their own values and evaluation. The process is essentially the same for prenatal tests and prenatal investigations like CVS or amniocentesis. The obstetrician accompanies the patient through the following steps:

Clarify values: When talking about the tests and investigations, we have to discuss very personal issues concerning the possibility of a handicapped child and the question of abortion. What are your feelings and attitudes about this?

Give information based on evidence in an understandable way

E.g. (Prenatal test) *Nuchal translucency and blood tests can provide a number, which describes the probability of a disease of the child. The advantage of this test is that it has no risk either for you or the child. The possible disadvantage lies in the fact that you only get a number and not a diagnosis. This means that, on the one hand, even with a low risk you cannot be absolutely sure that there is no chromosomal abnormality, and on the other, a high risk may raise a lot of unnecessary anxiety, because the child may well have no chromosomal abnormality at all.*

E.g. (CVS, Amniocentesis) *You have received a test which says that the probability of disease is 1: 100 and you consider now whether to undergo a CVS or amniocentesis. The advantage is that in 99 out of 100 investigations you get a clear diagnosis; the disadvantage is that the procedure entails the risk of a miscarriage in 1 out of 100 investigations. This means that a healthy child may be lost.*

Let patients evaluate the information and anticipate the effect

E.g. (Prenatal test): *Imagine you get a number which says that the probability of disease is 10 in 1000 or 1 in 100. What are your thoughts about this, do you think this number would give you a sense of security or would it raise anxiety? Do you think it would help you to make further decisions*?

E.g. (CVS, amniocentesis): *How do you personally value this information? What are your personal priorities and concerns? Would you need more information? Would it be important to discuss this with your partner? Would it be important that you have some more time?*

Breaking (bad, ambivalent news)

The general guidelines are:

- Preparation for the encounter. (Quiet setting, enough time, is all the information needed available? Does the patient come alone or accompanied by a family member or friend? What is the emotional situation of the physician?
- Introduction (Using a more personal issue for getting closer to the patient, a brief summary of the previous events and the objective of the consultation)
- Announcement (Unfortunately I have to give you bad news)
- Statement (Give the diagnosis in simple words)
- Waiting for the individual reaction of the patient (Stunned, paralyzed, confused, shocked, desperate, crying, stoic, denying, etc.)
- Response to the reaction (emotion handling, reflecting, summarizing)

- Encouraging questions and giving further information in small pieces
- Give hope (there is always something that can be done)
- Structure the near future (what is the patient going to do next, define next steps to be taken and give appointments)

It is especially important that obstetricians are aware that the diagnosis refers to the patient's child and that here again the relationship of the mother to the child is a very important determinant in coping with the diagnosis. The pregnant woman is confronted with the destruction of her hope to have a healthy child and she is at the same time aware that she has to take an active decision with respect to her child's existence, which eventually may lead to actively separating herself from her child. Thus the communication about the affected child has to be very empathic and respectful.

Caring for the women with an affected child

Pregnant women with an affected child are in a potentially traumatic situation. They have to decide about their own future, the future of their family's and their child's destiny. This goes frequently beyond the coping capacity of the women concerned.

Obstetricians should be able to accompany these women during their decision-making with respect to carrying on with the pregnancy or opting for abortion. It is important that women can discuss with their physicians the possible consequences of their decisions, that they are provided information about possible difficulties and consequences, and that possible ways of help are anticipated.

After the decision has been made, her strength and her ability to cope with anxiety, depression, guilt, anger, aggression, and many other possible emotional responses are required. The obstetrician's task is not to escape these negative emotions but to withstand them and stay with the patient. Together, they may look at different ways of coping and explore the possibilities of help.

Whatever the decision, it is important to acknowledge that the woman and her partner have to go through a process of mourning, which may be extremely difficult because of the fact that this experience is extreme and cannot be shared with others. Women who decide on an abortion do not often allow themselves to mourn, because they feel that they have actively contributed to the death of their child. For them it is even more important that they find empathic obstetricians, midwifes, and nurses who will accept their decision and encourage them that they also have the right to be sad and express their feelings.

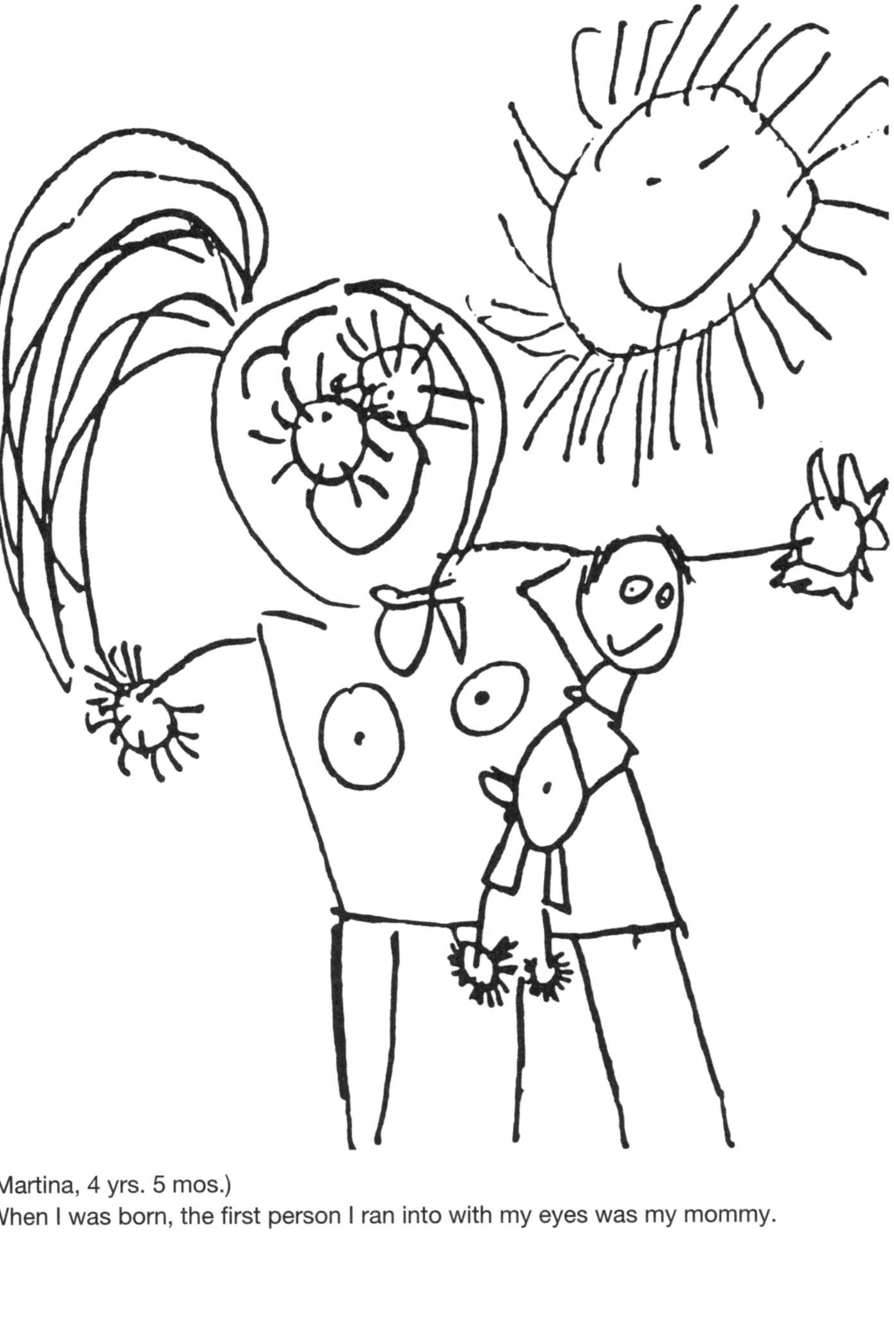

(Martina, 4 yrs. 5 mos.)
When I was born, the first person I ran into with my eyes was my mommy.

16. 'Care' in neonatal intensive therapy

Fabrizio Ferrari; Department of Neonatology, University of Modena and Reggio Emilia, Italy
Marisa Pugliese; Department of Mother and Child, Psychosocial Division, University Hospital, Modena, Italy
Natascia Bertoncelli; Mother and Child Department, Neonatal Division, University Hospital, Modena, Italy
Maria Federica Roversi; Mother and Child Department, Neonatal Division, University Hospital, Modena, Italy

During the last 25–30 years there has been a significant increase in the number of survivors amongst very-low-birth weight (VLBW, <1500 g) and extremely-low-birth-weight (ELBW, <1000 g) infants. Preterm delivery represents a risk for the infant's neuropsychological, emotive, and affective-relational development. Indeed, in spite of significant developments in neonatology, especially for VLBW and ELBW infants, we can observe important sequels in their neurological and neuropsychological development. Case histories show that 10–15% of VLBW infants develop neuro-motor deficiencies during early years. Behavioural difficulties, neuropsychological deficiencies, attention deficit, and learning difficulties also characterize a very high proportion (50–60%) of VLBW and ELBW infants (Marlow et al., 2005).

Recent studies have demonstrated that in addition to the neuropsychiatric consequence caused by cerebral injuries, there are some developmental disorders which can be attributed to neonatal intensive care unit (NICU). Current NICU conditions, in particular those of incubators, are in fact very far from ideal and cannot ensure the infant's psychophysical and affective-relational well-being. The newborn suddenly finds itself alone, projected in an environment full of lights, noises and odours, where it is disturbed from 82 to 132 times a day, whilst it is constantly kept away from its mother. Contrary to what was once believed, recent ample scientific evidence has demonstrated that infants are able to perceive, decode and memorize painful stimuli in all their intensity. The infant, even when born preterm, is capable of memorizing painful experiences: the limbic and diencephalic structures which are required by memory processes are well-developed and perfectly functioning (Johnston et al., 1996; Goubet et al., 2001; Mitchell, Boss, 2002; Puchalski, Hummel, 2002; Grunau, 2002).

The newborn in NICU undergoes many painful procedures: heel punctures, endotracheal intubations, mechanical ventilation, endotracheal aspiration, blood samplings from the arteries, insertion of central vein catheters, lumbar punctures, etc. Even procedures such as application or removal of electrodes or plasters, the positioning of the nasal-gastric tube, diaper change or bathing time can become a source of pain. In particular, some authors have demonstrated that even during a banal procedure such as diaper change, premature infants express a longer and more intense pain than full term babies, for whom pain is shorter and less intense (Morelius et al., 2006).

And yet, it is not just the pain produced by these stimuli we are concerned with. The infant, in fact, also experiences the anxiety and the pain provoked by its affective and relational isolation. It has recently been demonstrated that, in man, physical pain activates the same cerebral areas activated by psychological pain (Eisenberger et al., 2003). Furthermore, in many animals, the distress caused by separation anxiety from the mother shares the same sub-cortical circuits and the same neurotransmitters of physical pain (Panksepp, 2003). It was indeed possible to demonstrate that early separation from the mother is associated with a distinct increase in the percentage of apoptosis (approximately twice as much as in controls). Furthermore, studies carried out on cerebral plasticity, have emphasised that separation from the mother determines an over-expression of the NMDA receptors compared to the controls and that, even during separation, the ability to hear the mother's voice enables the newborn animal to reduce the over-expression of such receptors. Generally speaking, the exposure to an environment which could be defined as hostile from a sensorial and social perspective seems to cause a reduction in the proliferation of the progenitor cells of the cortical layers, and to lead to a reduction in the cortical and sub-cortical synaptogenesis (at the level of the hippocampus). We have by now gained enough scientific evidence to demonstrate that pain must be always considered as a somatopsychic entity, even more so during the neonatal period when the distinction between the body and the mind is even more artificial and unfounded. Hence, pain has an essential role in stress: pain is always stressful. The treatment of pain, then, must be a fundamental part of 'care', understood as the attention to, and consideration for, the primary needs of the infant and its family.

Recurring stress and pain determine the division of the infant's circadian rhythms, apnoeas, abrupt variations of the oxygen tension, sudden fluctuations of the infant's cerebral flux, hormonal unbalances which activate the hypothalamic-hypophyseal-adrenal axis, with the risk of causing micro-damages to the central nervous system. Experimental studies suggest that the exposure to recurring pain provokes an increased activity of the NMDA amino acids which determine an excitatory-toxic damage in the developing neurons. In addition, during the neonatal period, multiple metabolic traumas and/or the lack of social stimulation increase the physiologic apoptosis through the loss of activity of specific receptors (Bhutta, Anand, 2002). Some studies on volumetric magnetic resonance, which were carried out on premature infants without documented cerebral injuries at birth, have demonstrated that these subjects exhibited a reduced cerebral volume when compared to controls: this aspect is probably connected to the occurrence of cumulative 'micro-damages', mainly linked to small, but repetitive, variations of the infant's homoeostasis. 'Because it lacks inhibitory control', the infant's brain therefore appears 'far too sensitive, at the mercy of sensory information, and unable to limit the incoming flux' (Als, 1992; Als et al., 2004).

Besides the developmental risk caused by NICU, there are other factors which may be held responsible for the behavioural and neuropsychological difficulties experienced by premature children. These factors might be identified within the family environment and the relational aspects which determine the infant-parent relationship.

Preterm delivery, in fact, triggers an emotional crisis in parents, mainly as a result of their concern for the infant's survival, the frequent invasive treatment in the NICU, and the protracted separation from the child. In particular, many parents of ELBW infants manifest stress-induced post-traumatic reactions lasting even many years after the premature birth (Holditch-Davis et al., 2003; Miles, Holditch-Davis, 1997; Jotzo, Poets, 2005). The alteration of the parents' role, caused by the separation from their child and the sense of impotence they experience in the NICU, can affect the way they perceive their child (Allen et al., 2004; Miles, Holditch-Davis, 1997). These factors must therefore be taken into account during infant's care, as they might have damaging repercussions on the global development of the child.

The pain and the stress experienced by the preterm infant in the NICU, are not always easily recognized by their caregivers (doctors, nurses, physiotherapists). The recognition of signs of pain and stress, stress management, pain reduction, and the contact with the mother, as well as the family's involvement in the care of their child, thus become first priorities in the care of premature infants (Als, 1992).

The models which can meet the premature child's neurodevelopmental needs, and can therefore favour its psychophysical and affective-relational well being, rely on the Individualized Developmental Care, in particular the NIDCAP method (Neonatal Individualized Developmental Care Assessment Program), which focuses on the preterm infant's individuality and the respect for both the infant and its family (Als, 1999; Als et al., 1984; Als et al., 2003; Als et al., 2004; Als et al., 2005). According to this model, the course of the organism's development is necessarily determined by the constant interaction between the systems of which it consists (neuro-vegetative, motor, behavioural, self-regulatory, and interactive) and the environment in which they are placed or in other words, the NICU environment. The premature child's behaviour, in a totally inadequate and occasionally hostile environment, presents a wide range of signals which should guide the caregiver's attitude towards this fragile and lonely child. The attempts premature infants make to clear their discomfort are many: change of skin color, breathing irregularity, abrupt movements, sudden extensions of legs and arms, and crying. Furthermore, the infant also adopts many strategies to overcome destabilizing and stressful situations such as a simple diaper change or the application of electrodes. Amongst these strategies we can observe the movement of the child's hands towards its mouth or its face, its clinging onto the tube or sheet, and its sucking motion. Through the careful observation of preterm infants' behaviour in their incubator, the NIDCAP method enables caregivers to recognize immediately the signs of stress caused by routine care procedures and the signs of self-adjustment that infants might put into practice themselves.

The observation of the preterm infant's behaviour is so important because it enables deductions from the child's behaviour about the neurodevelopmental needs of that particular child at that particular stage of life. In practical terms, the acknowledgment of such needs determines the possibility of creating individualized and developmental care programs for premature infants, which should be closely connected to their development and clinical conditions. Premature infants thus become active partners in the care process in which they are involved. Through the communication of stress or well-being, the premature infant guides the caregiver and 'suggests' the most adequate way to follow its development.

The application of the NIDCAP method in a NICU necessarily entails a change in the type of assistance which is offered to the premature child: an assistance based not only on 'treating', but also on 'caring'. We thus move towards an assistance which we would like to define as 'relationship-oriented' (that is, assistance based on relationship and communication), thereby leaving behind more classic views based on the mere completion of duties, that is, 'task-oriented' views of assistance. The realization of this task requires, in the first place, a multidisciplinary approach which involves the participation and the involvement of the whole NICU staff: doctors, nurses, physiotherapists, psychologists, as well as auxiliary and technical personnel.

Various studies demonstrate that the adoption of the NIDCAP method in neonatal intensive care produces positive short and long term results. In the short run, this method reduces the number of days of mechanic ventilation and the need for oxygen, it favors early oral feeding, increases ponderal growth, reduces the incidence of intra-ventricular hemorrhage and broncodysplasia, reduces the days of hospitalization, enhances the staff's ability to evaluate the premature child's state, increases the family's involvement and their support, improves the NICU environment for the infant and its family, and not the least important – improves the work environment for the staff. In the long run, the application of the NIDCAP method improves the neuropsychological outcomes (Kleberg et al., 2000; Kleberg et al., 2002; Als et al., 2004; Westrup et al., 2004).

The NICU of the University Hospital of Modena has developed an individualized program of care which focuses on the child and its family. This also requires a preliminary meeting between doctors and psychologists which, whenever possible, takes place before delivery. The psychological support for parents helps them cope with the emotional trauma and with the process of becoming parents, and is an essential part of the care model adopted by the staff of the NICU.

References

Allen EC, JC Manuel, C Legault, MJ Naughton, C Pivor, TM O'Shea: Perception of child vulnerability among mothers of former premature infants. Pediatrics 113 (2) (2004) 267–73

Als H: Individualized, family-focused developmental care for very low-birthweight preterm infant in the NICU. Developmental Psychology 6 (1992) 341–388

Als H: Reading the premature infant. In: Goldson E (ed): Developmental Intervention in the Neonatal Intensive Care Nursery. Oxford University Press, New York 1999

Als H, G Lawhon, FH Duffy, GB McAnulty, R Gibes-Grossman, JG Blickman: Individualized Developmental Care for the Very Low-Birth-Weight Preterm Infant. Journal American Medical Association 272 (1994) 853–858

Als H et al.: A three-center, randomized, controlled trial of individualized developmental care for very low birth weight preterm infants: medical, neurodevelopmental, parenting and caregiving effects. Journal of developmental and behavioral pediatrics 24 (6) (2003) 399–408

Als H, FH Duffy, GB McAnulty, MJ Rivkin, S Vajapeyam, RV Mulkern, SK Warfield, PS Huppi, SC Butler, N Conneman, C Fischer, EC Eichenwald: Early experience alters brain function and structure. Pediatrics 113 (4) (2004) 846–57

Als H, S Butler, S Kosta, G McAnulty: The Assessment of Preterm Infants' Behavior (APIB): furthering the understanding and measurement of neurodevelopmental competence in preterm and full-term infants. Mental Retardation and Developmental Disabilities Research Reviews 11 (1) (2005) 94–102

Bhutta AT, KJ Anand: Vulnerability of the developing brain. Neuronal mechanisms. Clinics in perinatology 29 (2002) 357–72

Eisenberger NI et al.: Does Rejection Hurt? An fMRI Study of Social Exclusion. Science 302 (2003) 290–293

Goubet N et al.: Learning about pain in Preterm Newborns. Journal of developmental and behavioral pediatrics 22 (6) (2001) 418–424

Grunau R: Early pain in preterm infants. A model of long-term effects. Clinics in perinatology 29 (3) (2002) 373–94

Holditch-Davis D, TR Bartlett, AL Blickman, MS Miles: Posttraumatic stress symptoms in mothers of premature infants. Journal of Obstetric, Gynecologic, and Neonatal Nursing Online 32 (2) (2003) 161–71

Johnston CC et al.: Experience in a neonatal intensive care unit affects pain response. Pediatrics 98 (5) (1996) 925–30

Jotzo M, CF Poets: Helping parents cope with the trauma of premature birth: an evaluation of a trauma-preventive psychological intervention. Pediatrics 115 (4) (2005) 915–9

Kleberg A, B Westrup, K Stjernqvist: Developmental outcome, child behaviour and mother-children interaction at 3 years of age following Newborn Individualized Developmental Care Assessment Program (NIDCAP). Early Human Development 60 (2000) 123–135

Kleberg A, B Westrup, K Stjernqvist, H Lagercrantz: Indications of improved cognitive development at one year of age among infants born very prematurely who received care based on the Newborn Individualized Developmental Care Assessment Program (NIDCAP). Early Human Development 68 (2002) 83–91

Marlow N, D Wolke, MA Bracewell, M Samara: Neurologic and developmental disability at six years of age after extremely preterm birth. New England Journal of Medicine 352 (1) (2005) 9–19

Miles MS, D Holditch-Davis: Parenting the prematurely born child: pathways of influence. Seminars in Perinatology 21 (3) (1997) 254–66

Mitchell A, BJ Boss: Adverse effects of pain on the nervous systems of newborns and young children: a review of the literature. Journal of neuroscience nursing 34 (5) (2002) 228–36

Morelius E, L Hellstrom-Westas, C Carlé, E Norman, N Nelson: Is a nappy change stressful to neonates? Early Human Development (2006) Article in press

Panksepp J: Feeling the pain of social loss. Science 302 (2003) 237–23

Puchalski M, P Hummel: The reality of neonatal pain. Advances in neonatal care 25 (5) (2002) 233–44

Westrup B, B Bohm, H Lagercrantz, K Stjernqvist: Preschool outcome in children born very prematurely and cared for according to the Newborn Individualized Developmental Care Assessment Program (NIDCAP). Acta Pediatr 93 (2004) 498–507

17. Neurological development assessment of the newborn

Romana Negri; Infantile Neuropsychiatry, University of Milan, Italy

Meeting with Martha Harris was fundamental to my research on the assessment of newborns and babies, especially in their first six to twelve months. She supervised three of my Infant Observation cases carried out according to the Ester Bick method. Along with the meeting with Martha Harris, the Bobath course in London that I attended in 1979 and 1981 about neurological development in babies and the treatment of infantile cerebral palsy proved very informative.

In the case of a newborn infant, there is still a period in which its motor behaviour reveals significant phylogenetic residues; there is a marked latency from the time of birth to the maturity of appropriate neuronal and functional adaptation to the extrauterine environment. This usually takes place only after two to three months. At this stage, the baby has not mastered many abilities and is most definitely unable to cope with fundamental requirements of the extrauterine environment. This phenomenon is not as significant in other primates and seems to point to the higher significance of the role of the mother in the human development and growth.

For this reason, physical contact with the mother in terms of sensorial, tactile, kinaesthetic, olfactory, acoustic, and visual stimuli cannot be considered as merely the most suitable method to facilitate the integration and the development of motor action, but plays another significant role in a wider context for the perception and understanding of emotional communication which underlies the development of thought and symbolization, and therefore the self-integration of the baby.

The Bobaths consider the neurological and motor-sensory development of the baby from the ontogenetic point of view and their theories regarding the first period of a baby's life are much in line with Esther Bick and Melanie Klein's theories regarding mental processes. Bick speaks of a typical non-integration in the newborn period where the mother's care is seen as vital to the development of the baby. At the same time, (from a motor-sensory perspective) the Bobaths highlight a rather unstable situation which can be observed when the newborn is lying on its back and in an asymmetric position. The torso does not fulfill its role as central component and axial part as it should from 4 months onwards. In fact, only from this time does the baby maintain a symmetrical posture when placed on its back and is capable of holding objects with two hands, looking at them and taking them to its mouth. Such abilities are connected to the central part and axis, and superior abilities therefore assume the function of "psycho-motorial antennae" so necessary for the development of the baby and the acquisition of knowledge. After the fifth month, abilities include exploring the axial part, abdomen, and reaching for the shoulder of the opposite side of its body, etc.

It is known that from the fourth month, the baby's mental capacities are at the stage where, according to Klein, it individualizes, can live completely as an entity and prepare itself to face the "depressive position".

These demonstrative acquisitions of complete integration between mental processes and neurological development of the baby have allowed me to fully understand how impossible it is to separate physical, somatic, and mental components of the newborn.

From a neurological interpretation of "soft signs" to a psychopathological interpretation

There has been justifiable emphasis on the importance of the early detection of the premature symptoms of cerebral suffering in the newborn infant from neonatal and neurological points of view. The earlier the treatment is administered (even though it does not serve to repair the damaged central nervous system), the more the functional damage caused by the lesion can be reduced, ensuring the best possible development of the baby (Bobath, 1967; Bobath, Bobath, 1980; Negri, 1982, 1983a; Touwen, 1989). With this aim, a series of symptoms can be taken into account in the context of pediatric neurology allowing, in many cases, the formation of real symptoms-tables (Tables 1 and 2; Touwen, 1989). However, a strictly neurological interpretation of results is not completely predictive in terms of diagnosis, as clearly stated by Touwen when he points out that in a study of 161 newborns displaying some of these symptoms, a mere 10% turned out to be suffering from infantile cerebral palsy. This leads the author to believe that "not all the premature signs exist in cases of infantile cerebral palsy and that the same signs can lead to different prognoses. Thus, the presence of a certain symptom does not necessarily indicate a neurological disorder". Amiel-Tison and Dube (1985) identified correlations between "transitory anomalies" and Touwen's "soft signs" and learning difficulties at school-age.

It is clear that in many of the described symptoms (and I refer in particular to hyper-excitability, apathy syndrome, transitory dystonia, irritability, hyperactivity, tremulousness, various types of crying, sleep disorders, etc.), the interpretation would be inadequate if the importance of mental functions (which are active not only from birth but also in utero) was not taken into consideration – as confirmed in the psychoanalytical (Corominas, 1993; Delassus, 2001; Freud, 1925; Gaddini, 1981) and neuro-physiological (Dreyfus-Brisac, 1968, 1970; Jouvet, 1962, 1978; Mancia, 1980, 2004) fields, and more recently in the field of ultrasound research (Devries et al., 1982; Prechtl, 1984; Tajani, Ianniruberto, 1990; Negri, 1997, 2004).

The recognition of mental functions renders the pediatric environment even more difficult to interpret, because as I have previously mentioned, for reasons of a biological nature it is difficult to differentiate between somatic and psychological functions at such an early age. "The newborn feels with its own body and uses it to express itself" (Negri, 1983b). The newborn, therefore, uses all activity and physical potential at its disposal to express deep and extremely intense emotions. It is important to recognize the newborn's tendency to experiment with corporeal sensations when it comes to different types of emotions such as joy, suffering, well-being, unease, and illness. This is why neurologists speak of extreme variability in muscle tone which, in a newborn baby, is indicative of the postural situation.

However, in the case of a newborn at risk of psychopathology or infantile cerebral palsy, there is lack of variability and postural flexibility and the infant is seen to be extremely distressed which, in turn, incites defensive mechanisms characterized by stereotypy and hinders the consensual integration of the sensual organs. The infant at risk of psychopathology has, for the most part, spent the first period of its life in an incubator or by its nature appears rather disinclined towards integration. The infant who develops infantile cerebral palsy, often experiences a state of distress preceding the appearance of the neurobiological disorder, which causes suffering in the nervous system (which we can understand by considering how neurological maturation developes a containing function for primitive anxieties). The baby is left extremely traumatized after hospitalization due to isolation in the incubator or intervention techniques that are too invasive.

The infant at risk is therefore capable of demonstrating pathological characteristics through its mental activities at this very early stage of mental development. On the basis of my experience I have been in a position to draw up a "table of alarm symptoms" which indicates psychopathological risk (Table 1; Negri, 1998). The alarm symptoms can also be present in a healthy infant, albeit to a rather limited degree. In the case of the infant at risk, however, the symptoms are abundant. In addition, while the healthy infant may present some symptoms temporarily, the symptoms present in the infant at risk become a dominant character and can be seen in aspects of its personality which are repetitively expressed (Negri, 1998).

Loss of variability is often the first, or one of the first symptoms to manifest itself among recognizable signs of a disorder, e.g. an increase in stereotypy, decrease in adaptability and "coping", the ability to integrate adequately or "cope" with one's environment. "The concept of variability, as opposed to stereotypy, is very useful as a means of distinguishing between normal and deviant functioning in the early stage of brain disorder" (Touwen, 1989).

The "alarm symptoms" are thus so dominantly expressed that they hinder the consensual integration of the sensual organs or sensoriality of the infant. Sensorial components are vital to integration and need to develop so that they can strike a harmonious balance, aiding the cohesion of the relationship between the newborn and its mother, who at the early stages of development, is equipped to satisfy the newborn's needs.

Assessment

The neuropsychological assessment takes place when the pretern infant is in the minimum treatment ward, when it is near term and hospital discharge is imminent. In the hospitalization phases, neurological maturation and any possible central nervous system (CNS) damage can be assessed while the infant is already in its incubator. The clinical findings are compared with morphological symptoms and the functional activities of the CNS detected during instrumental examinations carried out during the hospital stay.

Neuropsychological assessments of pre-term infants, and more generally of newborns, are based on observation, an approach which is in keeping with recommendations from the major European and American schools (Cioni, Prechtl, 1988; Ferrari et al., 2000; Korner et al., 1987, 1990; Milani, Comparetti, 1982a, b; Prechtl, 1984; Touwen, 1990). The above authors attribute much importance to the quality and variability of movement, to the aims of spontaneous motility – that which Milani Comparetti refers to as the newborn's "propositive abilities". Even in the course of strictly neurological training (Cioni, Ferrari, Milani Comparetti, Prechtl, Touwen and others), the emphasis has been foremost on the value of observation as a means of examination, and in my opinion, this has been notably influenced by ultrasound research on fetal motility.

The significance of ultrasound observations has greatly reduced the importance of somewhat dated reflexology techniques which played a predominant role in the assessment of newborns until the onset of ultrasound (Saint-Anne Dargassies, 1972, 1974; Thomas, 1966; Peiper, 1961). Neuropsychological assessment of the baby prior to discharge from the hospital takes place in the presence of parents and nurses who have been with it throughout the hospital stay. In my opinion, this intervention is an important moment, catalyzing all activities previously developed in the ward. I attribute a therapeutic importance to the assessment highlighting the most positive features and characteristics of the baby to the parents also including any positive behavioral aspects that I, the nurses and the parents themselves would have observed while the infant was in the incubator (Negri, 1998, 2003). I underline the importance of holding the infant, looking him in the eyes and speaking to him in order to give a name to the distress experienced during the hospital period, in terms of the illness, loneliness, and traumatizing medical procedures. At this stage, therefore, I explain the possible reason why the infant might in the future be afraid to be undressed, to have its feet touched, or its head (the so-called "hat phobia"). During the examination, I clarify the reasons – in psychogenic terms – behind the baby's possible tremulousness, irritability or hypertonia. In these circumstances I also explain the importance of follow-up meetings after discharge from the hospital. Where there is serious neurological risk, it is advisable to arrange for a rehabilitation program at a very early stage and important that the parents meet with the physiotherapist prior to discharge, who will later be working with the infant.

The examination of the infant

In keeping with Brazelton, Korner, and Tronick in the area of neurological development assessment, I wish to emphasize the state of consciousness of the baby. The baby's responses to stimuli greatly depend on its level of consciousness and any interpretation of the responses needs to take this very much into account. Its ability to maintain control of reactions to internal and environmental stimuli is a highly important mechanism and reflects its potential capacity for self-control (Brazelton, 1973, 1984, 1995). Throughout the assessment it is important to note any changes in state, lability, and direction with regard to responses to internal and external stimuli. The criterion for determining state is based on studies carried out by Wolff (1966), Brazelton (1973, 1984, 1995), Aylward (1981), and Korner (1988). Once homeostasis has been achieved, the way in which the infant organizes or controls various states at around the forty-second week, is paramount from a prognostic point of view as far as the mental development of the pre-term newborn is concerned.

The states of the baby can be considered well under control as soon as it remains in a well-defined state for significant periods of time and with a smooth, gradual transition from one state to another. Sudden changes are identifiable from the vulnerability of the baby, which can be detected from its motor and postural behavior, and also this vulnerability affects its emotional stability (Wolff, 1966; Brazelton, 1973, 1984, 1995; Korner et al., 1988; Tronick, 1989). In agreement with Brazelton (1973, 1984, 1995), I reiterate the state of consciousness as being one of the most important elements to be taken into account in the neuropsychological assessment of the infant.

With the development of my neurological examination, I refer to important authors in the field such as Amiel-Tison and Grenier (1980), Brazelton (1973, 1984, 1995), Dubowitz V. and Dubowitz L. (1981), Ferrari F. (1984), Grisoni Colli (1968), Le Metayer (1989), Korner (1987, 1990), Milani Comparetti and Gidoni (1976), Paine (1960); Paine et al., (1964), Peiper (1961), Prechtl and Beintema (1964), Dargassies (1972, 1974), Thomas and Autgaerden (1966), Volpe (1987). I maintain that familiarity with the research carried out by the above authors is fundamental in identifying the potential of the neurological development of infants and detecting any deviance. In this context, my proposal of the infant assessment scheme is firmly based on experience.

As I have already highlighted, it is important to consider the state of the baby while being examined, taking care that the infant is as calm as possible and touching it carefully and gently to favor the best performance. Most importantly, the infant should not be crying, it should be awake and ready to participate. Minimum interference in the manipulation of the infant should be aimed for, allowing a better assessment of tone and spontaneous motility.

At the outset, I observe the baby in its mother's arms and I explore its functions and relational attitudes with the parents. It is important to observe how the parent (usually the mother) holds the baby and how it, in turn, feeling comforted, uses its organs of perception and performs movements to relate to the environment ("free motility", according to Amiel-Tison and Grenier, 1980). Subsequently, I ask the mother to lay the baby, still dressed, on the examination bed. I observe its reactions to my voice and I try to make eye contact, all while keeping my face about 50 cm from the baby. After evaluating the reaction and the attention the baby pays to my looking at him and the words I speak, I ask the mother to assume a similar role while I observe and assess the baby's responses once more.

At this point, I ask the mother to undress the infant and I move away from the examination bed. This procedure constitutes an important part of the assessment, as the mother that is left alone can create a sense of intimacy and begin to relate to the infant – while undressing the infant she speaks to and handles her baby inspiring emotions such as safety, confidence, fear and hesitation, and I can observe how she does this. At the same time it is also possible to observe the infant's reactions. It is particularly important to detect the reappearance of rhythmical vocal communication which characterizes the baby-mother relationship which has already begun within the uterus (this was recently discussed by Trevarthen, 2006). The experience reoccurs after birth when it is possible to observe how maternal verbal communication gets interrupted, rhythmically leaving spaces for pauses which can be filled by the baby as it utters its first phonemes. The recognition of this experience becomes extremely important and very beneficial from a prognostic point of view. In the case of the newborn at risk of psychopathology it cannot be identified as the baby very quickly develops stereotypy of sounds which cancel out the possibility of detecting and observing this melodic exchange. Another reason why the experience may not work could be due to the mother's inability to stabilize this familiar rhythm if she is extremely distressed or suffering from depression.

Once the baby has been undressed I observe it on its back and assess its spontaneous motility, tone, and its deep-tendon reflexes. I then elicit the use of traditional reflexology techniques, testing the Moro reflex (by gently tugging the little sheet on which the baby is lying), the cardinal points, symmetrical and asymmetrical tone reflexes, and hands and feet grasp. Then, placing two fingers in the baby's fists so it grasps tightly, I use a traction maneuver to bring it gently to a sitting position and assess the reactions of the head, trunk and lower and upper limbs. Subsequently, I hold up the baby by supporting it under the armpits with the soles of its feet touching the surface on the examination table. I assess the Thomas static straightening reflexes, the automatic step and the placing reaction. At this stage I gently assess the tone of the trunk with the "suspension in the left and right lateral positions" maneuver (Peiper, 1961) while the baby is still being held up.

Finally, I place the baby in the prone position and note its reactions and posture. The assessment format is very similar to those proposed by French researchers (Thomas, Autgaerden, 1966; Saint-Anne Dargassies, 1972, 1974) and those to which the Bobaths refer in their proposed rehabilitation program for child cerebral palsy.

As I have already pointed out, the baby needs to be handled extremely gently so as not to interfere with spontaneous tone or motility. It is for this reason that while testing the deep-tendon reflexes I place my finger between the baby's joint and percussion hammer. I take great care not to produce any nociceptive stimulus (instead this can be assessed during hospitalization with regard to perfusions, injections, and taking blood samples etc.), but I note the ability of the baby to control itself and remain calm on its back after it has been undressed and submitted to unsettling stimuli such as the Moro reflex and symmetric and asymmetric tone reflexes. If the baby is unable to console itself alone, I intervene by first stabilizing eye contact and then speaking to it. If this is not sufficient, I place a hand on its chest or ultimately I take the baby in my arms and whisper some words softly in its ear. For the most part my intervention works, but in cases where it does not, I then ask the mother to take the baby in her arms. I maintain that it is beneficial from a prognostic point of view that the baby is comforted in the arms of its mother. This is also demonstrated in the ability of the baby to recognize its mother through the senses – in particular the olfactory and auditory senses which are already active by the fourth month of prenatal life. Brazelton (1973, 1984, 1995) particularly highlights the importance of "consolability" as an item on his NBAS scale and suggests increasingly complex means of intervention to achieve this issue.

My assessment does not include the following items from Brazelton's NBAS:

- Response to light with closed eyelids
- Rattle (as auditory stimulus)
- Bell
- The gentle pin-prick
- Ankle clonus
- The Babinski response
- Passive movements with upper limbs
- Passive movements with lower limbs
- Crawling response
- The glabella response
- Cot sheet over face

In my opinion reflex tests such as gentle pinpricks, ankle clonus, the crawling reflex and covering the face with a cot sheet can have a distressing effect on the newborn.

The risk of excessive attraction with regard to sensorial stimuli

I do not subject the baby to stimuli with luminous or sonorous objects, I prefer to observe the spontaneous attention the baby pays to objects and people, and more generally that which surrounds the baby in the environment. On the other hand, all these babies in their first period of life are subjected to specific oculistic and audiometric examinations. It can actually happen that newborns who are fragile by nature, very preterm infants, or those suffering from cerebral pathology who had to undergo a long period of hospitalization, demonstrate excessive interest in objects or sensorial stimuli.

This attraction may interfere with the process of attachment (Robson, 1970) and lead to refusal in relations with the mother, parents and people in general, whereby the infant increasingly excludes itself from relationships. It has also been noted that these mothers have been traumatized by the experience of premature birth or by their baby's pathological state and are quite distressed. A distressed mother is not seen as such by her baby, but rather as a person concerned about herself, rejecting others, and hostile to comprehension and the relationship to her child. Such emotions are picked up by the baby who is highly vulnerable, thus leading to a sense of isolation in the baby.

In this context there is the risk of a baby developing a series of primitive defensive mechanism that are used to try and "protect" itself from experiencing emotions (regarded as intolerable) connected with establishing relationships, particularly with the mother. This may lead the newborn to favor autosensory behavior, manifesting itself in the form of stereotypy experiences with sound and movements (for example the repetitive protrusion of the tongue from the mouth) which offer the baby some sort of gratification on the sensorial level and "cancels out" any emotional strain which it finds intolerable and disturbing and hinders the baby from stabilizing an adequate relationship with its environment.

The same significance is attributed to the "obstinacy" often displayed by infants when they seek sensorial perceptions derived from the objects to which they are attracted because of their color, brightness, or their sound, which are often shown to the baby for calming or stimulating its interest.

There is also the risk that the mothers of these babies feel ancious to have their child recover the developmental stages as soon as possible and tend to stimulate them with the objects that they witnessed being used during the course of neurological or specialist examination or things that have been suggested by the physiotherapist caring for the baby after being discharged from the hospital.

This may have a detrimental effect on relations, empathetic emotional contact, and confidence with adults.

Relational difficulties other than heightened auto-sensorial behavior are mainly expressed through what I have called "alarm symptoms" (Robson, 1967; Table 1). In my assessment, therefore, I refer once again to Brazelton's NBAS scale and believe it is extremely important to assess the "cuddliness" of the baby, which Brazelton defines as the newborn's ability to snuggle into a position and relax in the limited space of someone else's arms, i.e. from the chest to the shoulder of the person carrying out the examination. The infant's readiness to accept and enjoy the dependency and protection on offer from the adult is, in my opinion, positive from a prognostic point of view. The relational attitudes of the baby are even more developed if the baby tries to grasp onto the clothing of the examiner, lays its open hand on the examiner's chest and maintains eye contact with him/her.

Table 1

Alarm symptoms
Avoiding eye-contact
Spying
Pretending to be asleep
No smiling
No crying
Forced rigidity
Lack of "cuddliness"
Abnormal responses to sounds and voices
Stereotypic sound and movement, repetitive index attitudes, etc.
Lack of rhythmical vocal communication in the mother-baby relationship
Excessive or strange movements of tongue in mouth, lip movements
Tremulousness (especially in the first two months)
Hiccups (especially in the first two months)
Restlessness
Postural anomalies
Postural retardation
Psychosomatic manifestations
Fear of being undressed
Other fears
Eating disorders (frequently annorexia)
Major changes in biological rhythms – often in the form of sleep disorders, irritability

In this way it is possible to get a thorough impression of the baby – not only the expression of biological satisfaction but at the same time the start of mental activity. By looking into the eyes of the examiner, the baby expresses a desire to see and to have contact with the source of its sense of well-being. With this test I conclude my assessment of the child.

In follow-up meetings, I do not follow a predetermined program, but prefer to fix appointments on the basis of what was discovered in my first assessment with regard to the extent of neurological deficit in the baby and its psychopathological condition. Naturally the extent of prematurity and possible damage to the central nervous system (assessed from tests which the baby underwent during hospitalization) are taken into account. The date of subsequent meetings is decided upon in conjunction with the parents.

In research on the consolability of babies, Brazelton (1973, 1984, 1995) suggests that the examiner use interventions of increasing complexity. At the beginning he just speaks to the baby, then he/she tries placing a hand on its abdomen. After this he tries to gather the baby's arms together on its median line, and failing this he takes the baby in his arms, snuggles it close and rocks it until he gives it its model. Brazelton scores the reactions differently depending on the maneuver needed to finally console the infant. He takes into account pre- and perinatal factors regarding the baby's performance under the various items in his assessment. In my estimation, however, the difference in the emotional stability of the full-term newborn, admitted to hospital for a minor disorder, and that of a seriously pre-term newborn is not sufficiently emphasized.

References

Amiel-Tison C, A Grenier: Neurological Evaluation of the Newborn and the Infant. Masson, New York 1980

Amiel-Tison C, R Dube: Signification des anomalies neuro-motrices transitoires. Correlations avec les difficultés de l'àge scolaire. Annales de Pediatrie 32 (1) (1985) 55–61

Aylward GP: The Developmental Course of Behavioural States in Preterm Infants: A Descriptive Study. Child Development 52 (1981) 564–568

Bick E: Notes on Infant Observation in Psychoanalytic Training. International Journal of Psycho-Analysis 45 (1964) 558–566

Bobath B: The Very Early Treatment of Cerebral Palsy. Developmental Medicine and Child Neurology 9 (4) (1980) 373–390

Bobath B, K Bobath: Student's Papers. Bobath Centre, London 1980

Brazelton TB: Neonatal Behavioral Assessment Scale. Spastics and Heinemann, London 1973

Brazelton TB: Neonatal Behavioral Assessment Scale. Spastics, London 1984

Brazelton TB, JK Nugent: La scala di valutazione del comportamento del neonato. Masson, Milano 1997

Cioni G, HFR Prechtl: Development of Posture and Motility in Preterm Infants. In: Euler C v, H Forssberg, H Lagercrantz (eds): Neurobiology of Early Infant Behaviour. Stockton Press, New York 1988

Corominas J: Psicopatologia i desenvolupament arcaics. Assaig Psicoanalitic 1993

De Vries JIP, GHA Visser, HFR Prechtl: The Emergence of Fetal Behaviour, I. Qualitative Aspects. Early Human Development 7 (1982) 301–322

Delassus JM: Le génie du foetus. Dunod, Paris 2001

Dreyfus-Brisac C: Sleep Ontogenesis in Early Human Prematurity from 24 to 27 weeks of Conceptional Age. Developmental Psychobiology 1 (1968) 162–169

Dreyfus-Brisac C: Ontogenesis of Sleep in Human Prematures after 32 weeks of Conceptional Age. Developmental Psychobiology 3 (1970) 91–97

Dubowitz L, V Dubowitz: The Neurological Assessment of the Preterm and Full-term Newborn Clinics in Developmental Medicine 79 (1981)

Ferrari F: L'osservazione comportamentale del neonato sano e malato: la scala di Brazelton. In: Bertolini M (ed): Atti del Congresso "La nascita psicologica e le sue premesse neurobiologiche". IES Mercury, Roma 1984

Ferrari F, N Bertoncelli, MF Roversi, S Cattani, C Gallo, G Gargano, M Pugliese, A Ranzi, MP Guerra, GB Cavazzuti: Posture, postural behaviour and spontaneous movement in low-risk preterm infants from birth to 3–4 months post-term age. Ebta Conference Verona (Italy) 6–9 sept. Book of proceedings 2000

Freud S: Inhibitions, Symptoms and Anxiety. S.E. (1925) 20

Gaddini: La vita psichica del feto. In: Zilli P, A Ianniruberto, FA Catizone: (a cura di) Motricità e vita psichica del feto. CIC, Roma 1982

Grisoni Colli A: L'assistenza educativa al bambino con paralisi cerebrale netta prima Infanzia. Capelli, Bologna 1984

Hafez ESE: The Behaviour of Domestic Animals. Ballière Tindal & Cassel, London 1975

Harris M: Thinking about Infants and Young Children. Clunie Press, Perthshire 1975

Harris M: Some Notes on Maternal Containment. In: "Good Enough Mothering". Collected Papers of Martha Harris and Esther Bick. Clunie Press, Perthshire 1987

Jouvet M: Recherches sur les structures nerveuses et les mécanismes responsables des differentés phases du sommeil physiologique. Archives italiennes de biologie 100 (1) (1962) 125–206

Jouvet M: Does a Genetic Programming of the Brain Occur during Paradoxical Sleep? In: Buser PA, A Rougeul-Buser (eds): Cerebral Correlates of Conscious Experience. North-Holland, Amsterdam 1978

Klein M: Some Theoretical Conclusions Regarding the Emotional Life of the Infant. In: Klein M, P Heimann, S Isaacs, J Riviere: Developments in Psycho-Analysis. Hogarth Press, London 1952

Korner AF, HC Kraemer, EP Reade, T Forrest, S Dimiceli, VA Thom: A Methodological Approach to Developing an Assessment Procedure for Testing the Neuro-behavioral Maturity of Preterm Infants. Child Development 58 (1987) 1478–1487

Korner AF, HC Kraemer, EP Reade, T Forrest, S Dimiceli, VA Thom: A Methodological Approach to Developing an Assessment Procedure for Testing the Neuro-behavioral Maturity of Preterm Infants. Child Development 58 (1987) 1478–1487

Korner AF, BV Brown, EP Reade, DK Stevenson, SA Fernbach, VA Thom: State Behavior of Preterm Infants as a Function of Development. Individual and Sex Differences. Infant Behavior and Development 11 (1988) 111–124

Korner AF, WA Thom: Neurobehavioral Assessment of the Preterm Infant. Psychological Corporation, New York 1990

Le Métayer M: Bilan neuromoteur (cérébromoteur) du jeune enfant. Encyclopédie Mèdico Chirurgicale, 26028 (B20-4) Paris (1989)

Lester BM, CFZ Boukydis, M McGrath, M Censullo, L Zahr, TB Brazelton: Behavioral and Psychophysiologic Assessment of the Preterm Infant. Clinics in Perinatotogy 17 (1) (1990) 155–171

Mancia M: Vita prenatale e organizzazione della mente. In: Ammaniti M: (a cura di) La nascita del sé. Laterza, Roma-Bari 1989

Mancia M: "Fonctions intégratives du cerveau et origine du psychisme foetal" Relazione al Colloque International: Anthropologie du foetus Lyon 26-27 Novembre 2004. In Press

Milani Comparetti A: Protagonismo e identità dell'essere umano nel processo ontogenetico. In: Ianniruberto A, FA Catizone, L Bovicelli: (a cura di) Giornate italo-americane di ultrasonografia. Monduzzi, Bologna 1982

Milani Comparetti A: Semelotica neuroevolutlva. Prospettive in Pediatria 48 (10–12) (1982) 305–314

Milani Comparetti A, EA Gidoni: Dalla parte del neonato: proposte per una competenza prognostica. Neuropsichiatria Infantile 173 (1976) 5–17

Negri R: L'evoluzione della teoria Bobathiana nel trattamento del bambino con paralisi cerebrale infantile. Giornale di Neuropsichiatria dell' Età Evolutiva 2 (3) (1982) 299–307

Negri R: Fisioterapie e rieducazioni precoci alla luce dei problemi dello sviluppo emotivo. Quaderni di psicoterapia infantile 8 (1983a) 82–98

Negri R: Introduzione al dibattito: il neonato in neuropsichiatria infantile. Giornale di Neuropsichiatria dell' Età Evolutiva 3 (1) (1983b) 59–70

Negri R: La vita prenatale e la strutturazione del pensiero. Psicoanalisi e Metodo 1 (1996) 68–86

Negri R: Quelques propos sur la "personnalité" du foetus. In: Que savent les foetus? Mille et un bébés. ERES 1997

Negri R: Il neonato in terapia intensiva. Cortina, Milano 1998

Negri R: La "memoria fetale" nella "care" del neonato pretermine in incubatrice. Ped. Med. Chir. (Med. Surg. Ped.) 25 (2003) 13–22

Negri R: Personalità e memoria fetale. Conferenza tenuta a Firenze, palazzo Strozzi, 29 Ottobre 2004. In Press

Paine RS: Neurologic Examination of Infants and Children. Pediatric Clinics of North America 4 (1960) 471–510

Paine RS, TB Brazelton, DE Donovan, JE Drorbaugh, JP Hubbell, EM Sears: Evolution of Postural Reflexes in Normal Infants and in the Presence of Chronic Brain Syndromes. Neurology 14 (1964) 1036–1048

Peiper A: Cerebral Function in Infancy and Childhood. Consultant Bureau, New York 1961

Prechtl HFR: Continuity of Neural Function from Prenatal to Postnatal life. Levenham Press, Suffolk 1984

Prechtl HFR, BJ Beintema: A Neurological Study of Newborn Infants. Clinics in Developmental Medicine 28 (1964)

Robson KS: The Role of Eye-to-Eye Contact in Maternal Infant Attachment. Journal of Child Psychology and Psychiatry, and allied disciplines 8 (1967) 13–25

Robson KS, HA Moss: Patterns and Determinants of Maternal Attachment. Journal of Pediatrics 77 (6) (1970) 976

Saint-Anne Dargassies S: Le dévelopement neurologique de nouveau né à. terme et prèmaturè. Masson, Paris 1974

Tajani E, A Ianniruberto: The Uncovering of Fetal Competence. In: Papini M, A Pasquinelli, BEA Gidoni (eds): Handicap, Rehabilitation: Practice and Theory. Excerpta Medica, Amsterdam 1990

Thomas A, S Autgaerden: Locomotion from Pre- to Post-natal Life. Clinics in Developmental Medicine 24 (1966)

Touwen BCL: Early Detection and Early Treatment of Cerebral Palsy: Possibilities and Fallacies. Giornale di Neuropsichiatria dell'Età Evolutiva 4 (1989) 31–38

Touwen BCL: Variability and Stereotypy of Spontaneous Motility as a Predictor of Neurological Development of Preterm Infants. Developmental Medicine and Child Neurology 32 (1990) 501–514

Trevarthen C: "Running with the natural motives of learning and teaching." Relazione al Congresso Internazionale-Education, a Determining Factor in The Life of Every Human Being- Athens 24–25 February 2006. In Press

Volpe JJ: Neurology of the Newborn. Saunders, Philadelphia 1987

Wolff PH: The Causes, Controls and Organization of Behavior in the Neonate. Psychological Issues, 5 (1966) 1–105

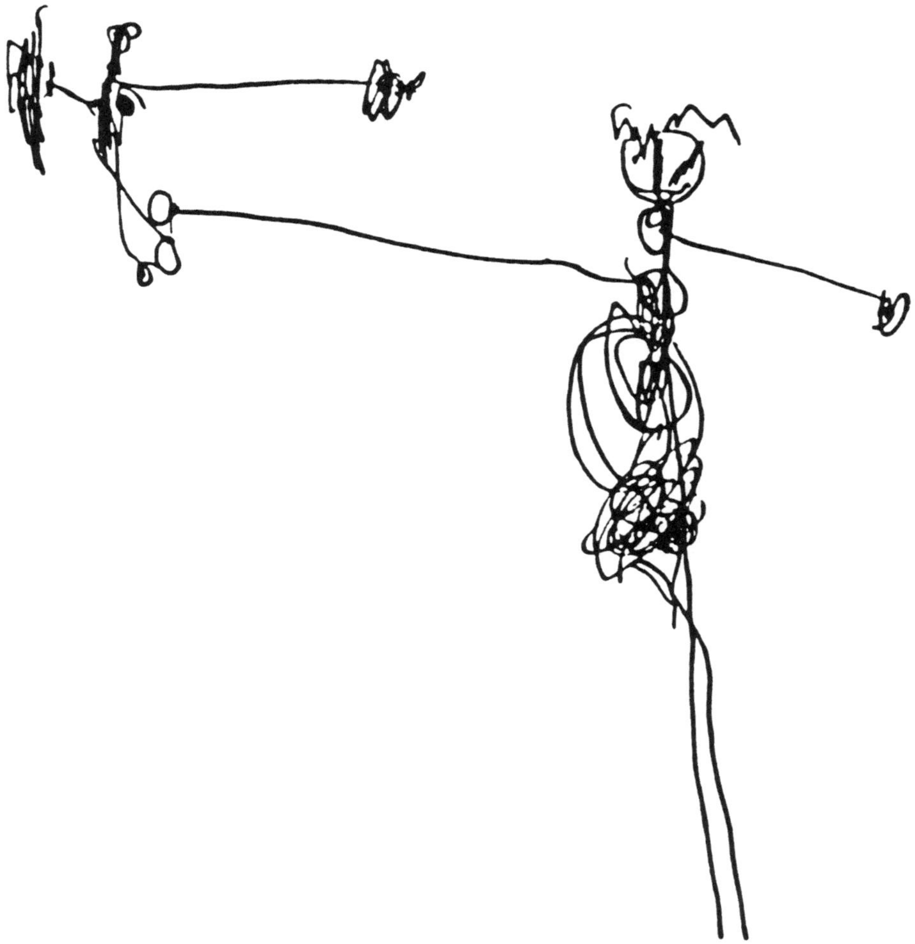

(Stevens, 3 yrs. 2 mos.)
I was a boy inside my mom's tummy, then the doctor gave me a name and I became a girl.
First I was a girl and then I got formed like a Stevens. Then the doctor said: "Keep the name Stevens", and so I stayed a boy.

18. Subjective perspectives on the maternity experience – A qualitative analysis

Vania Valoriani, Paola Benvenuti, Adolfo Pazzagli;
Department of Neurological and Psychiatric Sciences,
Faculty of Medicine, University of Florence, Italy

Maternity is an intensely emotional experience bringing with it internal and external changes and requiring the woman, partner and couple to adapt psychologically to their new situation.

What we define as "the job of becoming a parent", a mental development process involving a series of changes both internally and to external reality (Benvenuti et al., 1981), enables people to constructively overcome the crisis of becoming a parent for the first time.

Birth of a child, with its creative significance, also brings about a sense of loss. Nowadays, the process of having a child means renouncing some aspects of personal life such as the exclusive role of son/daughter, wife or husband while also experiencing new feelings and anxieties associated with this change. The future parents enter into competition with their own parents until they assume their role, bringing back into question the real and imaginary relationships they have with these figures. It implicates the loss of the previous relationship in which respective roles were very clearly set out.

Maternity is a time when affective and relational dynamics, be it within the family or outside, are changed. It also has significant social importance, i.e. the beginning of new family ties and the reorganisation of the woman in society and in her immediate and extended family. Birth of a child is currently an event that is not repeated many times in a couple's relationship. For this reason, when it does happen, it is even more important than in the past in terms of subjective experiences of the parents. At the present time, having a child is more a predetermined choice and often the sole one of its kind in the span of adult life. Becoming a parent, therefore, represents an apical stage in the adult's life cycle, an event which signals the development of personality which takes place in a determined period of time but should be included in the maturing process. From many points of view, it has been highlighted how birth of a child can be interpreted as a "developmental crisis" or "individual development phase" (Benedeck, 1959).

According to Erikson (1957), birth of a child, especially the first one, brings about the most significant developmental crisis in the adult because confronting their own procreative capacities means acquiring the ability to be responsible for taking care of themselves while also experimenting with their own creative powers as a further means of the development of their own identity. A different instinct emerges during pregnancy which provokes the woman to reassess her system of values, prioritising life and its continuation and therefore, ways of caring for and protecting compared to only having to refer to herself. New networks of relationships, sympathies for new causes, new relationships drawing on the early experiences of the development of the individual and relations with important figures in the person's life are all developed in this period.

During pregnancy, the mother experiences a type of "mental pregnancy", a psychic process which prepares her for the profound transformation of her identity that is about to take place and which will influence the relationship with her partner, her family relationships, and her own feeling of identity. In this phase the woman forms the image of the baby, of herself as mother figure, and her partner as father of her new family. It is a complex mental process which could be called the "genesis of the maternal personality", and can be considered the counterpart of organogenesis – the physical process that takes place during pregnancy. It is almost possible, therefore, to speak of two pregnancies, physical and psychic, which evolve in parallel and mutually influence each other until the time comes to give birth (Bennet et al., 1994).

Stern (1985, 1995) proposed that with the birth of a child (especially the first), the mother undergoes a specific psychic re-organisation, defined as "maternal constellation" and bringing about a series of new actions, tendencies, fears and desires. The reorganization of the woman's psychic characterizes a profound change in the representation of herself as a person, wife, daughter, and mother, who is activated during maternity, but it means also the stabilizing of the function of maternal mentality. According to the author, the realm of actions that are objectively detectable and the realm of subjective ones are in a state of constant interaction, in a process of mutual influence and modification.

Psychoanalytical perspectives of pregnancy have been extensively dealt with. According to Raphael-Leff (1980), pregnancy can be subdivided into three periods corresponding to the three phases in the mother-child relationship described by Mahler (1957), the (i) autistic, (ii) symbiotic and the (iii) individualism-separation phases. The first is the normal autistic phase and is characterised primarily by a state of vigilant inactivity. The symbiotic phase is where mother and child are submersed in a common confine known as "dual unity". In pregnancy, this is no illusion but very much a reality. The second, symbiotic phase involves premature individualism. Finally, the third phase which culminates at birth consists of real separation and extrauterine reunion.

In a study Lumley (1980) highlights how important the ability to form the image of the fetus as an individual is, in the emotional life of the woman. The earlier the images are formed, the stronger the emotional investment and the less ambivalence towards the idea of a new baby and the pregnancy itself. It is possible to say that the mother's imagining of her baby includes elements of ambivalence (Ferraro and Nunziante Cesaro 1985) and fluctuates between the mental representation of the "desired" baby which corresponds to the imaginary picture of childhood and the baby imagined during pregnancy (Lebovici, 1983; Soulè 1982) along with narcissistic and compensatory values and ideas that the baby is disturbing, it is an undifferentiable part of herself or an idealised or intrusive part of her sexual partner.

In the latter months of pregnancy a particular object relationship begins to set in due to fetal movements, inducing the characterization of the fetus as a real entity in itself. Bibring (1959, 1961) speaks of two major means of adaptation in relation to two stages of pregnancy. The first refers to the acceptance of the embryo and then of the fetus as an integral part of oneself – an experience of fusion with the fetus which lasts from the first months of pregnancy to the perception of fetal movements which breaks this narcissistic unity and determines the baby as a new autonomous object inside her own body. At this point, the means of adaptation involves the reorganisation of her own object relationships to prepare herself for the birth-separation of the baby.

Mental representation during pregnancy, or rather modifications to the representational world of the woman, is a topic which has been extensively dealt with in the literature. The concept of representation can be as one of the pivotal points in psychoanalytical theory and considered as a way the individual organizes and constructs with introjection and identification processes involving mental images of self and others. It deals with dynamic representations, with active constructions which operate subconsciously and include more than just simple cognitive patterns in the interpretation of reality. Freud (1915) associates representation with affection as a constituent part of the drive and at the center of the psychic life of the individual.

On the topic of maternal representation in pregnancy, Ammanti (1995) points out the existence of various maternal styles and types of caring which the baby receives. This means that the development of some types of representation during pregnancy may have the ability to predict the future mothering ("*maternage*") style. The author singled out three types of maternal representation during pregnancy: integrated representation, non-integrated representation and restricted or disinvested representation. The woman who has an integrated representation of pregnancy experiences it as a profound transformation of her normal, everyday life, climaxing at birth. Pregnancy completes the development process of female identity. The crisis aims to work out the past to enable future growth. The changes are not feared but, rather, are contentedly accepted so as to achieve a new balance. The woman experiences a period of orientation with herself. The maternity is an intense feeling, and the woman may attach "messianic" connotations to the baby. The woman gives in to regression and is contented with the family environment. She undergoes a discovery stage with her baby which helps with the process of differentiation.

Non-integrated representations of maternity correspond to experiences of ambivalence, to fears of losing the child and anxiousness for the future providing a backdrop for the attempt to deny them. Adaptation to change is only partial and is experienced with a sense of irritation. Fantasies about the baby often involve threatening presences and morbid feelings; fetal movements are not immediately recognized but denied. The ability to differentiate from the fetus is lacking and the relationship often has negative characteristics where the mother experiences the desire to attack and expel the fetus from her body.

Restricted/disinvested representations correspond to the fact that the pregnancy is considered as an obligatory step towards having a child. The waiting period though, has no investment, no function, and is not experienced as a maturing stage in her own identity. The rhythm of life stays the same as it was before the pregnancy and there is a lack of fantisizing about the baby and about her future role as mother. The inevitable regression is experienced with a lot of pain producing a defensive reaction of closure towards her internal world. There is an attempt to rationalize the experience, resulting in difficulty in creating the mental space for which the baby is competing.

The description of a woman who faces maternity merely as a transition period she needs to go through to fulfil her desire to become a parent, seems to correspond to the current cultural transformation taking place which calls for a more active role for the father in caring for the child, generally qualified as "maternal". The risk lies in the fact that women require more and more participation and sharing of experiences from their partners in the hope of receiving emotional and practical support – something which is often lacking in other social areas (e.g. the extended family in the past) and have expectations which risk moving the paternal role into the maternal arena. The maternal elements in the father are, of course, useful in caring for the little child but he gradually recuperates his specific paternal role (with some conflict) by facing the unpleasant task of separating the mother-child dyad and preparing the child for dealing with the impact of external reality (Argentieri, 1999). In this momentous phase however, a progressive homogenization of the two parent figures takes place, along with a converging of the two roles in the maternal area distinguished by indulgent, tolerant, understanding and protective characteristics.

According to some studies (Scopesi, 1994), becoming a parent also consists of traditional behavioral stereotypes, for example when future fathers often help out with the housework before birth in order for their partner to have more time for themselves, whereas afterwards they return to more traditional roles such as division of tasks in an attempt to reinforce gender identity. The arrival of a newborn compels the couple to face reality and reorganize space and time in their own lives, physically and mentally, so as to accommodate the baby and harmoniously transform themselves in an efficient and balanced way. The relationship between the couple can change in some ways, on one hand there is a decline in some aspects of "companionship" tied to the pleasure of "doing something together". On the other hand, the senses of belonging and support (the "partnership") are increased.

In order to understand what the woman goes through during pregnancy and the first period postpartum, a qualitative study model was used, allowing mothers to express their own emotions and beliefs either with regard to pregnancy and the period just after birth, or postpartum depression, the most frequent psychopathologic condition after giving birth.

Research

The subjective experience of maternity was the object of a qualitative study involving 5 Focus Groups (FG) with a total of 24 mothers from the Florence area who were contacted through the Department of Obstetrics at the Polytechnic University. All had babies aged 3–8 months who were healthy at birth and did not suffer from any developmental problems. The sample has an average age of 31 years, an average total of 14 years' education; 50% was employed and 62% were married (the remainder living with their partners); 92% were primiparas (*Table 1*).

Table 1 Characteristics of the sample.

Average age	in active employment	education	marital status	other children
31	37.5% work in the home 50 % employed 12.5% students	12% middle school (up to about 15 years) 54.16% high school diploma (up to about 19 years) 33.33% university graduates	62.5% married 37.5% living with partners	92% no

Every FG session was audio- and video-recorded and then transcribed *verbatim* so as to carry out computer-assisted qualitative analysis (QSR NUD°IST IV; Richards, 1995). With this methodology, the units of significance extrapolated were codified during the first subdivision of the text and subsequently inserted into lexical ties. Following the methodology of Grounded Theory (Strass, Corbin, 1990), the units were initially openly codified and then more specifically using a hierarchical system. Finally a selective codification was carried out whereby the contents of the lexical ties were identified according the focus of the study: fears, anxieties and in general negative emotions experieced by mothers during pregnancy, their attributional processes of causality and the perception of pregnancy and abnormalities in their experiences according to the social representation of the emotional difficulties tied in with maternity. A consensus among the researchers was reached as to suitability and individual significance in the determining of the emotions expressed.

During the FGs several topics were suggested which examined feelings of satisfaction and unhappiness during the pregnancy and after birth, knowledge of postpartum depression, and suggestions for the improvement of the quality of help during maternity. The subjects that came up throughout the sessions are illustrated in Table 2 as well as being reported in full in the text with some significant sentences transcribed from the Focus Group recording.

Table 2 Topics and points raised during focus groups.

FG topics	Points raised
satisfaction during pregnancy	partner support/movements of the baby unexpected event being at the center of attention
satisfaction after birth	partner support/breastfeeding recovery of independence relationship with baby
unhappiness during pregnancy	worries/fears an excess of analyses/tests conflict with partner
unhappiness after birth	feelings of inadequacy/loneliness having to renounce certain aspects of life lack of relationships with own family
knowledge of postpartum depression	reference to specific symptoms awareness of the complex nature of the pathology difficulty in adapting to social norms
suggestions	increase in relational and social supports refusal of therapeutical pharmacological treatment more information constant assistance creation of specific activities and structures

Satisfaction during the pregnancy

Women who participated in the study listed many factors that are attributable to the perception of happiness during pregnancy. Support from their partner was one of the main factors, followed by feeling the movements of the fetus inside their bodies. Also mentioned was unexpected pregnancy, the fact of being at the center of attention, the importance of physical looks, good health and the growth of the abdomen.

Support from partner

The importance of a supportive partner emerged as one of the central factors in the feeling of happiness during pregnancy. Women involved in the study consider the emotional support of their partners more important than practical support. Their desire is that their partners accept their pregnancy with full awareness and share the experience with them including accompanying them to prenatal classes or keeping themselves informed about all developments in the pregnancy, and that they be present during the entire period of the pregnancy, labor, and birth. To describe the results obtained we have chosen to cite the most significant statements made by the women for each topic proposed during the FG sessions.

"I believe that the most important thing is the relationship with one's husband or partner who is experiencing the same thing and to feel more or less united."

"My husband's support helped me greatly during my pregnancy."

The partner emerges as the most important reference figure throughout maternity, even compared to other figures who could fulfil similar roles such as the mother, female friends and relations. Women's expectations of their partners seem very high, as if they are the only person who can help them in fulfilling their maternal role and consequently they invest great responsibility in the partner.

In the current socio-cultural climate, women experience a certain detachment from their own families as if proving their own independence. At the same time, they turn to their partners with expectations and responsibilities which are beyond the actual possibilities of support he can provide. If this investment in the partner figure is not satisfied it can cause great unhappiness and disappointment. The hypothesis is that the women experience feelings of loneliness once they detach themselves from their own families and therefore ask the partner to fill an emotional gap caused by an unsatisfactory or conflictual relationship with her own parents.

Unexpected pregnancy

Quite surprisingly, unexpected pregnancy emerged as a major topic in our focus groups. In the past few decades, maternity has profoundly changed in Italy, with one of the lowest national birth indices in the world and with the age of first pregnancy significantly on the increase. As a result, we could hypothesize that many women have experienced a certain conflict between their desire to become pregnant and pressure, either internal (e.g. the desire to fulfil oneself as a person, fears of being an inadequate mother …) or external (e.g. conforming to social norms, difficulties in finding employment and accommodation) which tends to delay the event of having a child. It seems that unexpected or not deliberately-planned pregnancy can avoid the problem of making the decision, representing an apparent solution to this type of conflict.

"I felt a very physical, natural thing – and thought – see how well the hormones work ... because actually the pregnancy was not planned, it just happened, and in the beginning I was quite anxious. I was delighted but I didn't really think I'd get pregnant, we weren't trying, we were being extra cautious."

Being at the centre of attention

Another topic refers to the value of maternity as a factor in personal, familial, and social affirmation. The women felt extremely gratified by the attention they received from people around them during pregnancy. The physical changes accompanying pregnancy are seen as testimony to their ability to procreate and the attention of people is usually drawn to the growing abdomen.

"Everyone sees you in a different way, you're constantly at the center of attention among all the people around you. You have the sense that the world around you is protecting you, and this gave me a lot of comfort."

"And then there's the attention you get from everyone, you rarely encounter hostility but usually find people with big smiles when you have a pregnant tummy."

Satisfaction after birth

The main topics that emerged from the focus groups were support from the partner, relationship with the baby and breastfeeding, along with becoming an autonomous person once more.

Support from the partner

In keeping with the points previously raised regarding the support of the partner, the ability to share changes which take place in the couple's relationship after the birth, emerges as the main factor in the happiness felt by the woman.

"I associate happiness with my little baby girl but also with the rediscovery of a new relationship with my husband. The birth of the baby completely changed the relationship we had before and it was also quite difficult."

Relationship with the baby and breast-feeding

As predicted, the stabilizing of the relationship with the baby and the pleasure of breastfeeding and seeing the baby grow are the main reasons why women feel gratified after birth. The satisfaction the mother feels in undertaking these functions compensates for any difficulty in caring for the child in its first phase of adaptation to the world.

"The origins of happiness were definitely the baby herself, seeing her grow and the progress she makes every day. Seeing how she gradually learns to recognize and get attached to you. This gives satisfaction despite the tiredness; my baby still wakes up during the night. However, when I go to her, she smiles at me and I'm already gratified."

"If I were to recall a particular moment of gratification, it was one time that after breastfeeding she looked up at me and smiled, not just a reflex, but a real smile. And it's also so great how every day she discovers something and seeks participation and protection from me and my husband."

Recovery of independence

It seems that while on the one hand women express a desire to get back to their personal activities, on the other they feel anxious and uncertain about being away from their babies, experienced as irreparable separations.

"Actually I think I'm much more calm and serene now that I'm back working and have space and daytime for myself. I also get on better with my little baby girl."

"I still have to understand how the relationship will be with myself once alone again – I don't know what is going to happen to me. And my poor little girl, nothing will happen to her, but she's also had constant contact with me, it won't be easy to interrupt that."

To fulfil their requirements women turn to their own families, in particular their mothers, from whom they expect eminently practical help and complete abstention from interfering with how they care for the baby, with their emotions, and issues involving their partner. It is as if they fear the risk of having an identity crisis when confronted with the maternal model. In analyzing the main factors in feeling gratification after birth, some sources of conflict clearly emerge, showing the ambivalence of maternal feelings and the need to face maternity with a full sense of awareness.

Unhappiness during pregnancy

Feelings of unhappiness during the pregnancy are linked to the presence of fears and worries with regard to the development of the pregnancy itself, conflict with the partner and, rather unexpectedly, to the series of what women consider excessive diagnostic tests they have to undergo.

Fears and worries

The majority of the women referred to the fears and worries they felt regarding the health and development of their baby, the uncertainties about the ability to bring the pregnancy to term and the possibility of harming the baby in some way from certain types of daily behavior (such as food choices, physical activity, sporadic use of symptomatic medications), the fear of being abandoned by their partner after birth.

"I felt entirely responsible for the little being that was inside me, so... there were certain foods I couldn't eat ... for example at the beginning of my pregnancy, when I didn't really know ... I took some medicine, which made me feel really bad... and also for the fact that the little baby might have problems."

Conflict with partner

The difference in attitude towards the pregnancy between women and some of their partners who showed a lack of understanding and uncertainty about accepting them turned out to be an important issue in the overall topic of unhappiness during pregnancy.

"While I was enthusiastic... my husband needed time to take in the whole situation, and at the beginning this really got to me."

The woman, as previously described, attributes a great importance to the enthusiastic participation of the partner in the maternity experience and to his ability to emotionally support her. Consequently, misunderstandings and disputes which can arise in the couple's relationship and the difference in attitude towards the pregnancy can cause unhappiness and loneliness which the woman seems to experience in an extreme way, as if unable to evaluate the reality surrounding her and the possible reasons why the partner might be feeling or acting in this way.

Excess testing

The National Health Service provides a specific diagnostic protocol for all pregnant women who have the role of primary and secondary prevention of illness in their babies and birth complications. The tests set out in the protocol are considered to be excessive by women and viewed in a negative light overall, they are seen as the over-medicalizing of a natural, physiological phenomenon such as pregnancy and creating problems for women instead of being reassuring. Such observations have highlighted the divergence between the opinions of the health organization which justifiably considers this protocol responsible for the drastic reduction in perinatal mortality and the subjective views of the women who undergo the series of tight periodic diagnostic tests.

"For me the tests were really annoying, this never-ending series of tests, beginning with amniocentesis – all my female friends urged me to make sure I got it done along with a whole load of tests which for me were way over the top."

"Yeah, there were a little too many, I was also surprised at just how many there were... and all of us were considered as being in a non-risk category, instead the health service sets out this protocol with so many tests, there seem to be so many of them ... because in reality we're young people, if at the first check-up the blood test shows that everything is more or less under control, at the worst lacking in a bit of iron."

Unhappiness after birth

The main issues that emerged under this topic were feelings of inadequacy and solitude, having to renounce certain areas of their lives and some conflicts with their own families.

Inadequacy and solitude

Women expressed unease linked to feelings of inadequacy in their fulfilment of the maternal role, connected to taking on new responsibilities towards caring for and looking after the wellbeing of the newborn. The uncertainty about the mother's own maternal abilities stems from the feeling of being left alone in caring for the child, especially by the partner or assistance structures.

"Immediately after birth, I felt depressed, at home I didn't know what to do, I would say to myself – you'll never make it as a mother, I felt like a failure... then these feelings passed ... after the obstetrician came, maybe, it felt like one more means of support ... everything got a bit better, but at the beginning I felt so alone in caring for my little one ... and also maybe it was a type of abandonment crisis ... I felt like I was abandoned and by myself, as if the life of this tiny girl depended only on me, that everything rested on my shoulders ..."

Having to renounce certain aspects of their lives

This came up as a sub-topic under the women's feeling of unhappiness after birth in attempting to recover their independence. The feeling of having to give up certain major aspects of their own lives leads to frustration and unease which provokes the desire to find their independence and free time once more, accompanied by guilt due to feelings of needing to leave the baby in order to do so.

"I decided to leave some time to myself and I would leave the baby, on returning however I felt so guilty and feel quite ambivalent."

"I was pleased that my husband urged me to set aside some space for myself. When I'm with my baby I try not to burden him, I play and I joke with him, but I don't really feel like one of those mums from TV ads."

Conflict with their own families

A certain competition with the original mother figure seems to emerge towards the way the baby should be cared for and interacted with. Any possible advice or suggestions given are not accepted by the new mother and are taken as unwanted interfering and considered intrusive. The women stress that the relationship with their partners is much more important to them compared to their own parent figures and they refuse any attempt of interference they might make in the relationships with the baby and the partner.

"I was very sure I was doing well in a certain way and when sometimes they began saying "but when I was in your position I did such and such..." I would reply saying that the pediatrician told me to do it in that way, and blamed the pediatrician, even if it wasn't true, but this meant they wouldn't dare to contradict."

"My mother used to tell me not to say anything to Giovanni, "not to burden him with the situation", but I needed to tell him what was going on, such as one time when I didn't have enough milk, or when the baby was crying."

Knowledge of postpartum depression

In general, women were aware of the existence of postpartum depression and had been mainly informed through the mass media and from communicating with other women about their experiences. Some considered the condition normal, or at least, so they were told, but didn't seem to be able to differentiate between the "maternity blues" and postpartum depression. They listed only a few symptoms of the depression such as sadness, tiredness, or crying for no reason.

Women thought that postpartum depression had a multi-factorial etio-pathogenisis and highlighted in particular the vulnerability felt by the individual as a determining factor. They also mentioned other possible causes of psychosocial problems, such as a lack of support from their partners, tiredness from the burden of domestic duties, excessive interfering from their own families or mother-in-laws' expectations of them or the loss of their independence. They also pointed out the importance of biological factors such as hormonal and physical changes.

"Maybe the family doesn't really understand how a mother could be sad when she has a brand new baby."

"There's the hormonal element, and then the tiredness. And I remember I just wanted to cry for no reason."

"For me it was the culmination of several things – with my baby I've no problems. It was more external factors like selling my house and finding a new one. I went through a really tough period linked to external factors. I don't know whether it was these external factors that lead me think in the morning as soon as I woke up how on earth I'd find the strength to make it to the end of the day or whether it was linked to my new condition. Maybe it was all of the factors put together, I'm in great doubt about what I did and am still confused."

The importance of the partner clearly emerged based on the experiences of the women – they referred to the fact that they felt it was fundamental that the partner be informed about the pregnancy and everything regarding maternity and that he be emotionally involved and capable of providing reassuring practical and emotional support.

"The closeness of my partner. It's the thing I felt the most and would have wanted him to have been closer to me."

The women also referred to support coming from members of their own families, especially from parents, particularly important for the practical organization of their daily life. Support and being able to share the experience with other women was considered very helpful, as was being able to speak to psycho-pharmacological experts. However, the women denied the possibility of undergoing psycho-pharmacological treatment in the case where depressive symptoms develop. *"In my opinion the approach towards psychology and the psychologist is quite behind the times in Italy, at least as far as I can see... Anyway, to get in contact with a therapist, to open a dialogue, to speak... I think it's the best way to go. But taking a pill in the morning and evening is much quicker and straightforward."*

Other topics which came up regarded the recovery of independence, learning to ask for help, and the early recognition of psychological problems.

Suggestions

All of the women who participated in the FGs offered the same suggestions for improving the health system regarding maternity. Preparatory courses were considered as being too focussed on pregnancy and the birth, whereas they should have provided more information on and preparation for the postpartum period and depression. Partners and other members of the family should have been more involved either by participating in the courses or with the provision of relevant information.

The women pointed out the need for a specific service dealing with problems in pregnancy and the postpartum, a service to which women can turn for advice on various problems they may be having, with the aim of improving constant assistance throughout pregnancy, birth and postpartum. They also indicated the importance of having the same obstetrician during pregnancy and at birth and the possibility of maintaining contact with some of the staff after birth, who provided assistance during their pregnancies along with receiving home visits by obstetricians. They also expressed the desire for the availability of semi-formally structured women's support groups with the presence of a professional figure in order to share their experiences and lessen the anxiety of the postpartum period.

Some interviews conducted with clinicians in this period with regard to their knowledge of postpartum depression and its treatment confirmed the need for more attention and information about it and the distinct lack of services specifically for this condition. Some of them believed such services to be unnecessary and indicated basic medications (which were not at all mentioned by the women) as the key to managing postpartum depression, whereas often the woman turns to the pediatrician for advice pertaining only to the health problems of her child.

Conclusions

Women appear to be focussed primarily on emotional aspects of the pregnancy, birth and the postpartum period whereas the practical aspects regarding the birth of a child were left in the background. The partner emerged as the main figure of reference for the organization of an event which the woman feels incapable of handling by herself. If in previous times women relied on their partners for financial support, these days it is emotional support and the sharing of the pregnancy experience that the woman needs from her partner. Women experience feelings of ambivalence about the baby, anxiousness and doubt about their role as mother and their ability to take care of the newborn, leaving them in an emotionally vulnerable state. The partner, therefore, becomes the central figure in the expectations of the women and his affective behavior is pivotal in determining their happiness or unhappiness either during the pregnancy or after birth. They actually wish to receive all the support that they require exclusively from him, to the exclusion of their own families. The partner is also identified as the main confidant, a figure which, in their imagination, replaces the family and friends as being able to fulfil a "nutritional" role for the woman as well as protective one for the baby. It is obvious that it is not always easy to satisfy such expectations and women can become disappointed, especially if the man experiences difficulty and personal conflicts with regard to becoming a father himself.

Maternity tends to be considered an event to be experienced within the relationship of a couple, to the exclusion of the couple's own families who are almost only called upon for practical support in caring for the child and help with recovering some of the mother's own independence. In general, the role of the family was to tie in family traditions with the needs of subsequent generations, whereas nowadays the experiences of their parents are not considered sufficiently viable parenting models, and situations of conflict can actually arise if the mother or mother-in-law overstep their mark in terms of the practical help they are required to give.

The very critical attitude that the diagnostic tests included in the national protocol for pregnancy are excessive and disturbing was revealed. In the years of demographic increase, the organization of the health service was orientated towards using standardized protocols for screening the woman and fetus and yielded positive results. However, as previously illustrated, the prescribed diagnostic tests are considered as the over-medicalization of a natural, physiological event making the pregnancy almost seem like an illness. The women would prefer health assistance based more on their own personal needs.

In a survey conducted by the Italian National Statistics Institute (*Istituto Nazionale di Statistica*; ISTAT) (Sabbatini, 2001), on a sample of 2,500,000 women, results emerged that were in accordance with our research findings. Pregnancies are rarer and later (in our group of women only 8.33% were on their second pregnancy), awareness of problems related to maternity is high, participation of partners in prenatal classes and their involvement at birth is on the increase – especially in the central north area; use of public structures is high (90%) and the over-medicalization of pregnancy emerges as an issue. A rather contradictory situation thus emerges regarding the use of health services – besides the obvious processes (99% of the women consulted with a doctor, 93% of births were in the ninth month), there was an elevated number of ultrasounds and cesarean births and extensive and wholesale use of diagnostic tests which indicate the medicalization of pregnancy corresponding exactly to the subjective experience referred to by the women.

The women's criticism of our health system highlights the discrepancy between the assistance they receive during the pregnancy and what they receive after birth. Women actually receive a lot of medical care during pregnancy but significantly less afterwards and it is as if personal problems are being denied. In fact, there are no classes for parents after birth nor are there any mother-baby units in hospitals or day hospitals to assist women with psychological and relational difficulties.

Very symbolic was the statement of one woman who expressed the sensation that maternity was a tough challenge "with only ourselves to rely on for help". This feeling of loneliness which women may feel after birth may correlate with the current crisis in the traditional maternal model and the "disappointment" they feel when assigning to their partner a form of maternal support. The partner is not equipped to fulfil this model of maternal care both for historical reasons and due to personal experiences and also because he is just as much inexpert at parenthood as the woman is. Consequently, this attempt at "maternalization" risks transforming the partner into a failed or inadequate mother-substitute who is incapable of fulfilling the role of psychological support provider (Stern, 1995) needed by the woman to carry out her main duties. This type of support had always been provided by a female and maternal network and the care of babies was traditionally the realm of women with the men kept at a safe distance and only gradually allowed to approach. The relative disappearance of the extended family, the lack of benefits from other social units and the desire for independence and self-fulfilment risk making maternity too difficult a task to take on for many women. Paradoxically, it seems that women would like to receive assistance and support from health workers – information, assistance and support that women traditionally received from their mothers and other maternal figures in their lives.

Knowledge of postpartum depression coming from various sources (mostly from mass media and prenatal classes) was, at least on an informative level, widespread among our sample of women taking part in the FGs. We need to ask ourselves, however, how much information about puerperal psychopathology can actually be useful to women and their close ones if it is not accompanied by advice for the couple on how to work through and share the anxieties and insecurities that emerge throughout pregnancy and after the birth.

The fact that clinicians have a limited interest in problems associated with the postpartum period and particularly the risk factors of depression, seems to point out that in mass education, maternity is treated in a conformist way. The exploration of problematic aspects is avoided, of which the women are all too well aware and, furthermore, the techniques used in dealing with them have the same prejudices as the people involved with maternity.

It is possible to conclude therefore, that maternity represents a symbol of the psychosocial transformation which has taken place in our culture where the tendency is towards the disownment of the traditional mother figure, leaving a gap which causes generational conflicts, fears, and powerful fantasies about the ability to compensate for this, on the one hand by delegating the maternal supportive role to their partners and, on the other, by investing high expectations in the health system and health workers. It emerges that women show substantial helplessness/insecurity when it comes to self-reflection, being aware of their own identity, and the need to share the psychological process with their partner. In other words, it seems the thought prevails among women regarding parenthood that there is some sort of magical scotomization of the entire world and its vicissitudes while denying any conflicts or problems which belong to the normal psychological working of the individual and stigmatizing any signs of unease as mental illness without performing a comprehensive and interpretative diagnostic check of clinical phenomena.

References

Ammaniti M, C Candelori, M Pola, R Tambelli: Maternità e Gravidanza. Studio delle rappresentazioni materne. Cortina, Milano 1995

Argentieri S: Il padre maternio da San Giuseppe ai nuovi mammi. Meltemi, 1999

Bennet S, I Sackler-Lefcourt, W Haft, P Nachman, DN Stern: The activation of maternal representations. Infant Mental Health Journal 15 (4) (1994) 336–347

Benvenuti P, A Pazzagli, M Rossi Monti, C Rogari: Il lavoro del diventare genitori: difficoltà e fallimenti. Rivista di patologia nervosa e mentale 102 (1981) 241–68

Bibring GL: Some considerations of the psychological process in pregnancy. The Psychoanalytic Study of the Child 14 (1959) 113–121

Bibring GL: A study of the psychological processes in pregnancy and the earliest mother-child relationship. The Psychoanalytic Study of the Child 16 (1961) 9–13

Erikson E: I cicli della vita. Continuità e mutamenti. Armando, Roma 1999

Ferraro F, A Nunziante Cesaro: Lo spazio cavo e il corpo saturato. La gravidanza come "agire" tra fusione e separazione. Angeli, Milano 1985

Freud S: Trasformazioni pulsionali, particolarmente dell'erotismo anale. In: "Opere", 11. Boringhieri, Torino 1979

Lee Shapiro J: Il padre in attesa. Età Evolutiva 95 (1989) 33–37

Lumley JM: The image of the foetus in the first trimester. Birth and Family Journal 7 (1980) 5–14

Mahler M, F Pine, A Bergman: La nascita psicologica del bambino. Boringhieri, Torino 1978

Raphael-Leff J: Psychotherapy with pregnant woman. In: Blum BL: (a cura di) Psychological Aspect of Pregnancy, Birthing and Bonding. Human Sciences Press, New York 1980

Richards T, L Richards: The QRS NUD•IST Qualitative Data Analysis System. Qualitative Sociology 14 (1991) 307–324

Richards T, L Richards: Using Computers in Qualitative Research. In: Denzin NK, YS Lincoln (eds): Handbook of Qualitative Research. Sage, Newbury Park 1994

Sabbadini L: Gravidanza e parto: una nuova coscienza femminile, un nuovo protagonismo maschile. ISTAT, Roma 2001

Soifer R: Psicodinamica della gravidanza, parto e puerperio. Borla, Roma 1975

Soulè M: L'enfant dans la tête. L'enfant imaginaire. Sa valeur structurante dans les échanges mère-enfant. In: Brazelton Th, B Cramer, L Kreisler, R Schäppi, M Soulé (eds): La dynamique du nourrisson. E.S.F., Paris 1982

Stern DN: Representation of relationship experience. In: Sameroff AJ, RN Emde: (a cura di) Relationship Disturbance in Early Childhood: A Developmental Approach. Basic Books, New York 1985

Stern DN: The Motherhood Constellation. A Unified View of Parent-Infant Psychotherapy. Basic Books, New York 1995

Strauss LA, J Corbin: Basic of qualitative research. Sage, Newbury Park 1990

Strauss LA, J Corbin: Grounded Theory Methodology: An Overview. In: Denzin NK, YS Lincoln (eds): Handbook of Qualitative Research. Sage, Newbury Park 1994

19a. Reciprocity and psychic growth: The neglect of neglect

Graham Music; The Tavistock and Portman NHS Trust, London, United Kingdom

Both authors of these two linked papers, Lynda Miller and myself, work at the Tavistock Clinic in London where we attempt to integrate the traditions of developmental psychology research and psychoanalysis, and our title reflects this, with 'reciprocity' being a concept derived from Brazelton's (1974) developmental work, and 'psychic growth' a psychoanalytic concept from the tradition of psychoanalysts such as Wilfred Bion and Donald Winnicott. We hope to focus on a particular group of children, those who suffer a degree of emotional neglect, through the lens of two explanatory disciplines that both originated at the Tavistock at about the same time, attachment theory and psychoanalytically informed infant observation. Esther Bick (1968) developed the model of psychoanalytic infant observation at the Tavistock in the late 1940's, in the same period that Bowlby (1979) was developing the attachment theory. At the time, adherents of these two ways of thinking were rather rivalrous and oppositional; Bowlby seemed to be interested more in external behaviors, and was treated with suspicion by psychoanalytic colleagues who were more interested in the inner world and the unconscious. Today, we have placed these divisions in the past, and developmental psychology and neuroscience and psychoanalysis seem to exemplify reciprocal growth. In this paper, I will look at some of the research on the broader group of children who might be considered emotionally neglected, and will use a psychoanalytically informed view of attachment theory and developmental psychology. In her linked paper Lynda Miller will then use infant observation to discuss a small subgroup of those children who can be 'pushed' towards premature development and independence.

My focus is on children who suffer a degree of emotional neglect, and I will allow the term 'neglect' to cover a broad spectrum ranging from examples of relatively mild neglect to the extreme examples seen, for example in children brought up in horrifically unstimulating orphanages. Ironically not only do neglected children receive less attention than other children from their parents and carers, but often also from professionals. I am not talking about the children who are traumatized, who suffer overt abuse or violence, whose often uncontrollable behavior evokes huge worry for professionals, as I think these children get lots of attention and can become the focus of huge worry for teachers, social workers, therapists, and others. But children whose emotional and psychological lives are more neglected, who for whatever reason need to manage more 'on their own', and who become more self-sufficient, often precociously so, present us with real problems. The developmental trajectory following emotional neglect is often quite different from overt trauma, and in some ways the prognosis for the more emotionally neglected child can be very poor, but can be hidden from view, as they often seem to be 'fine on their own' and they cause so little trouble. The worry that they stir up is often of a very subtle and quiet kind.

I do most of my clinical work in two contexts; in the Tavistock fostering and adoption team, where we see many children adopted after early neglect, whether experiencing profound deprivation in British homes, or those adopted from orphanages in Eastern Europe, and these children present very different worries to the more traumatized ones. I also deliver therapeutic services to schools in London where all too often it is the acting out, behaviorally disturbed children that make the schools and their staff feel worried' anxious, angry, upset, and useless. Yet often there are many 'neglected' children in each of these classes who are learning little, who struggle with social relationships, cannot concentrate, yet who do not receive the attention of mental health and other professionals. On meeting these children clinicians often are struck by the 'desolate' nature of their inner worlds, and by a mental 'flatness' and lack of more ordinary lively human interactive capacities.

Humans are born as social beings, with an evolutionary history of living in packs or tribes, who have developed not just language, but an innate potential to be sensitive to the feelings of others, their moods and states of mind (e.g. Trevarthen, 1993). Yet it might be argued that western society is moving in a direction where there is an increasing value placed on individuality, autonomy, freedom, the self, and much less on the social, on the common good, on community, on altruism. The anthropologist, Clifford Geerttz (1973), for example, distinguishes 'ego-centric' as opposed to those 'socio-centric' cultures in which the whole is more important than the individual person, and children and adults learn to play an assigned role and to conform strongly to social norms. The Japanese have a concept called Amae (Doi 2005), which seems to have no translatable word in western languages, and seems to mean partly an 'expectation to be loved', but also 'to love others', to be cared for; amae is a need, an emotion, a cultural value, an action, all at once. This describes not just a fine attunement between mother and infant, a wish to love and be loved, the wish to be cared for and to care, that has features which some in the west might less kindly call 'indulgence' or 'spoiling' one's child.

There is obviously a continuum of degrees of neglect, and the continuum is very wide, from institutionalized orphans to the many milder forms of neglect that we see in other contexts, such as children of preoccupied parents who have little time for their children, or even the children of depressed mothers that Lynne Murray (e.g. 1991) has taught us so much about, who do not receive much lively attention or attunement. The spectrum is wide, with different kinds of neglect giving rise to different development deficits and different trajectories.

Some groups of children are not easily compared to others; for example children of depressed mothers have a different experience from children of emotionally 'cut-off' parents who are unaware of their own and their children's emotions; similarly many avoidantly attached children have been neglected emotionally, but not all neglected children end up as avoidantly attached (for example, some institutionalized children who are then adopted might show massive emotional impairment as a result of neglect, but might not quite fit the usual picture of avoidant attachment, as Zeanah et al. (Smyke et al., 2002) point out. Despite this I think that there are enough commonalities for us to usefully think of a continuum and so I hope I can be forgiven for the 'broad sweep' of this presentation, which ranges between research with different groups and traditions.

At the most extreme end are the tragic cases of children adopted from institutional care, many of whom are now being brought to the clinics where we work, often by adoptive parents who are struggling to make sense of their children, or to get close to them. Much of the research on the Romanian orphans has been widely publicized. Those removed earlier, and those who suffered less chronic neglect and abuse, most definitely fared better (Rutter, 1998). Scans of the brains of these Romanian orphans show that their temporal lobes have atrophied significantly, indicating that profound social deprivation can induce equally profound alterations in the physical architecture of the brain. Canadian research showed that many problems such as social disinhibition persisted in many such children after adoption (Chisholm et al., 1995). Similarly Rutter found that a disproportionate proportion of the children in his sample adopted from Romanian orphanages manifested autistic symptoms, they showed preservative movement, lack of empathy, and much more.

Other studies showed that, compared to the control group of children brought up in ordinary families, these children do not seek proximity to caregivers, nor even respond to efforts to interact (Zeanah et. al., 2003). Interestingly these children have been shown not to release oxytocin, the 'love hormone', when they are cuddled by their adoptive parents, something that generally happens between birth parents and children. They can struggle to express emotion, and can also be hard to 'warm' to, let alone love. Such recent research corroborates earlier studies of the effects of institutional care, such as those of Hodges and Tizard (1989a, b), who followed children up to age 16 who had spent their first few years in an institution, and found persisting differences in the quality of peer relationships, even in children who had later been adopted into well-functioning families.

Although these studies consider extreme cases, they nonetheless cast light on the desultory effect of neglect. We know that we are a species primed for social interaction and researchers such as Trevarthen have long described us as social creatures from birth, something that the psychoanalyst Wilfred Bion (1962) described as the baby having a preconception of the breast. We know that babies can imitate only minutes after birth (e.g. Meltzoff, 1985) and that they do not imitate non-communicative gestures like sneezing. These observations highlight how sensitive the majority of newborns are to other people. These early experiences are vital, and are the building blocks for later relationships, and our expectations of the social world, our internal representations of other people. We know about how the human brain is experience dependent (e.g. Schore, 2001; Pally, 2000) and is structured according to its particular experiences; we know from Rizzollatti (2004) and his colleagues about mirror neurons and how we begin to learn about other minds.

We also know from researchers such as Tronik (1998) that in good-enough mother infant relationships we do not see perfect attunement, but rather a constant movement between disruption and repair in interactions, and that well functioning mother child dyads are attuned only 30% of the time. Other researchers such as Beebe and Lachman (2002) have also stressed that it is the capacity to *repair* disrupted interactions that is so crucial in good mother-infant relationships.

Coming from the Tavistock, where attachment theory was born, it seems sensible to use the attachment categories as a conceptual tool for thinking about neglect, the social, the unsocial, and the asocial. The familiar categories of attachment theory divide children into secure, or insecure, and that insecure attachment can be divided into at least 3 categories, primarily the anxious-ambivalent, the anxious-avoidant and the disorganized. There is of course now a mass of scientific evidence for the usefulness of these categories, backed up by lots of ongoing research. The human infant is an incredibly adaptable creature, and adapts to its emotional and psychological environment. In evolutionary history we have needed to adapt to an enormous range of environments, the frozen climates of the Arctic to the Sahara, from abundance to drought, from fish to meat to vegetarian diets, and the same is true of our capacity to adapt to emotional environments. A securely attached infant is adapting to an environment where the parent/carer is thoughtful, able to be in touch with their own and others emotions, able to make sense of what might be going on in the psyche of the child, will be able to accept the need of the child to be dependent and needy, for example. Other children have to adapt to less favorable environments.

Bowlby's colleague, Mary Ainsworth (1978) developed the Strange Situation Test in the 1960's to examine how infants of about a year reacted to the stress of separation from their mothers. They were classified according to how they reacted to the separations, and the children classified as avoidant, generally children who have lacked a parental figure empathically attuned to their emotions, act as if they do not care when their mother leaves the room, and barely react on her return. It is easy to see how people can imagine there is nothing much to worry about in relation to the avoidant children; they can 'look fine'. Watching an avoidant child in the strange situation can cause less upset in us than seeing the secure child who cries when its mother leaves. The physiology of the avoidant child gives them away, as their heart-rates and cortisol levels show that they become extremely stressed, but if the observer would not notice; this is maybe typical of such children, we often do not notice their distress, but maybe more interesting is that they too do not seem to know they are distressed, and they seem to have lost the ability to read their own bodily signals, such as the raised heart-rates.

The next phase of attachment research which spawned a host of further research was spearheaded by Mary Main (1985) and her colleagues who developed the Adult Attachment Interview (AAI), which measures the states of mind of carers. There has been shown to be a huge association between the states of mind of carers and the attachment status of their children. The AAI aims to 'surprise the unconscious', to bypass the rational mind, the left hemisphere, and get to 'the heart' of an adult's expectations about relationships. Research has shown that carers who are thoughtful, reflective, who have a coherent narrative about their own life, tend to bring up their own children to be secure. For example, Fonagy (1991) and colleagues found that the AAI status of a pregnant mother predicted the attachment status of a child at a year with 70% accuracy, and others have replicated these findings. Research at the Anna Freud centre has shown conclusively that the AAI status of an adoptive parent impacts on the likely success of an adoption, and the attachment status of the adopted child. The carers of avoidant children often have the so-called 'dismissing' state of mind; when describing their own lives their narratives are minimal, often lack information, and at times are not coherent. They might idealize their own parents, might say '*my parents were the best*' but not be able to think of anything good their parents actually did, and indeed often when pushed, give examples of quite harsh parenting (e.g. '*yes my mum was very caring*', yet in the next sentence say '*there was the time when I fell out of a tree and broke my arm and no-one noticed for 4 hours but that's ok*'). The not remembering does not appear to be repression, in the classical Freudian sense; it is *not* about traumas that are pushed out of consciousness. Professor Alan Sroufe (2005) and the Minnesota study group, who have recently published results of a massive longitudinal study, suggest that an avoidant attachment at 1 year might give rise to dissociative patterns throughout childhood and beyond, and the research points to what we might call a 'dis-avowing' of mental life.

These children and adults are 'hard to reach'; we rarely feel they make contact with us or us with them. Their inner worlds can feel rather dead or flat; they often have little fantasy life, little capacity to play, as well as little ability to empathize. They maintain homeostasis by blocking out the other, by not allowing connection. Colozino (2002) suggests that in neuroscientific terms right brain, more emotional functions, might be dissociated from and not very connected to left brain, more rational and logical thinking. These children might be very logical but have little emotional depth. In therapy we often find that they ignore what we say, however empathic or accurate, and just carry on with what they were doing anyway. The children who are avoidant seem not to need social contact, and often make us feel that we are not needed, superfluous.

Sroufe et al. (2005) found mothers of avoidant infants to have negative feelings about being a mother; they tended to be tense and irritable, and engaged in care-giving in a perfunctory manner. Feeding was not adapted to the infant's pace, they were less responsive to the infant's distress, much caretaking was described as routine and unemotional, and they often avoided physical proximity with their children. Decades earlier, Ainsworth had found that these mothers held their children as much as other mothers *except when the infants wanted to be picked up, and then they turned away.* Sroufe and his colleagues have found that the avoidant group showed the most behavior problems at pre-school. They had less capacity for empathy, did not comfort other children in distress in school and nursery, initiated less contact with other children and were less popular. Two securely attached children together rarely fight or indulge in bullying, but there often is bullying when an avoidant child is involved.

It seems likely that, in neuroscientific terms, the avoidant child has a 'dampened down' system, a low level of emotional expression, heightened parasympathetic nervous system, which fits with children who are socially withdrawn, explore less and seek little support from others. As Schore and others argue, early emotional regulation and attuned interactions with caregivers contributes to the organization and integration of neural networks and the consequent capacity for self regulation.

Colozino argues that the securely attached child has a higher degree of neural integration between the emotional and cognitive processing aspects of the brain. There does seem to be some neuroscientific evidence now to this effect; Field (2004) reported research which showed that depressed mothers have high EEG activation in their right frontal parts of their brains, but more startling, that infants as young as one month old show the same pattern. Such EEG patterns also linked with difficult sleeping patterns and more negative affect.

Daniel Siegel (1999) has also attempted to understand avoidant and dismissive patterns in neuroscientific terms. Autobiographical memory is dependent on the frontal cortical regions of the brain, parts of the brain that undergo rapid growth and change in the first few years of life. Rich tales, stories and narratives about their lives can become prominent in more secure children by the third year of life in families. Such autonoetic or autobiographical memory seems to be underdeveloped in dismissing individuals, which makes sense of why these children can so often seem unimaginative and flat, the tapestry of their lives much poorer than those who have easy access to narratives about themselves and their family. Siegel suggests deficits in the right orbitalfrontal region, a brain area that is central to attachment patterns, which also co-ordinates social communication, empathic attunement, emotional regulation, and autonoetic consciousness.

We all of course tend to remember events which have emotional meaning; the dismissive children and adults who are more cutoff from their emotional lives will not 'red-flag' events to be remembered in the same way. Gross and Richards (2000), for example, asked 57 volunteers to watch an emotive film about a surgical procedure and then asked them about how they were feeling, how much effort they put into hiding their emotions and how much they remembered about the film. The people who said they had put the most effort into hiding their emotional response to the film had the worst recall for what they had seen.

It is maybe worth flagging up a differentiation between 2 different groups of children who suffer emotional neglect. Tiffany Field's research (2004) on mothers who are depressed distinguishes between children of more intrusive mothers, which maybe linked to cases Lynda Miller describes, as opposed to the children of more withdrawn depressed mothers, who I am focusing on. Unfortunately, of the two samples, Field found that the withdrawn mothers interact in ways that are less likely to foster both emotional and cognitive development than the intrusive ones. These mothers were less likely to have insight into or awareness of the effect of their interactions. Intrusive mothering led to more abuse, whereas withdrawn mothering led to more neglect.

Even looking at neonates, those of withdrawn mothers did worse on most scores. All the depressed mothers had higher than average cortisol levels, but the withdrawn ones had lower dopamine levels, and also their newborns had lower dopamine levels than the intruded upon! Low dopamine and high cortisol is also a risk factor for premature delivery, and so can make the cycle worse. The withdrawn mothers and their infants also had lower serotonin levels.

Interestingly, the infants of intrusive mothers spent 55% of their time avoiding their mothers, whereas the infants of withdrawn mothers watched their mothers less than 5% of the time. The laboratory research showed that infants of the withdrawn mothers were inactive and spent a lot of time staring, whereas the infants of intrusive mothers fussed a lot. Boys were seen as particularly vulnerable to the lack of parenting as they are less able to regulate themselves and seem to need more input. These babies who are inactive and stare can become the children who get lost at school and who teachers and others barely notice.

Furthermore, infants of intrusive parents generally showed more exploratory behaviour than their withdrawn counterparts at one year, and also did better on most developmental tests. By 3 years old the children of withdrawn carers were not showing empathy, were showing more internalizing behaviors (compared to the externalizing behaviors of the children of intrusive mothers) and their form of non-empathy is more passive and withdrawn, compared to the aggressive lack of empathy in children of intrusive parenting.

These infants lack stimulation, as well as suffering from dysregulation, and they are stimulated less than the intruded upon ones, who did better cognitively. So what is happening here? This is a different form of tragedy from that suffered by abused children. These children have not been regulated by others, and have to protect themselves by, as Beebe found, doing much more self-regulation; other categories of children, such as anxious ambivalent ones, expect a continuation of the inconsistent caring they have often received, and have to regulate other people, and take care to prevent intrusion, impingement, even attack, to ensure they are safe and not overwhelmed.

Beebe found that these avoidant infants did not manage positive affect well, and when interactions with their mothers were more positive, the avoidant infants would be 'cocked for escape', and indulged in much more self-soothing. They are over-aroused by positive interactions and so energetically self-regulate, or in ordinary language they could not experience much pleasure without being overwhelmed. This contrasted with secure infants who held the gaze of caregivers without looking away or self-soothing. The avoidant ones self-sooth much more when distressed, but also need to maintain more self-soothing behaviors when in contact with their mothers, in order to maintain the contact and Beebe found that self-regulatory disturbance at 4 months predicted insecure attachment at a year and less responsiveness to mothers' vocalizations at 2 years. As they are less responsive to the others' language, Beebe suggests that their language will be imbued with less dyadically shared meaning. Beebe sees the strategies adopted by avoidant children as a compromise between the need to maintain engagement with a partner and a need to protect what she calls 'organismic integrity', and to manage arousal levels.

This partly explains why these are the children who become more passive, with less belief in their capacity to make things happen, and less sense of their own agency. In Tronik's classic 'still-face' experiment, when mothers interacting ordinarily with their infants suddenly are told to become still and not interact, their infants show distress and try hard to woo their mothers back. Field showed that, unlike the normal samples, infants of depressed mothers hardly reacted at all. The withdrawn infants expect less from others, are less interested in other people so will also not develop skills at imitation, or at being socially responsive.

To conclude, early relationships hugely influence a child's developing brain and personality. Attuned caregivers who are in touch with a child's emotional states, who help children feel safe while exploring and discovering new things, are laying a strong foundation from which their children can grow up to be happy, confident adults. Conversely, caregivers who are absent emotionally, or who offer little to help infants and children manage both enjoyable or stressful situations, can be laying the foundation of future problems, for these 'doubly' neglected children.

References

Ainsworth MDS, MC Blehar, E Waters, S Wall: Patterns of attachment: A psychological study of the strange situation. Erlbaum, Hillsdale, N.J. 1978

Beebe B, F Lachman: Infant research and Adult Treatment. Analytic Press, New Jersey 2002

Bick E: The experience of the skin in early object relations. International Journal of Psycho-Analysis 49 (1968) 484–6

Bion WR: Second Thoughts. Heinemann, London 1967

Bowlby J: The making and breaking of affectional bonds. Tavistock Publications, London 1979

Brazelton TB, B Koslowski, M Main: The origins of reciprocity: the early mother-infant interaction. In: Lewis M, LA Rosenblum (eds): The Effect of the Infant on its Caregiver. Wiley, New York 1974

Chisholm K, M Carter, E Ames, S Morison: Attachment security and indiscriminately friendly behaviour in children adopted from Romanian orphanages. Developmental and Psycho pathology 7 (1995) 285–294

Colozino L: The neuroscience of psychotherapy. WW Norton, New York 2002

Field TM: Early interactions between infants and their postpartum depressed mothers. Infant Behaviour and Development 25 (1) (2002) 25–38

Field T: Prenatal depression effects on the foetus and neonate. In: Nadel J, D Muir (eds): Emotional Development: Recent Research Advances. Oxford University Press, Oxford 2004

Fonagy P et al.: Measuring the ghost in the nursery: a summary of the main findings of the Anna Freud Centre. Bulletin of the Anna Freud Centre, London 1991

Geertz C: The Interpretation of Cultures. Basic Books, New York 1973

Richards JM, JJ Gross: Emotion regulation and memory: The cognitive costs of keeping one's cool. Journal of Personality and Social Psychology 79 (2000) 410–424

Hodges J: The natural history of early non-attachment. In: Bernstein B, J Brannen (eds): Children, Research, and Policy. Taylor and Francis, London 1996

Main M, N Kaplan, J Cassidy: Security in infancy, childhood and adulthood: A move to the level of representation. In: Bretherton I, E Waters (eds): Growing points in attachment theory and research. Monographs of the Society for Research in Child Development 50 (209) (1985)

Meltzoff AN: Immediate and deferred imitation in fourteen- and twenty-four-month old Infants. Child development 56 (1985) 62–72

Murray L: Intersubjectivity, object relations theory, and empirical evidence from mother-infant interactions. Infant Mental Health Journal 12 (3) (1991) 219–232

Pally R: Mind-Brain relationship. Karnac, London 2000

Rizzolatti G, L Craighero: The mirror-neuron system. Annual review of neuroscience 27 (2004) 169–192

Schore AN: Neurobiology, developmental psychology and psychoanalysis: convergent findings on the subject of projective identification. In: Edwards J (ed): Being Alive. Building on the work of Anne Alvarez. Brunner-Routledge, London 2001

Siegel DJ: The developing mind: toward a neurobiology of interpersonal experience. The Signal. Newsletter of the world association for infant mental health 6 (3–4) (1999) 1–11

Smyke AT, A Dumitrescu, CH Zeanah: Attachment Disturbances in Young Children. I: The Continuum of Caretaking Casualty. Journal of the American Academy of Child and Adolescent Psychiatry 41 (8) (2002) 972–982

Steele M, J Kaniuk, J Hodges, C Haworth, S Huss: The use of the Adult Attachment Interview: Implications for assessment in Adoption and Foster Care. http://www.annafreud-centre.org/baaf.htm

Sroufe LA, B Egeland, E Carlson, WA Collins: The Development of the Person: The Minnesota Study of Risk and Adaptation from Birth to Adulthood. Guilford Publications, New York 2005

Tronik E: Dynamically expanded States of Consciousness. Infant Mental Health Journal 19 (1998)

Trevarthan C: Playing into reality: conversations with the infant communicator. Winnicott Studies 7 (1993) 67–84

19b. Psychic growth and reciprocity: Psychoanalytical infant observation and socio-cultural factors

Lynda Miller; The Tavistock and Portman NHS Trust, London, United Kingdom

It is generally accepted today by professionals involved in the study of infants from a variety of theoretical perspectives that the healthy emotional and cognitive development of a baby is dependent upon a nurturing environment at both physical and psychological levels. Recent research in the fields of neuroscience, of developmental psychology, and of psychoanalytically informed infant observation studies all point in this direction.

Sue Gerhardt (2004), a psychoanalytic psychotherapist and co-founder of the Oxford Parent Infant Project brings together findings from the fields of neuroscience, psychology, and psychoanalysis. She explains why parental love is essential for healthy brain development in infancy, and how interactions between babies and their parents have a major impact in this respect. Gerhardt writes: "… the poorly handled baby develops a more reactive stress response and different biochemical patterns from a well-handled baby." (p. 15). The psychic growth of an infant can only be convincingly understood in the context of a dependent, reciprocal relationship between a baby and its parents.

I will focus upon infants raised in a middle-class western cultural context and draw attention to current socio-cultural trends that tend to undervalue what we know about the importance of dependency and reciprocity as being essential for healthy infant development.

Pamela Sorenson (2005) of the Under Fives Study Center, Virginia, USA writes about basic cultural assumptions that may underlie parental views of what is important for positive emotional and cognitive development of children in the USA, and I think her ideas are also applicable to some countries in Western Europe. I will use material taken from infant observations presented in seminars that I have led in both Italy and the UK, which have been carried out using a psychoanalytic framework of thinking.

In her description of North American society, Sorenson (2005) writes: "Americans value autonomy, independence and self reliance … The imagery associated with this mentality persists and permeates American culture." Sorenson describes the way in which there has been a surge in the marketing of toys and videos which teach without the need for human contact, adding that "… the idea of the autonomous learner is idealized in American culture". I think that there has been a similar promotion of such toys in western Europe, accompanied by an increase in TV programs aimed at a very young audience, with a distinctly 'educational' emphasis. This cultural trend, in that it encourages independence (or one could argue, pseudo-independence) from a very early age, runs in direct opposition to the notion, borne out by scientific research and observation, that dependency on a reliable, protective, receptive care-giver is the salient requirement for sound development.

Wilfred Bion's (1962) concept of the 'container and the contained' provides us with a psychoanalytic model of the mind in which reciprocity is the basis of all learning, both emotional and cognitive. In this model, the infant's states of mind, his desires and frustrations, are communicated to a receptive and understanding parent, initially at a primitive level then later verbally. The containing parent receives and processes these raw communications in her mind, and conveys them back to the baby, now imbued with meaning and in a tolerable form. I hope to illustrate, using infant observation material, different modes of reciprocity in play situations, in which the parent is either predominantly receptive or containing in relation to the baby, or by contrast seems to be pushing the baby towards independence, tending to deny dependency needs. All the extracts are from observations carried out by students in the UK and in Italy, as part of their pre-clinical training.

The first example is of baby Harriet and her mother Susan, using two extracts of observations, the first from when Harriet was five months old, then at age nine months. In this observation Harriet, at five months, had just awoken from a sleep. The observer wrote:

"*Harriet grabbed a rattle and shook it then dropped it and reached for a soft fabric ring that she also shook. The ring didn't make a noise and she dropped it and tried another, larger ring, which did make a noise. As she did this, she looked up at me and smiled, and I felt she was enjoying her newfound skills. Susan rejoined us and told me that the rings were part of a new stacking toy. Apparently Harriet had not liked the toy, although Susan wondered if she had been tired, as she had been introduced to it just before her sleep. Susan sat down next to Harriet and by this time Harriet was smiling, laughing and talking, and looking from one of us to the other, tending to linger longer on me. Harriet reached out towards the base of the toy, and Susan passed it to her. Susan then picked up all the stacking pieces putting them near Harriet. Some of the rings made a crunching noise when squeezed, others a rattling noise when shaken. Harriet seemed to become increasingly frustrated when handling the rings, making a cry-like noise and looking to Susan. Susan did not seem to feel (as I did), that this was frustration, wondering instead if Harriet was uncomfortable in her nappy. She decided to change her.*"

In this observation, Susan lets the observer know that Harriet had not initially liked this 'educational' toy (stacking rings in order of size) yet she can enjoy playing with it in her own way, when mother left the room. On her return Susan has another attempt at introducing the stacking toy to Harriet who now (according to the observer who attends carefully to Harriet's cries) again expresses her frustration with this toy. Susan does not seem to register this.

Here is Harriet again, four months later, aged nine months. The observer wrote:

"Susan picked Harriet up out of her chair and took her over to the enclosure. She sat her down on the sheepskin next to the toy box. Harriet reached into the box and pulled out a beany toy, a dog. Susan found the rabbit that she had bought for Harriet. Harriet held up the dog next to the rabbit before taking the rabbit from her mother. It felt as if she was comparing them. She offered the dog to Susan and then to me, but withdrew her hand almost immediately; Susan said 'it's the thought that counts!' Harriet found an empty tennis ball tube. She banged on the lid, turned it round and used her fingertip to explore the other plastic end. She kept turning it round from one end to the other. She banged it again and Susan gave her the little drums. Harriet copied Susan hitting the drums and then returned to the tennis ball tube. Eventually, she put it down and found a ball, carefully putting her fingertip onto the valve where the pump would connect."

In this observation a more reciprocal two-way interaction between mother and baby is evidenced, involving mirroring and imitation. Maria Rhode (2005), professor of child psychotherapy at the Tavistock Clinic, differentiates between developmental imitation of this kind, and mimicry which is non- developmental.

Susan allows Harriet the freedom to choose which toys she wants to play with, and in which way, that is not necessarily for the purpose for which they were designed. Her play is creative and experimental. Susan follows her daughter's lead, offering similar toys to those Harriet has chosen (the rabbit, the drums) perhaps with an educational intention in that drums are made for banging, tennis ball tubes are not, but Susan joins in with Harriet, interacting with her without coercing or forcing her own agenda. It seems to me that Susan is able to locate her natural wish to educate her child, that is for Harriet to develop emotionally and cognitively, in the reciprocal relationship between parent and baby in which the mother can be sensitive to her infant's need to experiment and to explore, at the same time as leading her onwards by providing a stimulating environment.

In 1988 Meira Likierman, a consultant child psychotherapist at the Tavistock Clinic, wrote a paper about maternal love and positive projections. She wanted to draw attention to "*... an aspect of maternal love which has not been emphasized in psycho-analytical theory, and which represents the mother's projections of her own loving emotions rather than her ability to receive her infant's projected feelings*". For the purpose of our current theme, I want to differentiate between the value of positive projections as evidenced in the reciprocal relationship between Susan and Harriet, and negative maternal projections. Likierman (1988) points out that a mother has a need to express her own loving emotions and to have these valued and confirmed by her baby. She adds that the mother's self-expressive needs in fact contribute to infant development, and that this is part of a mother's function in a reciprocal relationship, alongside her capacities to receive, contain and feed back in a more manageable form, her infant's communications. Returning to the infant observation extract above, Susan needs to participate in her baby's play as a means of expressing her love and her desire for her baby to develop healthily. This is entirely different from a mother's need to forcefully intrude into, direct and control her baby's play, which it can be argued is based on a negative maternal projection. Of positive projections, Likierman (1988) writes: "*…the mother's primitive transferential love for her infant has the important function of transmitting to it positive feelings which are not his own, and which he has not demanded by crying. They do 'intrude' into him, but offer a pleasure that is not of his own making, an unexpected gift, as it were. It gives the infant an experience of receiving, as opposed to the experience of earning and demanding pleasure*".

In the infant observation material that follows, I think it is possible to see a complex mixture of positive and negative projections from the mother, Claudia, towards her baby, Laura. The observer described this mother as warm and friendly, yet also very needy. The mother talked to the observer about her own feelings to the extent that the task of observation sometimes became very difficult, the observer's attention being torn between mother and baby. Claudia was clearly delighted by her daughter Laura; her intelligence, her impressive capacity to learn and to achieve her milestones early. Claudia confided that she herself had been 'a boring baby', apparently her own mother's words, and Claudia was determined that Laura would be quite the opposite.

The following observation took place when Laura was one and a quarter years old. The observer wrote: "*Laura picked up a toy which was a box with four geometric holes and four geometric squares. With great concentration she picked up a square and tried to put it in a wrong hole, while Claudia was looking at her to see if Laura could do that. She helped Laura to put it in a correct hole and said 'She knows how to put the circle in a correct hole'. Claudia then gave Laura a circle and she placed it correctly.*"

In discussing this observation the seminar group thought that mother's neediness is reflected in her wish for Laura to perform, to show her intelligence and to be successful. This could be understood in terms of mother's internal view of herself as the boring baby of a critical mother. A negative maternal projection would arise if mother felt that Laura was a boring baby. This would be intolerable to Claudia, who has constantly to prove to herself and to the observer that this is not so.

The next extract from the observation of Laura is from when she was one and a half years old. The observer wrote: "*Mother said 'Laura, let's go to show J your new pair of shoes'. Laura quickly left Claudia's room, went to her own room and opened the bottom drawer of her chest of drawers and picked up a pair of smart red leather shoes. Claudia proudly said 'Well done Laura'. Laura tried to put on one shoe. Claudia said 'No Laura, they are too big for you. Don't use them yet, you need to wait longer'.*"

Mother's need for Laura to be unrealistically clever is also evident; she expects her to understand that the new shoes are too big and that she should not wear them yet, rather than being able to respond to Laura's pleasure in the new shoes.

Here is a final extract from the observation of Laura when she was nearly one and three quarter years old: "*Claudia stood up, turned off the TV and said that she would put on music from a CD. When she turned off the TV Laura started to whimper and Claudia told her that she would have nice music because the Tweenies was boring. Laura whimpered and stared at her mother. Claudia picked up a big plastic bag that contained building blocks and said 'Lets go to play with this Laura'. Claudia put them on the floor and started to build something with the blocks. Laura looked at her mother's building, trying to do the same. She put her blocks onto Claudia's and her mother said 'We are building a very high construction'. As the building grew Laura stood up and was still adding blocks when the construction fell on the floor and Laura laughed. She started another one, pushed it over and then repeated the operation. Claudia said 'Laura, let's try to separate the blocks by colors'. Laura stared at her mother who was teaching her the colors of the blocks. While she was doing this Laura was putting the blocks in the bag and trying to separate them in the same way as her mother, but unsuccessfully.*"

In this observation an immediate link comes to mind; the Tweenies is Laura's favorite TV program yet Claudia switches it off and says it is boring. Claudia's anxiety that Laura will be a boring baby, just as her own mother reportedly described Claudia's infancy, drives her to try to make sure that Laura plays educational games that will develop her intellect. Claudia also of course loves her daughter and allows her space to knock the building block tower over and enjoy doing so, but Claudia cannot resist directing and organizing her play.

At the end of this extract Laura is trying to imitate her mother. This raises the question as to whether this is a "developmental imitation" (Rhode, 2005) or a kind of conformity brought about through a feeling of being under pressure.

It will be apparent that in neither of the mother-baby reciprocal relationships described above does there exist a pure culture of either positive or negative projections but rather two different mixtures of both. I suggest that it is only problematic for development if negative projections predominate, and especially if prevailing cultural norms foster the tendency in parents to control and pressurize their babies.

A brief comparison of Western and Eastern cultures with regard to parent-infant relationships adds another perspective on different attitudes and practices. Aronson (2004), writing on the subject of the differences between Asian and western culture cites research carried out by cultural psychologists, Markus and Kitayama, who identify a strong emphasis on connection, relatedness and interdependence in family patterns in Asian countries. By contrast they found that in North America and in many European countries high value is placed on individuation, a process whereby people strive to achieve autonomy, independence and self-reliance. Aronson quotes an example of this distinction noted by Kim Insoo Berg, family therapist: in Korea, with its emphasis on social connectedness, children are punished by being put outside the house – an enforced separation from the family, whereas in the West, where the emphasis is on independence, the favorite punishment of children in our times is to be 'grounded', that is, to be kept inside the home with the family!

In Asian countries, except in large modern cities where Western values increasingly tend to predominate, the involvement of the extended family in child rearing is in stark contrast to the nuclear family of the West. In an infant observation carried out in London, a student presented to the seminar group her observations of a family in which a white English woman had married an Indian man, who felt strongly that their children should be raised in a manner that incorporated traditional Indian family values. His parents arrived from India shortly before the birth of their first child, a son, and stayed with the new parents for six months in their tiny apartment. The grandmother played a dominant role in nurturing the baby and the seminar group empathized with the mother, who seemed to be doing her best to manage the situation, yet clearly found it difficult. She would retreat to another room to breast-feed her son, and this was the only time she had alone with him. The weekly observations were filled with accounts of grandmother cuddling and playing with the baby, whilst mother cooked traditional Indian meals for the family, and returned part-time to work in order to pay the rent (her husband was a student).

When the grandparents returned to India the seminar group breathed a sigh of relief, thinking that at last the mother would be able to get to know her baby. This indeed was the case and the baby seemed to have made a close bond with his mother in his early life, despite spending so much time with his grandmother. Then father announced that he would be taking the little boy to India for six weeks, so that he could be with his grandparents and extended family for his first birthday. Mother would have to stay behind to earn money. Again the seminar group felt very concerned about the impact of this separation on mother and baby.

During the six weeks absence the observer visited the mother who missed her son and her husband very much and seemed depressed. The seminar group anticipated that the re-uniting of mother and baby after the trip might give rise to complex, perhaps conflicting feelings. We wondered if the little boy would be confused in light of the attachments he had made to his mother and to his grandmother, and whether the loss of each of them in turn would leave him unsure about who was his main caregiver. It was a salutary experience for the seminar group to find that on his return to London this little boy had no difficulty in re-establishing a close, loving relationship with his mother, but had reportedly also loved being with his extended family in India. Doubtlessly he had missed both his mother and his grandmother when separated from them, but this did not have a detrimental effect on his capacity to sustain a secure attachment.

Leng (2005) gives a moving account of filming an infant observation in a Hindu family in rural Nepal. This formed part of a research project led by Barnett based on cross-cultural observation videos and studying emotional development. Leng writes: "... *individual identity remains a Western concept and family identities in Nepalese culture differ from those in the West*". She describes the way in which the baby, a girl, was usually held by members of the extended family and she writes: "*Hindu child rearing is reliant on the support of the extended family and other family members are readily on hand to hold the baby. She grew to be a very sociable baby and her stimulation came from being touched, held and included*". Leng reflects on the mother's role in this traditional village community: "*To the extent that individual identity remains a Western concept, I had never felt her to be the maternal centre around which this family gathered*".

This baby was the fourth girl in a family with as yet no boys, so her birth would be seen as inauspicious in a society where sons are valued more than daughters. This may have been a factor in the mother's observed depression following the birth. Here it seemed that a baby could benefit from the warmth and liveliness of the extended family that may also be a support for a depressed mother.

As a final example of cultural differences in the child-parent relationship I will turn to a biographic source. In his autobiography "Freedom in Exile" the fourteenth Dalai Lama of Tibet describes a painful and unhappy period of his life when aged three years he had to leave his parents and his family home, in accord with cultural expectations, to begin life in a monastery. He writes: "*It is very hard for a small child to be separated from his parents.*" but later he adds "*When I was very young, I developed a close attachment to the Master of the Kitchen. So strong was it that he had to be in my sight at all times, even if it was only the bottom of his robe visible through a doorway or under the curtains which served as doors inside Tibetan houses. Luckily, he tolerated my behavior. He was a very kind and simple man, and almost completely bald. He was not a very good storyteller, nor an enthusiastic playmate, but this did not matter one bit. I have often wondered since about our relationship. I see it now as being like the bond between a kitten or some small animal and the person who feeds it. I sometimes think that the act of bringing food is one of the basic roots of all relationships.*"

In conclusion, attachment considered in a non-Western cultural context needs to include the model of the child in a large extended family and even in a monastic community. This can be interestingly contrasted with attachment patterns in the nuclear family and single parent family characteristic of Western society. Returning to the main theme of this paper, psychic growth and reciprocity, it can be argued that a flexible use of the term attachment needs to be adopted in order to encompass child-rearing practices of other cultures. Furthermore, in the more affluent parts of the USA and of Western Europe, attention needs to be given to the phenomenon of "pseudo-independence" arising out a culturally endorsed situation in which independent learning is promoted by parents at the expense of adequately meeting an infant's dependency needs.

References

Aronson HB: Buddhist Practice on Western Ground. Shambala, Boston 2004

Bion WR: Learning from Experience. Karnac, London 1962

Dalai Lama: Freedom in Exile. Abacus, UK 1992

Gerhardt S: Why Love Matters. Brunner-Routledge, E. Sussex 2004

Leng M: Against the Odds: An account of filming an infant observation in rural Nepal. In: The International Journal of Infant Observation and its Applications 8 (2) (2005)

Likierman M: Maternal Love and Positive Projective Identification. Journal of Child Psychotherapy 14 (2) (1998)

Rhode M: Mirroring, imitation, identification: the sense of self in relation to the mother's internal world. Journal of Child Psychotherapy 31 (1) (2005)

Sorenson PB: Changing positions: helping parents look through the child's eyes. Journal of Child Psychotherapy 31 (2) (2005)

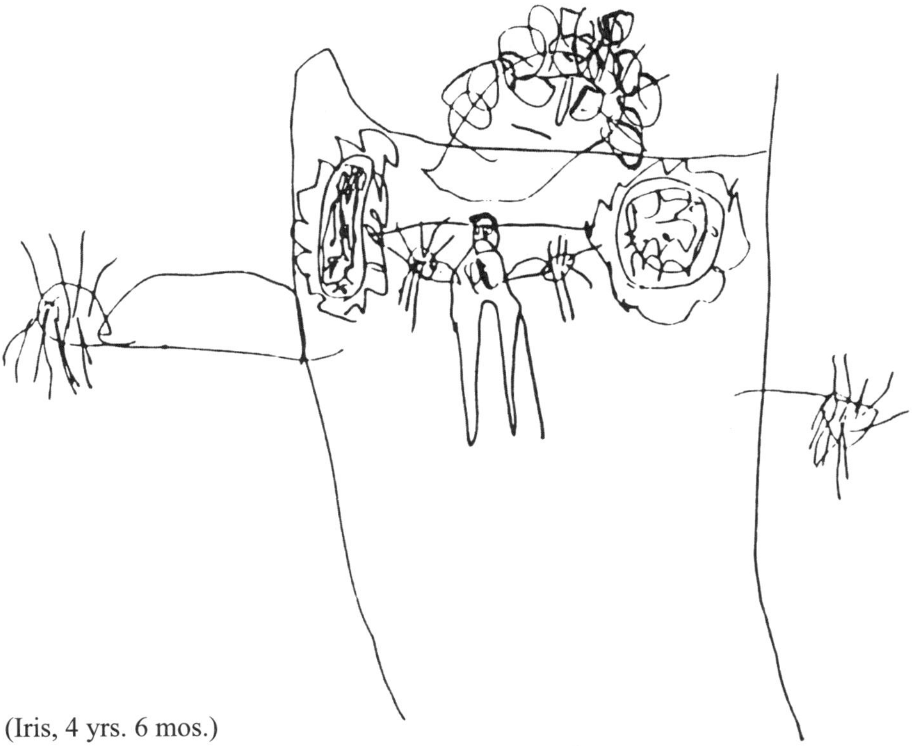

(Iris, 4 yrs. 6 mos.)
Mommy was soft, and I was born because I wanted my mommy.

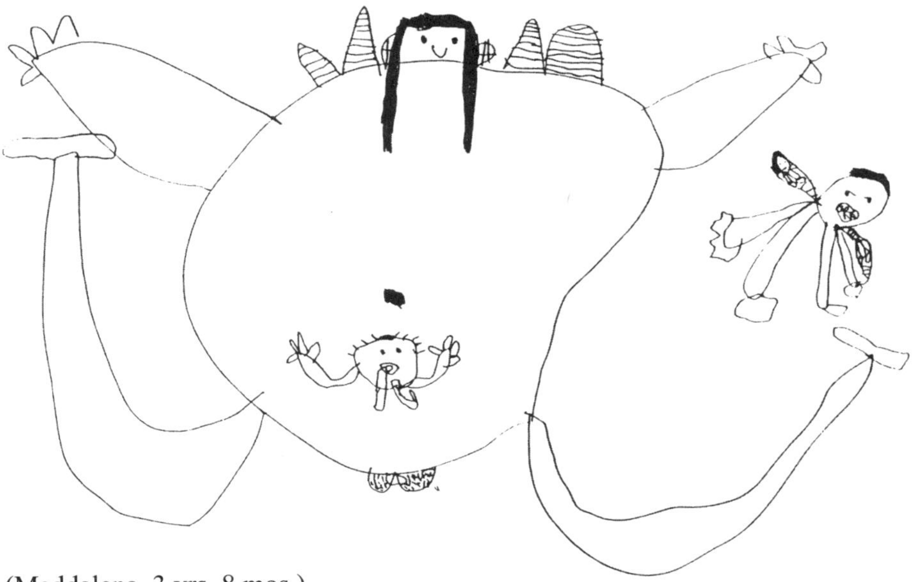

(Maddalena, 3 yrs. 8 mos.)
One day when I was inside her tummy, I smelled the perfume my mommy put on when she got married to my daddy.

20. The complexity of birth: The Cesarean section

Fiorella Monti; Faculty of Psychology, University of Bologna, Italy
Piergiuseppina Fagandini; Department of Motherhood and Infancy, S. Maria Nuova Hospital, Reggio Emilia, Italy
Francesca Agostini; Department of Psychology, University of Bologna, Italy
Daria Vettori; Parma, Italy
Giovanni Battista La Sala; Department of Obstetrics and Gynaecology, S. Maria Nuova Hospital, Reggio Emilia, Italy

Time present and time past
Are both perhaps present in time future
And time future contained in time past
(Thomas Stearns Eliot)

Pregnancy and birth

Parenthood, or the psychological process of becoming a parent, is connected to the parents' infant experiences, to family and social contexts as sources of support, of stress, and to the baby's characteristics which can make parental duties either easier or more difficult.

The birth of a baby undoubtedly inspires memories and emotions associated with the relationships with one's own parent figures, which can hinder or foster their new role. On the other hand, parenthood is linked to both the couple's relationship and the socio-cultural context to which they belong. It is a time for "starting afresh" where the plans of having a baby, of becoming mother and father, involve a long period of developmental crisis in the quest for new balances: maturation crises of identity and psychological readjustment.

For the woman, it is obvious that the biological and psychological reality of pregnancy involves a transformation of her body image, "the real body and the lived body", and her self-identity. The enormous fluctuation in the defensive system leads to a maturation crisis as well as a twofold self-individualization process, "as a daughter to her own mother and a mother to her own child" (Racamier, 1986), and at the same time, the acceptance of the baby which is separate from herself. This double process also takes place in the man who is the son of his own father but is also becoming a father, even if he does not experience the physical and psychological changes and the intense and complex anxieties linked to body transformation and birth. He has the challenging task of supporting the pregnancy in all its stages and then facilitating the mother-baby relationship and the subsequent explorative behavior of the baby by means of supporting the woman, cooperation, and caring.

Pregnancy, therefore, signifies a type of crossroads: genetic code, individual and family history code, and cultural code – all intertwine and influence each other. Thus maternity crosses the imagery in more ways than any other human emotional experience going beyond social changes and cultural adjustment. In the complex course of maternity, if the symbiotic (being mother, mother-baby unit) and individualization-separation (creating a baby, imagining the baby separate from herself) elements integrate, the integrity of her own body is confirmed against fears of damage and starts the tuning of mother-baby affections. If however, they do not integrate, but remain divided, they recall negative affective states, increase genetic (Fornari, 1981) and role anxieties which can permeate the early relationships in an asynchronous and therefore distorted way. "Everything regarding heredity and procreation defines a violently fragile inter-human zone where the most archaic anxieties become fixed and the way is made for the most enigmatic beliefs" (Kaes, 1995).

Pregnancy and birth involve, therefore, the events of the unique communication at the basis of the mother-baby relationship which forms the premises for realizing future relationships and interpersonal transactions: "the effects of the bio-psychological experience in the uterus are seen after birth and they keep and reveal themselves after the birth" (Soulè, 2000). Apart from the mother-fetus interaction influenced both by real and symbolic maternal activity and fetal initiatives, the fundamental nucleus of the psychological and emotional experience of every individual and the basis for subsequent development are formed; as a result, both a biological program and an affective and mental world are transmitted by the mother and adapted by the fetus and then by the newborn, according to its proactive competencies.

Throughout the course of pregnancy, the woman creates physical and mental space for the unborn baby, a space for the mental representations she has of herself as a mother and of her partner as a father for the future baby. The psychological organization which develops during pregnancy or "motherhood constellation" (Stern, 1995), "involves a combination of tendencies, of sensitivity, fantasies, fears and specific desires. It corresponds to three issues: the mother's relationship with her own mother, in particular with her mother as mother of herself as a child, the mother's relationship with herself and the mother's relationship with her baby" (Houzel, 2005). The experience of a pregnant woman with her own baby is very particular in that it is not about perceiving or representing a "being in itself" but a "being inside herself". The tendency to conserve this unity with her child, the instinctive desire to keep it within or with her, accompanies the fear of emptiness or loneliness. Identification with the baby which takes place throughout the entire course of pregnancy creates the fear of separation from the baby not only in terms of "*I'm about to lose the baby*" but also "*the baby's about to lose me*" (Lebovici, 1988).

The biological separation involved with the birth is complex and at times traumatic, from the much expected pregnancy-maternity to the actual birth-maternity, the difficult confrontation with the imagined baby and the real one, and between the imagined parental role and the subsequent real role. The way in which the birth takes place will be remembered (often intensely) even in years to come, particularly the beginning of labor, the breaking of the membranes, the arrival at the hospital, the actions of doctors and obstetricians, the birth and the first contact with the newborn. Therefore, it is likely that this moment is engraved in the mother-baby relationship, at least at the beginning and especially if different conditions than those imagined emerge. "Popular imagery transmits the idea of idyllic and perfect happiness connected to the birth and subsequent period. One should be at the height of happiness and instinctively find the way to become a good mother figure … This imagery does not allow for the presence of elements which contradict it. From the beginning it censors any disappointment, ambivalence or frustration which may be felt." (Cramer, 2000).

The discrepancy between parental aspirations and the psycho-social reality of the post-natal experience and the complexity of neonatal care cause unresolved infantile issues to re-emerge and hinder the transition to parenthood. "The exposure to emotions, touch, smell, sound and taste of every little baby is extremely intense, especially when the caregiver feels vulnerable and hypersensitive. The irresistible nature of this closed contact with a newborn is immediately tricky (...), there is an immediate impact with the inner mother with the eruption of inexplicable emotions, passion, desire, fear, desperation, anger" (Raphael-Leff, 2000).

Such a complex situation often risks being trivialized, idealized or medicalized, and may result in the psychic maternity being unattended to, misunderstood, lonely, and hindering the transition of the mother and father to parenthood.

The development process has to be seen through to the end;
any interruption, any gap left distorts something,
anything rushed or delayed leaves a scar
(Donald Woods Winnicott)

Cesarean section

"Hospital maternity is the modern formula of a universal custom, the place appointed for the birth to take place ... In ancient Jewish customs the baby would be born on sacred stones known as birth bricks. In Rome, in rich, aristocratic families, a part of the house was kept especially for births and when the time came, the husband would give his wife the key at the onset of labor. For the Oceania Arapesh people, the birth takes place in a special village cabin which is different from the normal living huts. The same tradition can be found among the Comanche Indians... in Australian culture, at the first signs of labor, the mother isolates herself in the women's camp accompanied by two female cousins" (Bydlowski, 2004).

Nowadays due to the advancement of obstetrics and changes in social and family structures, the hospital has become the place where the vast majority of births take place. According to recent statistics (ISTAT) (Sabbadini, 2001), almost all Italian women give birth in hospitals: 88.9% in public hospitals, 6% in accredited hospitals, 4.8% in private and only 0.3% at home. A figure emerged revealing the high frequency of Cesarean sections performed on Italian territory, with an average of 35% of births in southern Italy and 38% in in the islands. In private hospitals the proportion reaches 50%, almost double the figure for public hospitals, 27.3% or in accredited hospitals, 30.6% (Sabbadini, 2001). Thus data confirm "a large trend to the medicalization of pregnancy and the excessive employment of the diagnostic checkup" (Sabbadini, 2001).

There is a similar situation in the majority of the so-called "civilized" world. Research carried out by Walker et al. (2004) shows how there was an increase of 35% in Cesarean sections from 1990–2000 with a rate of 23% Cesarean births. There was a similar increase (of 33.34%) over the years 1995–2001 in Taiwan (Tang et al., 2006). In the United States, the New York Maternity Center Association (2004) reported a similar increase: "About 3 women in 10 now give birth by major abdominal surgery. The increase is due to many medical, legal, social, and financial factors, including *defensive medicine* and changing attitudes and values of caregivers and pregnant women"; and in Latin America, especially in Brazil, the percentage exceeds 25% (Barrett et al., 2005). "In some parts of Latin America, Cesarean section by custom or demand is becoming the norm, but in North America and Europe the phenomenon is also growing" (Klein, 2004): between 10%–98% in some regions of Latin America, 26% in United States and Australia (Walker et al., 2004). The rate of Cesarean sections performed has therefore increased by 13% compared to the highest rate fixed by the WHO in 1985 (World Health Organization, 1985). In Italian obstetrics resorting to Cesarean section is routine in the case of breech presentation and previous Cesareans (Signorelli et al., 1995). Neonatal mortality and morbidity factors attributable to the Cesarean section, irrespective of the risks linked to superimposed maternal-fetal pathologies, could relate to neonatal respiratory distress for the inhalation of amniotic fluid and a distorted absorption of alveolar fluid risking persistent pulmonary hypertension in the newborn (Henderson, Love, 1995; Lydon-Rochelle et al., 2000). Some authors confirm an increase in health risks for the mother and baby after the Cesarean birth, especially in the case of inappropriate indication. The use of analgesics and anesthetics which directly reach the placenta can decrease breathing of the newborn and the ability to suck. At best, these behavioral anomalies, generally irrelevant, can have only slight relational consequences, but if the health of the newborn is in any way precarious or the parents are highly stressed about the experience, inadequate interaction between mother, father, and child can develop.

On the basis of studies carried out, the Maternity Center Association (New York, 2004), highlights that a Cesarean section rather than a vaginal birth increases risk for the following problems: *longer hospitalization at the hospital*, *infection* (women with Cesarean generally receive routine antibiotics to try to prevent infection), *pain* (more intense and longer-lasting pain in the first days and weeks after birth), *poor birth experience* (unplanned Cesarean is worse than planned Cesarean), *less early contact with her baby*, *psychological trauma* (unplanned Cesarean poses high extra risk in comparison with planned Cesarean for having traumatic symptoms and for meeting criteria of PTSD, Post-Traumatic Stress Disorder). Besides, a woman who has had a Cesarean may have ongoing pelvic pain, possibly due to scarring and the growth of "adhesion" tissue and she may develop intestinal complications in years after surgery as a result of scarring and abdominal "adhesion" tissue. The physical or emotional problems of mothers as a result of a Cesarean birth may interfere with their ability to take care of their babies. In addition, it is possible to find a higher risk for the following problems in the babies: surgical cuts, respiratory problems, problems in breastfeeding, and asthma. The caregivers may propose a Cesarean for some non-medical reasons: concerns about pelvic floor disorders, profound fear of childbirth, to avoid perineal trauma and to protect sexual function after childbirth. The research does not support these assertions. Outcomes reported by Barrett et al. (2005) provide no basis for advocating Cesarean section, either elective or emergency, for a protective effect on sexual function after childbirth. Furthermore, there is a strong debate about the role of epidural analgesia as a contributor (or not) to the steady increase in the Cesarean section rate: "We knew that early use of epidural analgesia before the fetus was well engaged in the pelvis could cause extension of fetal head, or not allow for flexion, thereby interfering with rotation and descent … It has even led to the suggestion that, since childbirth is already "so unnatural", Cesarean section on request is not such an unreasonable idea, a surgical solution for a non-surgical problem" (Klein, 2006). An American study reported a troubling 63% decline in the rate of vaginal birth after Cesarean delivery from 1996 (28.3%) to 2003 (10.6%) (Lydon-Rochelle et al., 2006).

Psycho-social studies on Cesarean birth show that the procedure cannot just diminish the positive experience of birth but also can elicit negative psychological consequences (Fisher et. al., 1990). Some studies (Prezza et al., 1984) indicated how women, who have major anxieties and fears about birth accumulating in increased stress levels, request a Cesarean section without medical necessity. In a small number of cases this was provoked by the previous experience of a difficult birth. More often than not, these situations underpin the maternal fear of being unable to bear the pain or the fear that birth might cause the severe physical lesions to herself and the baby. "Fear of childbirth is often based on painful, frightening images as portrayed in popular TV programming. And birth, as a normal family-supported event, has been lost in the increasingly isolated nature of modern life" (Klein, 2004). An investigation (Walker et al., 2004) in an Australian community demonstrated that Cesarean section, independent of socio-demographic variables, was perceived as an easy, convenient way of giving birth. But, "Cesarean on demand is not a solution. It is a symptom of a problem. Women are not biologically defective or broken. Rather than spending precious community dollars on a surgical fix for a basic human and deeply personal experience, health professionals need to recognize the central importance of support and the contribution of doulas to improved maternal and newborn outcomes" (Klein, 2004).

Another element which seems to be important in determining the psychological impact of Cesarean is the level to which women believe it to be necessary. A study (Hillan, 1992) of women three months after Cesarean birth revealed that 20% of them did not know the reasons for which they underwent a Cesarean or the reason given was completely misunderstood. A further 16% had only part of the picture. Other studies have been carried out indicating a significant association between male physicians and the high socioeconomic status of patients who requested Cesarean delivery: "Male physicians were more likely to agree to a patient's request for Cesarean delivery than female physicians" (Ghetti et al., 2004).

On the increase of the medicalization of birth and use of Cesarean, the WHO published a series of "Recommendations about birth" (1985–97) highlighting the importance of a support network for the birth event, taking into account familial fears of giving birth and the promotion of the mental health of the unborn and its family: necessity of psychological support during the birth with the possibility for the woman of choosing a trustworthy figure to accompany her during delivery, active participation of the woman both with respect to inherent decisions required during birth and the choice of the most appropriate position to assume during delivery and birth. The maximum rate of Cesarean deliveries should be 15%, to be carried out only in cases of necessity.

The importance of natural birth in recognizing the newborn as child is indirectly confirmed by the greater difficulty encountered by women who have undergone Cesarean sections, especially under general anesthesia. Concrete signs of birth-separation are lacking and women with Cesarean section may be left fantasizing about an incomplete pregnancy, as if they had reached no conclusion (Vegetti Finzi, 1990).

Undoubtedly, Cesarean birth may seem to ease the intense and pervasive emotions surrounding labor and delivery, in the form of a "serene" birth in the expulsive phase, but the "price to pay is often an impression of absence or even extraneousness. Without pain, the birth risks becoming associated with unreality"

(Bydlowski, 2004). Research carried out by Brazelton (1987) had already highlighted that the mother may feel disorientated even if there was a natural birth, but after a Cesarean, especially an emergency procedure and general anesthesia, "not only does her body feel violated after the operation, but there is the impression of being robbed of her own baby". Kendell et al. (1987) indicated how a high number of women undergoing Cesarean sought help from psychological services after the birth, and more recently other authors have confirmed an increase in depression (Edwards et al., 1994) and psychological distress (Reichert et al., 1993; Francome et al., 1993), especially in cases where the Cesarean section was performed under general anesthesia compared to epidural. A metanalysis regarding psychological effects of the Cesarean section (Clement, 2001) indicates in 11 studies major signs of depression in women after Cesarean birth as opposed to natural birth.

An Italian study (Monti et al., 2005) highlighted the psychological consequences of natural and Cesarean birth shortly after the birth also taking into account primiparas and pluriparas. Women who had given birth naturally fared better than women who had undergone a Cesarean in the realm of obsessive-compulsive behavior and phobic anxiety. The pluripara women, on the other hand, who had undergone Cesarean section displayed more depressive and somatic symptoms and paranoid ideation. Often in the case of pluripara, the "active" natural birth is favorable and is a protective factor as opposed to the "passive" Cesarean section which instead becomes a risk factor.

The traumatic connotation of Cesarean section may lead to its definition as an event of multiple stress which only serves to worsen the feelings of inadequacy and anxiety, possibly hindering the first mother-baby encounter and having a negative effect on the "sensitive period" in the attachment phase. The Cesarean is not an "irreversible primary event" but involves a stressful impact on the "planning stages of a relationship in terms of its epigenetic stability" (Holmes, 1993); furthermore, especially if it is an emergency Cesarean performed under general anesthesia, it can increase anxieties and depression experienced by the woman, hindering interaction with the baby and the synchronic development of the mother/baby rhythm and as a result, of the behavioral system involved with attachment.

"The interesting part ... is not ...
the description of a state ... but of a process ...
the "birth" ... in the sense of "taking place";
an event which...may be referred to for all one's life
as a continuous series of "births" and "rebirths",
of eternally becoming, transforming, changing
(Giuliana Giovanelli)

Research

The research undertaken is still in progress and aims to compare couples expecting their first child from the point of view of natural or Cesarean birth. Much literature exists on the impact and consequent psychological experiences but little in the way of couple analysis and over sustained time periods, not just limited to the immediate pre- and postpartum but also taking into account the first few months of the baby's life. The idea for the research to focus on these two aspects comes from the reflections on how (taking a wide range of variables into account) psychological dynamics connected to Cesarean section can be best explored, the frequency of which is unfortunately quite high in Italy.

Methodology

At the current stage of the research, the sample consists of 186 subjects, 67 couples plus additional 52 women for a total of 119 women and 67 men, with an average age of 32.85 years (women 31.9, men 33.8). The subjects were enrolled from the outpatient clinic of the Department of Obstetrics and Gynaecology (Divisione di Ostetricia e Ginecologia) of the Santa Maria Nuova Hospital in Reggio Emilia (Italy) at the 20th–24th pregnancy week. By the time of birth, the average pregnancy period was 39.8 weeks (35 to 42). Of the 119 women, 72.3% had natural births, 27.7% Cesarean sections (18.5% emergency cases and 9.2% planned) for the following reasons:

Emergency Cesareans: 40.9% lack of dilation, 50% fetal distress, 9.1% gestosis; Planned Cesareans: 36.3% breech presentation, 27.3% maternal disease, 9.1% prenatal diagnosis of bradycardia, 27.3% explicit psychological reasons. Only 2 of the women resorted to epidural anesthesia during natural birth whereas all the women who underwent Cesarean section had an epidural apart from one woman who was put under general anesthesia. There were obstetric complications in 22.2% of the births (e.g. lack of dilation, fetal distress, hemorrhage, gestosis, etc.): 15.9% in the case of emergency Cesarean, 2.5% in planned Cesarean and 1.7% in natural births.

53.4% of the newborns were girls. A recovery period was necessary for 5.1% of the newborns but only 3.6% reported a serious pathology requiring prolonged hospital stay.

The *control sample* of this ongoing research consists of women who gave birth naturally and their partners, when present (136 subjects: 86 women + 50 men). The *study group* consists of all women who had Cesarean births and their partners (50 subjects: 33 women + 17 men). Analyzing the main socio-demographic characteristics of the sample and comparing the couples in which the women had natural births and those in which the women had a Cesarean section, no significant differences emerge with regard to the place of origin (majority coming from northern Italy), marital status (majority married), education (many had a degree and high school diploma), profession (over 50% dependent workers), participation in prenatal classes (majority attended). All couples were followed from the 20th–24th week until 3 months after birth.

The first stage was to contact the outpatients of the Department of Obstetrics and Gynaecology (Divisione di Ostetricia e Ginecologia) of the Santa Maria Nuova Hospital in Reggio Emilia during the 20th–24th week of pregnancy. At this point, along with signing an informed consent form, each participant compiled one questionnaire about depression and another about anxiety. Between the 30th and 32nd weeks, the same psychologist met with the subjects again, giving them the same questionnaires on depression and anxiety, and carried out an interview of the mental representations of parents during pregnancy – the IRMAG (maternal representations) and the Ra.Pa.G (paternal representations).

Within the first 5 days after the birth, the psychologist who handed out the questionnaires contacted the subjects at hospital. The last meeting took place at home 3 months after the birth: the above mentioned questionnaires and the interviews on maternal and paternal representations after the birth (IMARP and Ra.Pa.G, respectively) were handed out.

These steps were chosen on the basis of various psychological aspects of pregnancy in association with hospital organization. The 20th–24th pregnancy week corresponds to the time when the morphological ultrasound takes place, which allows the fetus to be "seen" during the period when fetal movements begin to be felt. The mother "with the ultrasound, humanizes the baby's photograph with her uncertain surroundings with fantasies and memories" (Bydlowski, 2000). Furthermore, the couples often attend the morphological ultrasound together and there is the possibility of introducing the research project and, once agreed upon, the tests can be given out. Subsequently, the couples are contacted again around the 30th–32nd week, coinciding with a hospital check-up for the beginning of the third trimester. At this stage there has been no "invasion" of anxieties about the birth and if there are no psychopathological situations, this period is characterized by the narration of representations, the imaginary baby who has a place in the body and mind of the mother. The third meeting usually takes place at the hospital, or definitely in the first few days after birth, where the meeting with the real baby is shadowed by maternity blues, the normal biopsychological reaction to the experience of birth. The last meeting, at 3–4 months after birth, is at home or at hospital, allowed the registering of the parental representations, the comparison between imagined and real baby, the period in which the normal "retirement" phase should have come to an end and the mother-baby proto-conversation begun.

The research tools included the semi-structured interview carried out between the 20th–24th weeks which provided information as to nationality, age, education, profession, etc. the EPDS, ASQ-IPAT, and the interview on representations. The *Edinburgh Postnatal Depression Scale (EPDS)* by Cox et al. (1987), is a self-evaluation questionnaire for the "*screening*" of the symptoms surrounding postnatal depression (PND). The validated Italian version (Benvenuti et al., 1999) uses a cut-off of 8/9, for the screening and detection milder forms of symptoms, whereas the 12/13 cut-off is used for the research and detection of major depression, which then needs to be diagnosed by means of psychiatric or clinical interview. The ASQ-*Ipat Anxiety Scale* by Krug et al. (1976), is a self-compiled questionnaire that provides information about the general levels of anxiety, latent anxiety, and manifest anxiety. *The interview on maternal representations in pregnancy* (IRMAG, Ammaniti et al., 1995) and that on the *paternal representations in pregnancy,* modeled on IRMAG (Ra.Pa.G, Giannone et al., 2002), are structured in a way suitable for the period between the 28th and 32nd weeks' gestation. They include 5 lists of adjectives which allow a guided description of the representation by means of assessing the significance attributed by the mother/father with regard to 5 concepts or characters: the baby her/himself, the partner, her/himself as mother/father, her/his own mother/father. These lists constructed on the model of semantic differential are presented in the form of a graphic scale, consisting of pairs of adjectives of opposite meanings. The first three adjective lists consider the individual characteristics of the baby, of the woman and partner, including 17 adjective pairs referring to "aspects of personal functioning, interpersonal style and affective orientation" (Ammaniti et al., 1995). The other two lists, which refer to the maternal/paternal characteristics of themselves and also of their own mother/father, consist of 17 adjective pairs referring to affections, personal functioning, parental role, and parental sensitivity, allowing the revelation of how much the mother and her partner wish to resemble the maternal and paternal roles already experienced or differentiate them, creating their own "parental style". In the current research only the semantic differences in the data regarding IRMAG and Ra.Pa.G are presented. At the end of the finding of possible differences between the Natural Birth (NB) and Cesarean Section (CS) groups, the data obtained from EPDS (the exact Fisher test and log-linear analysis) and ASQ-IPAT through ANOVA were compared.

Results

Depressive symptoms

Due to the fact that the research is yet incomplete (currently the numbers in the CS group are too low), only some aspects are analysed. The results relevant to the depressive symptoms between the NB and CS groups are briefly discussed below. At the first meeting, at the 20th–24th week, 22.1% of the NB group have some depressive symptom as opposed to only 2% of the CS group ($p < 0.0005$). The log-linear analysis conducted took the gender of the parent into account, with 23.5% of women showing these symptoms as opposed to 4.5% of men, irrespective of the groups.

At the second pre-partum meeting, the NB group has a 25% depression rate compared to 2% of the CS group ($p < 0.0005$). Again the log-linear analyses show a rate of 25.2% among women compared to 7.5% of men irrespective of the study groups. The change occurs postpartum: in the first few days after birth, 25.7% show signs of depression in the NB group compared to 16% of the CS group, of insignificant difference. Log-linear analyses detect depressive symptoms in 31% of women compared to 9% of men, irrespective of the groups. At the final follow-up meeting, 20.6% of NB subjects are depressive compared to 10% of the CS group, an insignificant difference. Again the women emerge more depressive in general terms (22.7% vs. 9%), irrespective of the groups.

Apart from the data regarding the global sample, it was interesting to analyze the difference between women who had a natural birth or Cesarean section. In this case, the distinction was between mild (cut-off EPDS 8/9) and severe (cut-off EPDS 12/13). Comparing the NB and CS women based on mild depressive symptoms, there is a significant difference between the two groups at the 1st and 2nd meetings, where the NB women report more depressive symptoms (Figure 1).

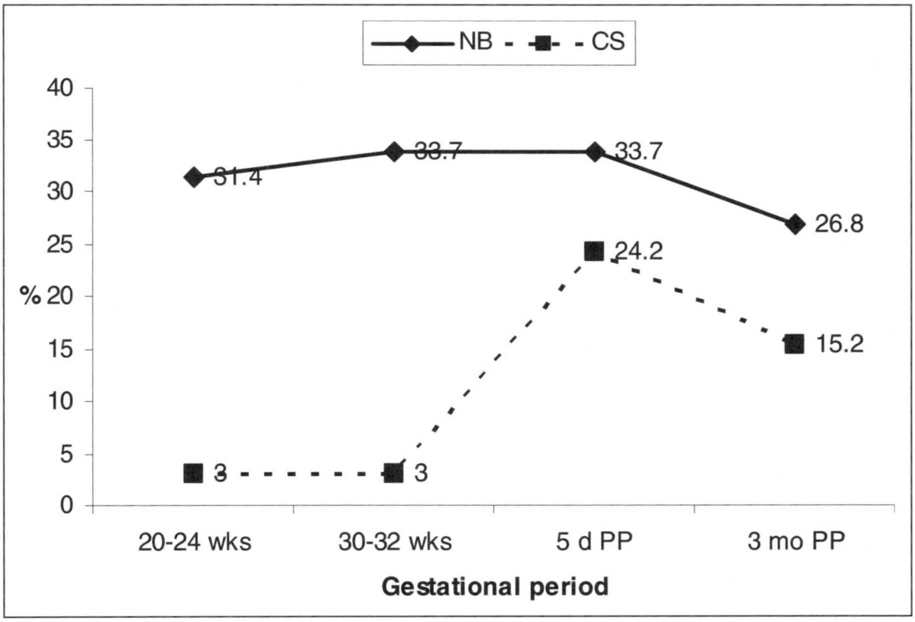

Figure 1. Proportion of depressed women (EPDS cut-off 8/9).
CS = Cesarean section, NB = natural birth, PP = postpartum

In the postpartum period there is a definite increase in the percentage of CS women with mild depressive symptoms without a significant difference between them and the NB women, even at the fourth meeting. If the women with more

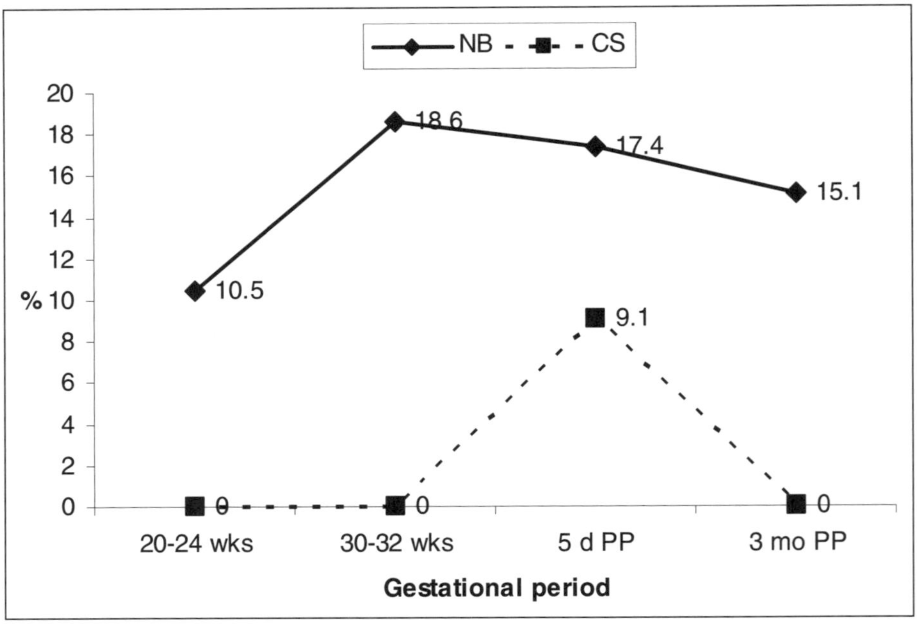

Figure 2. Proportion of depressed women (EPDS cut-off 12/13).
CS = Cesarean section, NB = natural birth, PP = postpartum

severe depressive symptoms are analyzed (cut-off EDPS 12/13; Figure 2), it is possible to detect how during the antepartum stages, there is a distinct difference between NB women (higher proportion of depression) and CS (none of the women had a severe depressive symptom) is maintained; in the postpartum period, the marked increase in the proportion of CS women with severe depressive symptoms can be seen, which after 3 months however, returns to the antepartum levels.

In the women-only sample, the CS group can be further divided into emergency and planned CS. Comparing the NB women and the emergency CS women, at the 3rd meeting, a significant increase emerges in the percentage of depression in the emergency CS women, reaching a similar value to the NB women (Figure 3). At the 3 months stage this percentage decreases, not reaching the antepartum values. As regards severe depressive symptoms (Figure 4) the percentage of depressive CS women clearly increases at the 3rd meeting, reaching the antepartum values at the 3rd month.

Comparing NB women with planned CS women, the number of CS women with mild depressive symptoms increases between the 2nd and 3rd meetings and 3rd and 4th (Figure 5). In the case of severe depressive symptoms, however, no CS woman displays any results as opposed to the NB women (Figure 6).

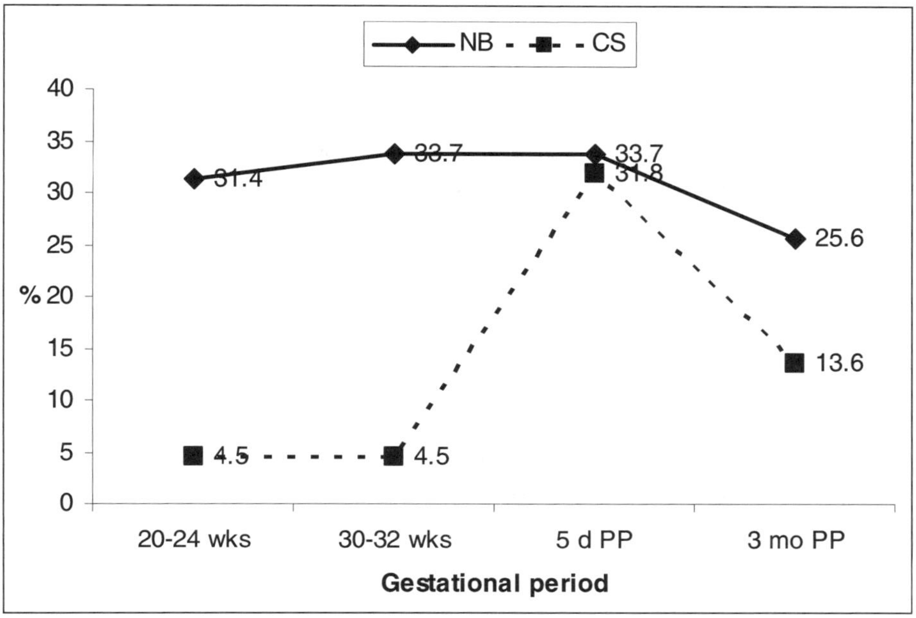

Figure 3. Proportion of depressed women (EPDS cut-off 8/9), having emergency CS. CS = Cesarean section, NB = natural birth, PP = postpartum

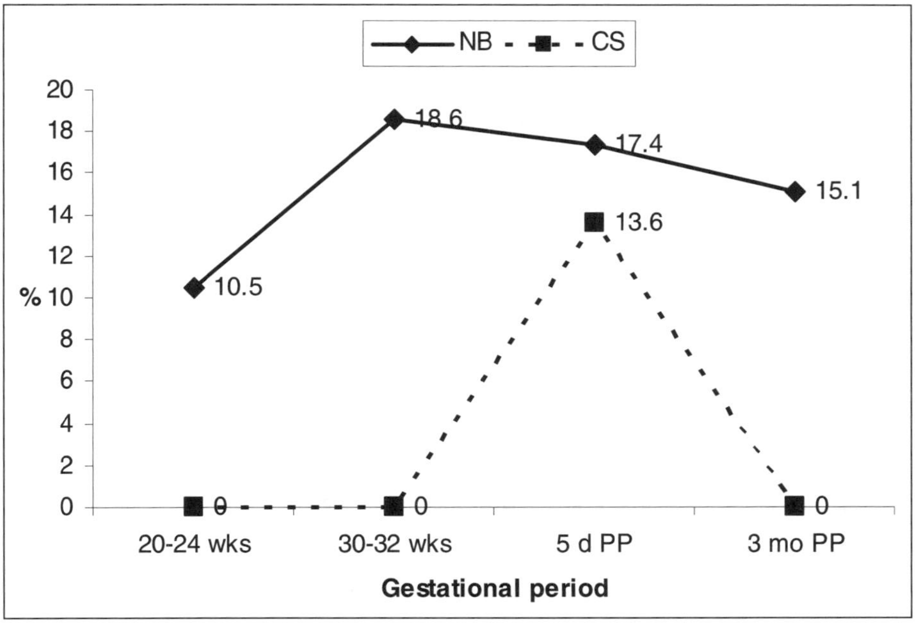

Figure 4. Proportion of depressed women (EPDS cut-off 12/13), having emergency CS. CS = Cesarean section, NB = natural birth, PP = postpartum

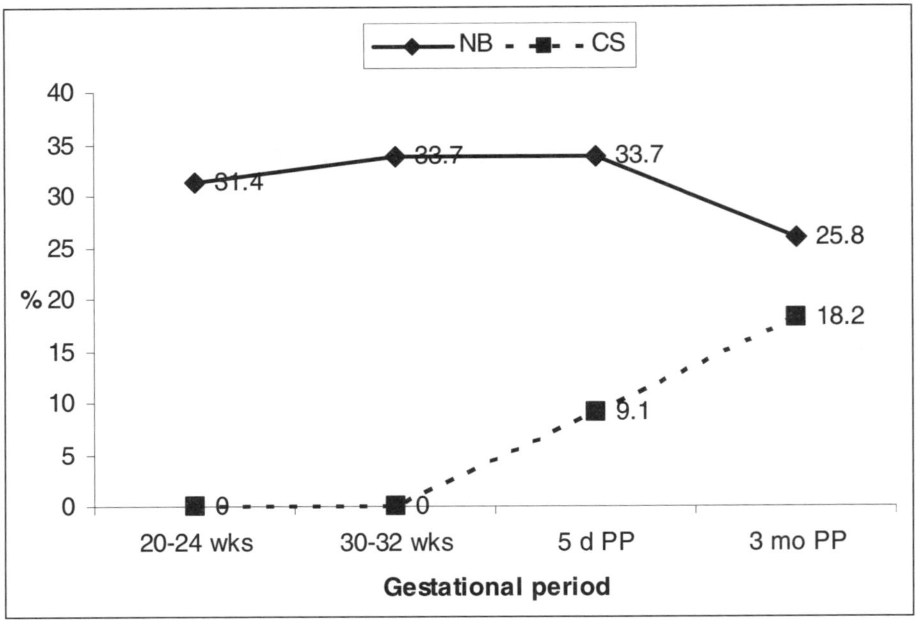

Figure 5. Proportion of depressed women (EPDS cut-off 8/9), having elective CS. CS = Cesarean section, NB = natural birth, PP = postpartum

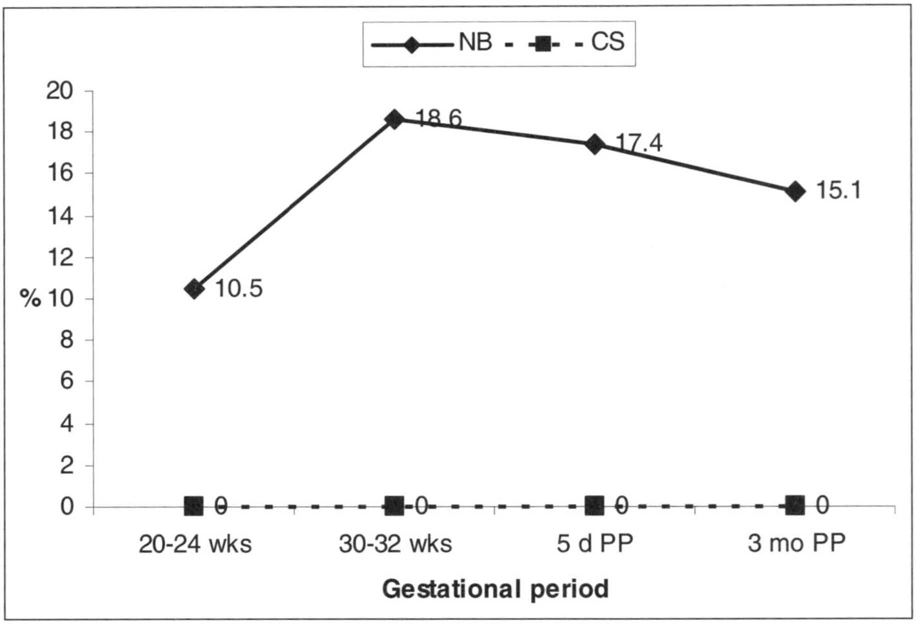

Figure 6. Proportion of depressed women (EPDS cut-off 12/13), having elective CS. CS = Cesarean section, NB = natural birth, PP = postpartum

Anxiety symptoms

The results are presented related to the ASQ-IPAT questionnaire scores comparing the NB and CS groups. Concerning *latent anxiety*, the NB group has a significantly higher score than the CS (13.49 vs. 11.64, $p = 0.04$), women scoring significantly higher than men (13.99 vs. 11.22, $p = 0.004$). At the second antepartum meeting, the NB group reports a higher anxiety score (12.81 vs. 10.04, $p = 0.003$) and women scored higher than men (13.05 vs. 10.29, $p = 0.003$). At the postpartum meeting, the only significant difference is regarding gender: a higher score for women compared to men, irrespective of whether they belonged to NB or CS groups (12.67 vs. 10.15, $p = 0.004$). At the final meeting, the high score of women is the only significant difference (12.17 vs. 9.39, $p = 0.004$).

With regard to *manifest anxiety*, again the only significant difference at the 20th–24th week is between genders: 11.38 anxiety score for women compared to 7.73 for men ($p < 0.0005$). At 30–32 weeks, the NB group has a higher score than the CS group (9.85 vs. 7.6 $p = 0.02$) and women had higher scores than men (10.7 vs. 6.6, $p < 0.0005$). Even a few days after birth, the NB group scores higher than the CS group (9.49 vs. 7.48, $p = 0.04$) and women scored higher than men (10.34 vs. 6.42, $p < 0.0005$). At 3 months after the birth, the only significant difference is the higher score among the women compared to men (9.35 vs. 6.51, $p = 0.001$), irrespective of whether the mode of delivery.

Regarding *global anxiety*, at the first meeting no significant differences between the NB and CS groups were found, but women scored higher than men (25.37 vs. 18.94, $p < 0.0005$). At the second meeting, the NB group has a higher score than the CS group (22.74 vs. 17.6, $p = 0.003$) and women scored 23.82 as compared to 16.89 of men ($p < 0.0005$).

A few days after birth, the NB again scores higher than the CS group (21.68 vs. 18.12, $p = 0.04$) and the women scored significantly higher than men (23.02 vs. 16.57, $p < 0.0005$). At the final meeting, the only significant difference in the global sample is the difference in scores between women (21.51) and men (15.91, $p = 0.001$).

In overall anxiety terms (latent, manifest and global) it is interesting to compare the scores of only women from the NB and CS groups, and also between NB women and emergency CS women and NB and planned CS women. In the case of *latent anxiety*, the comparison between NB and CS women shows a significant difference at the second meeting ($p = 0.008$), where the NB women score higher (Figure 7); this difference can also be noted if the scores of NB women and emergency CS women are compared (Figure 8): at the 2nd meeting the NB women score significantly higher ($p = 0.008$), whereas between NB and planned CS women (Figure 9) there are no differences.

Observing the levels of latent anxiety over time and keeping the NB and CS women groups separate, it is possible to detect a significant decrease in anxiety

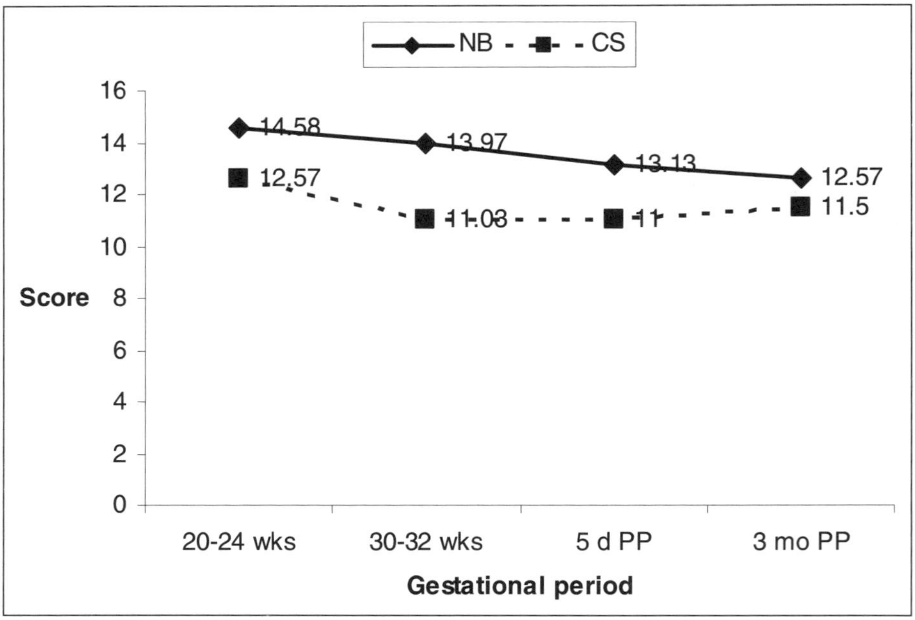

Figure 7. Latent anxiety scores, global (ASQ-IPAT).
CS = Cesarean section, NB = natural birth, PP = postpartum

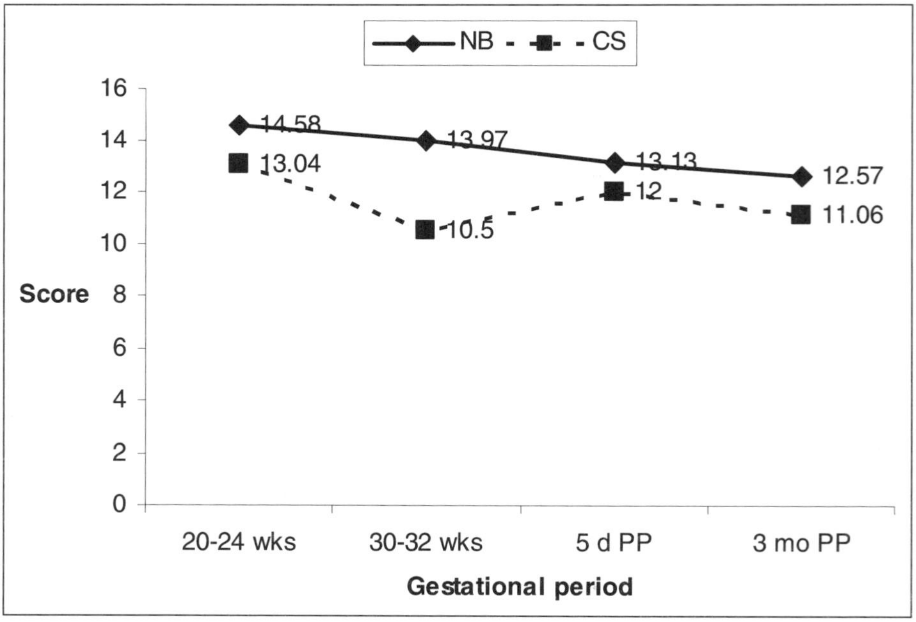

Figure 8. Latent anxiety scores (ASQ-IPAT), emergency CS.
CS = Cesarean section, NB = natural birth, PP = postpartum

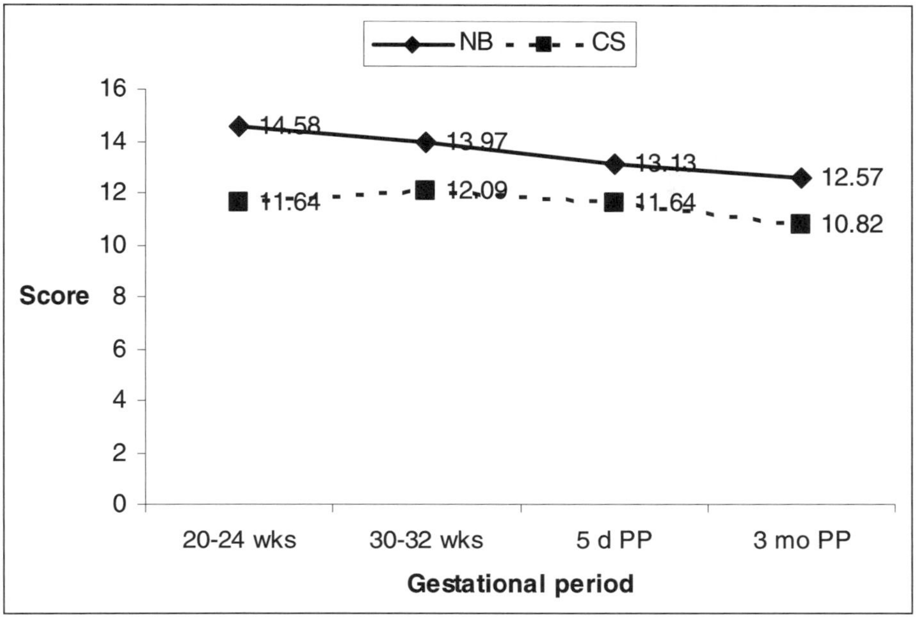

Figure 9. Latent anxiety scores (ASQ-IPAT), planned CS.
CS = Cesarean section, NB = natural birth, PP = postpartum

levels only in emergency CS women from the 1st to the 2nd meeting ($p = 0.001$). Regarding *manifested anxiety*, the NB-CS comparison (Figure 10) shows differences that are significant only at the 2nd meeting, where NB women score higher ($p = 0.04$); in the NB-emergency CS comparison there are no significant differences throughout the 4 meetings (Graph 11). However planned CS women score much lower compared to NB women at the 2nd and 3rd meetings ($p = 0.03$; $p = 0.01$; Graph 12).

Observing the levels of manifest anxiety over time, the only significant decrease to emerge is the scores of NB women from the 3rd to the 4th meeting ($p = 0.001$).

From the point of view of *global anxiety scores* the NB-CS comparison (Figure 13) shows how the NB women score significantly higher at the 2nd meeting ($p = 0.01$); in the NB-emergency CS comparison (Figure 14) the NB women emerge with higher anxiety scores at the 2nd meeting ($p = 0.04$), whereas there are no differences in the NB-planned CS scores (Figure 15). Taking into account the time factor in the global anxiety scores, it is possible to detect a significant decrease in the scores of emergency CS women between the 1st to 2nd meeting ($p = 0.01$) and NB women from the 3rd to 4th meetings ($p = 0.003$).

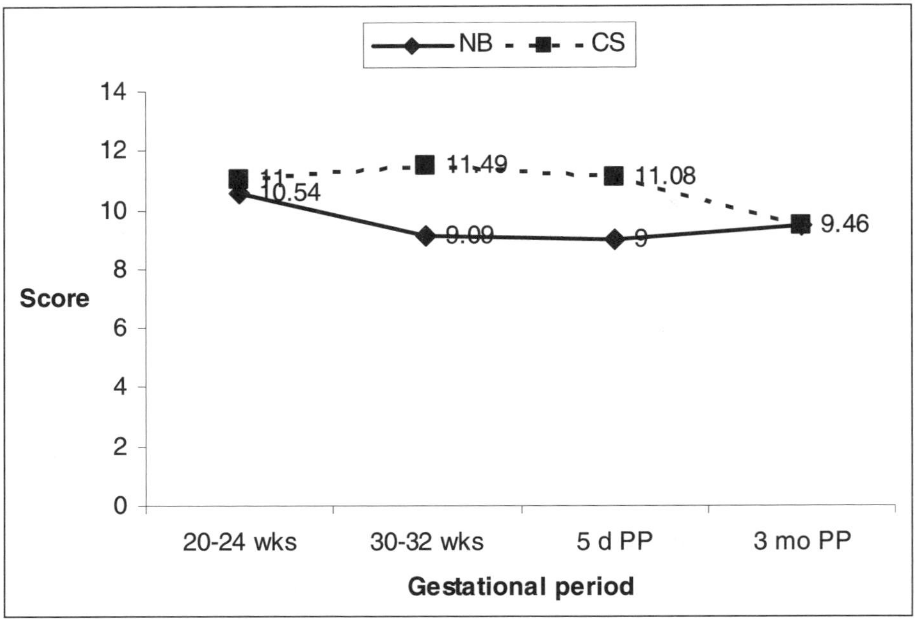

Figure 10. Manifested anxiety scores (ASQ-IPAT), global.
CS = Cesarean section, NB = natural birth, PP = postpartum

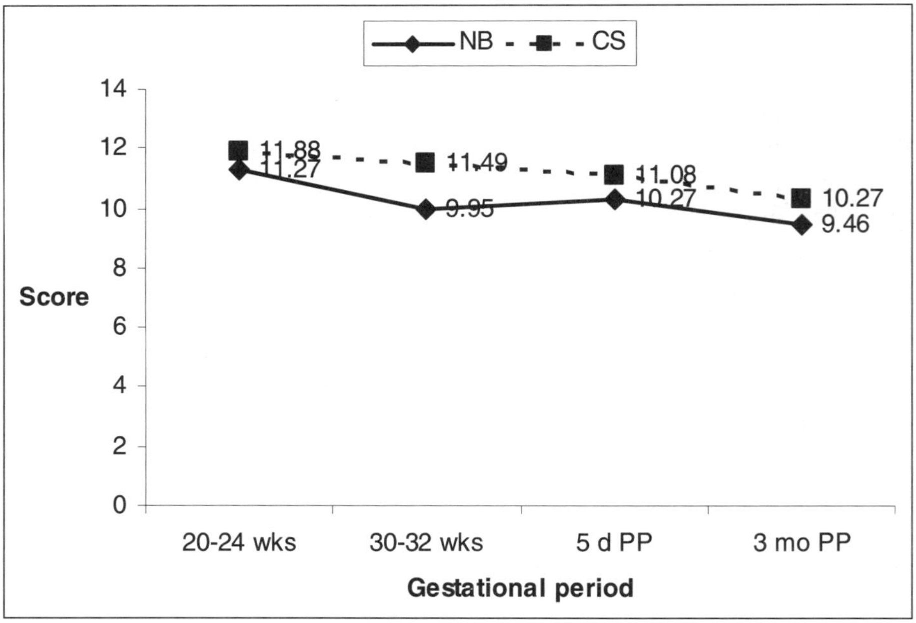

Figure 11. Manifested anxiety scores (ASQ-IPAT), emergency CS.
CS = Cesarean section, NB = natural birth, PP = postpartum

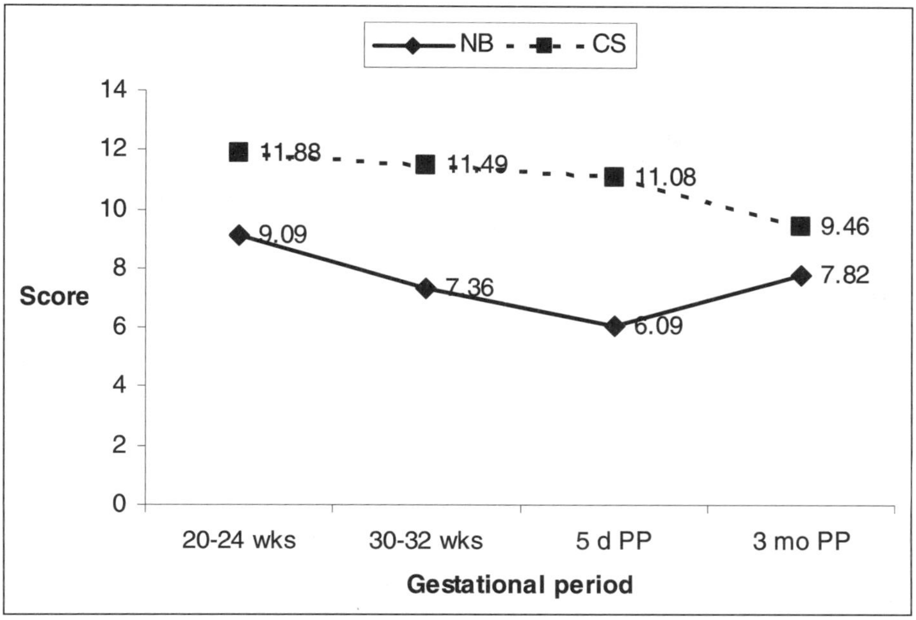

Figure 12. Manifested anxiety scores (ASQ-IPAT), planned CS.
CS = Cesarean section, NB = natural birth, PP = postpartum

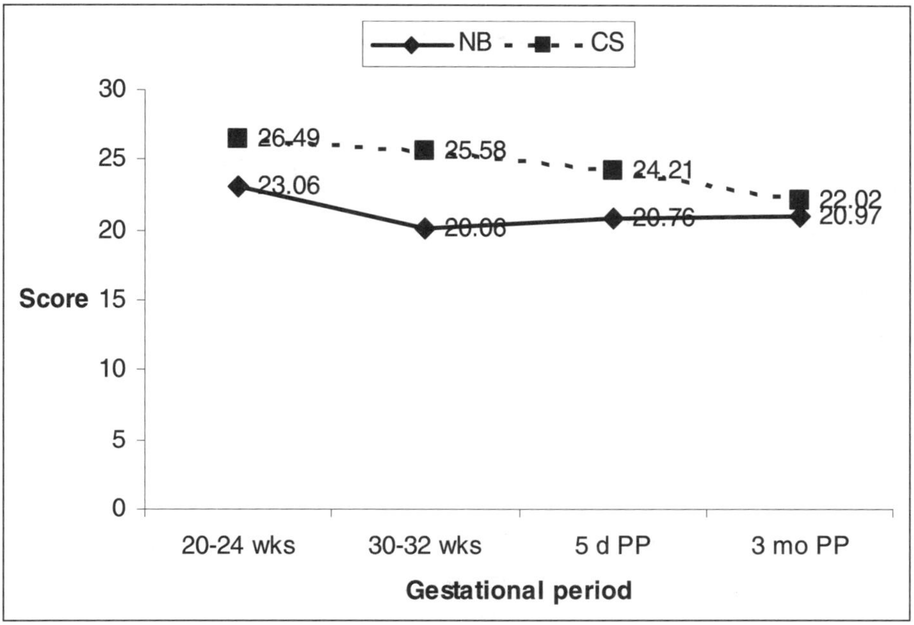

Figure 13. Global anxiety scores (ASQ-IPAT).
CS = Cesarean section, NB = natural birth, PP = postpartum

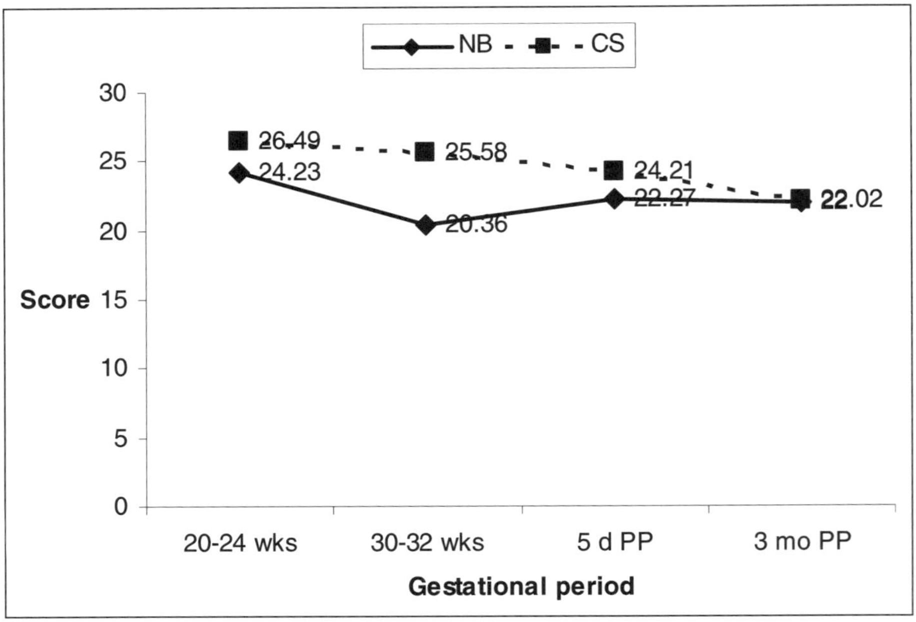

Figure 14. Global anxiety scores (ASQ-IPAT): NB-emergency CS comparison. CS = Cesarean section, NB = natural birth, PP = postpartum

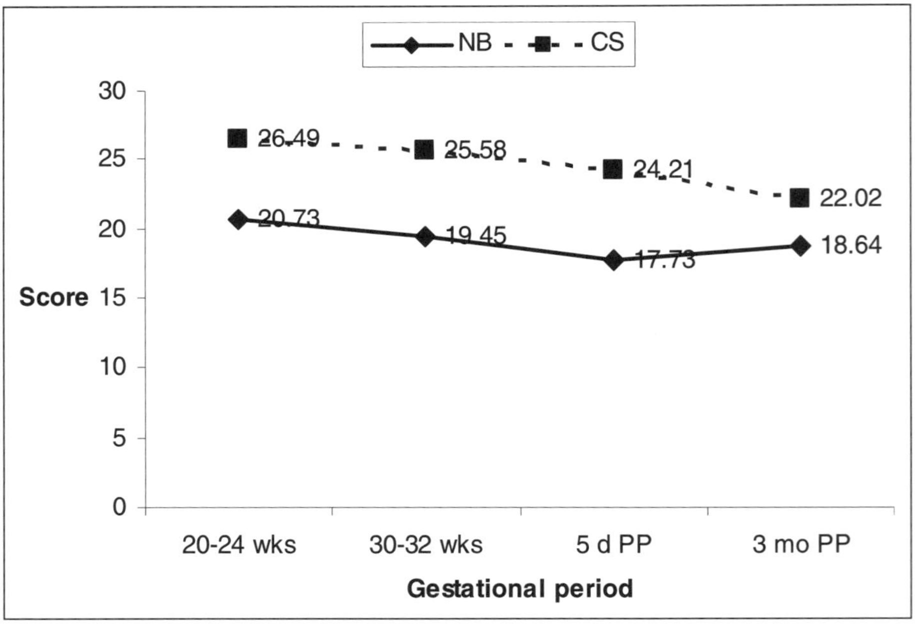

Figure 15. Global anxiety scores (ASQ-IPAT): NB-planned CS comparison. CS = Cesarean section, NB = natural birth, PP = postpartum

Maternal and paternal representations in pregnancy

Individual characteristics of the baby, of the self, and of the partner

The ANOVA tests were conducted on the whole sample using the semantic differential adjective pairs, taking the character in question into account (baby, self, partner) and the type of birth (NB or CS). Many adjective pair scores differ according to the type of birth. The CS group (including men and women) have representations of the baby, themselves, and their partner as more active, sociable, accepting, affectionate, resolute, and livelier compared to the NB group. Only in the representation of the baby as "very happy" there were no differences between the groups. Nine out of 17 adjective pairs showed a significant difference between the scores of the three characters (baby, self, partner), irrespective of the NB or CS groups. Both groups tend to represent the baby in the most positive terms (more sociable, proactive, cleaner, livelier, and more trustful) compared to themselves and their partners. Furthermore, the partner and baby are represented as more easy-going, more intelligent, and stronger compared to them.

Taking into consideration the type of birth and gender of parent as variables, 6 out of 17 adjective pairs (e.g. excited/calm, sad/happy, dependant/independent) show significant differences between mothers and fathers in as far as women tend to have a more negative self-representation (less calm, less excited, less strong, etc.) compared to men, and a more positive representation of their partner (e.g. calmer, more trustful, and happier).

Examining the results of the mothers and fathers separately, the women of the CS group have a representation of the character as more sociable, proactive, accepting, lively, and decisive compared to their NB group counterparts. The CS women also consider their baby as more "messy", whereas the two groups of women have the representation of themselves and their partners as "clean".

Women were compared taking the difference between emergency and planned CS into account. The emergency CS women have representations of the three characters (baby, self, partner) as much more proactive than themselves compared to the NB women. Both groups represent the baby as more sociable than themselves and their partner, livelier than themselves, the baby and partner more trustful and stronger than themselves, of themselves cleaner than the baby and the partner more independent and calmer than the baby.

In the case of planned CS, women represent the 3 characters as more active, sociable, proactive, happier, accepting, more resolute, livelier, and stronger than the NB women. The NB women see the baby as cleaner than the planned CS women, whereas both groups see themselves and their partner as very clean. The CS women see their partner as much easier-going compared to the NB women while both see the baby and themselves as relatively easy-going. Both groups see the baby and partner as more intelligent and trustful than themselves, and the partner as more excited and more independent than the baby.

The CS men have much more trustful representations than the NB men while both groups describe the baby as very happy. The CS men see their partners as very happy whereas the NB men less so. As the test sample still has not reached its full sample size, the comparison between men only of the emergency CS and planned CS groups was not carried out.

Maternal/paternal characteristics of the self and own mother/father

In regards to the representations of selves as parents and the representations of own parents, all subjects from both NB and CS groups see themselves as more affectionate, available, protective, flexible, playful, patient, active, satisfied and happier than their own mothers/fathers. The CS group present themselves as more affectionate and satisfied than the NB group, but also more anxious.

Considering the gender of the parent, out of 6 adjective pairs it emerged that women tend to associate more positive adjectives to themselves as mothers compared to men (e.g. more flexible, playful, relaxed).

Analyzing the results separately, based on the gender of the parent, both groups of women see their own mothers as sufficiently playful, the CS women represent themselves as much more playful than the NB women and have much more relaxed representations of themselves as mothers and of their own mothers. Distinguishing between the emergency and planned CS groups, the women of the former have representations of the two characters as much more satisfied than the NB women. The two groups of women tend to present themselves better than their own mothers (more affectionate, playful, available, flexible, active, more confident and happier). The planned CS women consider themselves much more positively in terms of the adjective pairs "confident/unconfident" and "anxious/relaxed" and their own mothers in a more negative light, whereas the NB women have positive representations for both characters. The planned CS women present themselves as more playful and happier parents than the NB women. Both NB and planned CS women present themselves as more affectionate, flexible, accepting and satisfied than their own mothers.

The CS men have representations of themselves as calmer and more active as compared to the NB men ($p = 0.02$). Again, due to the sample sife, the comparison between men in the emergency CS and planned CS groups was not carried out.

Maternal and paternal representations after the birth

Individual characteristics of the baby, self and partner

The CS group has representations of selves, baby, and partner as more sociable, affectionate and stronger compared to the NB group. Whereas both NB and CS groups consider themselves as relatively clean, the CS group represents the baby as messier and the partner cleaner compared to the NB group. The two groups represent the baby as very happy whereas the CS group represents themselves and their partners as happier than the NB group. Both groups present the baby as hungrier, sociable, pro-active, dependant, livelier, and messier compared to themselves and their partner. Similarly the baby and partner are imagined as more easy-going and intelligent than themselves.

From the point of view of the parent's gender, significant differences emerge from the analysis of 7 adjective pairs indicating how the women tend to represent the 3 characters as more easy-going and resolute and their partner stronger and more independent than how men consider them, but, at the same time, sadder and more untidy whereas the baby is considered as stronger but also more dependant.

Analyzing only the women's scores, we see that the NB women represent the baby as cleaner compared to the CS women. The CS women, however, see themselves as happier than the NB women even though both see the baby as very happy, and the NB women imagine the baby as tidier. Distinguishing between emergency CS and planned CS, the NB women have a cleaner image of the baby compared to the emergency CS women. However, the emergency CS women see their partners as cleaner. Both groups of women tend to represent the baby in a more positive way than themselves or than their partners: more resolute, sociable, happier, and livelier. Baby and partner considered as more pro-active, easy-going, and more intelligent than themselves, and both groups of women consider themselves as tidier than the baby and the partner. They see their partner as more trustful and stronger than themselves and the baby.

The planned CS women present themselves as more pro-active and themselves and their partners as happier. The NB group, however, present the 3 characters as tidier. The two groups of women have similar images of the baby as messier, more easy-going than themselves, more dependent than themselves or their partners, and more fearful than the partner.

The CS men represent the 3 characters as more sociable, happier, more intelligent, tidier, affectionate, livelier and stronger compared to the NB men.

Maternal/paternal characteristics of the self and own mother/father

Both NB and CS groups represent themselves more positively compared to their own parents (more affectionate, available, flexible, protective, patient, accepting, generous, satisfied, happier, and more active). In their representations of themselves as parents, the CS group see themselves as more playful, relaxed, satisfied, and happier than the NB group.

Analyzing the women only, those in the CS group see themselves as more relaxed than the NB group and see their role as easier, while the NB women have representations of themselves as more protective compared to the emergency CS women. Comparing the NB-emergency CS women, the NB women consider themselves as more possessive than the emergency CS women. However, they have representations of themselves and their own mothers as being more playful. Both groups see themselves as better mothers than their own, describing themselves as more affectionate, available, flexible, accepting, relaxed, more satisfied, happier, and more active.

Comparing the NB and planned CS women, both groups consider themselves as very affectionate, flexible and playful, but those in the NB group perceive their own mothers as more affectionate, flexible, and playful compared to the planned CS women. The NB women represent themselves and their mothers as more protective. The planned CS women consider themselves as more relaxed and happier mothers compared to NB women who are more or less consistent in their two representations. The CS women consider the maternal role as easier compared to the NB women. Both groups represent themselves as more available, more accepting and more satisfied than their own mothers.
The CS men have more affectionate, available and accepting representations than the NB men and the CS men present themselves as being more generous than their NB counterparts. However, both groups present their own fathers as relatively generous. At the end, the CS men have happier representations than the NB group and consider their role as father as being easier.

"... and while we are looking, we should allow
ourselves to recognize the meaning of what lies beyond"
Wilfred Bion

Discussion

At first reading, it should be kept in mind that the data are incomplete because of a limited sample size and the use of psychological measures based on self-evaluation questionnaires and therefore "subject to defensive processes difficult to check" (Solano, 2005). Secondly, regarding the link between emotions expressed and health, the questionnaires on anxiety and depression measure the affective state as it is expressed externally but do not tell us that a depressive tone of humor is negative, unless the cut-off indicates a probable risk. The pregnancy-birth event brings about grand physical and psychological changes along with complex emotions unless there is an emotional or psychopathological withdrawal. On the one hand, if the "psychological transparency" during pregnancy favors access to internal representations and therefore to future constructions of new bonds, on the other hand, it highlights the psychological "vulnerability" in the face of normal psychobiological turbulence. Expressing these non-pathological levels of anxiety and depressive symptoms (as possibly indicated with the tests employed in this study) could show "more a measure of the ability to construct and express anxiety rather than its actual presence. At this point, we have no reason to expect an inverse correlation between these scores and the state of health (the higher the anxiety scores the worse the health) but perhaps the opposite" (Solano, 2005). It is therefore important to analyze whether the emotional expression is inadequate (either minimal or excessive) with regard to the complexity of the observed phenomenon and to take into account, for prevention and thus for public health, that if an emotional process normal for the specific context is not dealt with properly, this triggers psychophysical uneasiness.

From the current research it appears that women show a significantly higher level of depressive symptoms (EPDS) and anxiety (ASQ-IPAT) than men, irrespective of the mode of birth or when the test was taken (either before or after birth). The results show the positive correlation between the complexity of psychobiological process linked to the pregnancy-maternity project and genetic and role anxieties and how a non-clinical group of women are able to express the connected emotional turmoil. It still needs to be examined whether the socio-health institution favors this expression and supports it or underestimates it by ignoring or medicalizing the problem. In comparing the NB and CS women, it appears that the latter show a clear increase and appearance of depressive symptoms in postpartum, whereas these emotional expressions hardly exist just before birth. This could point to the traumatic effect of Cesarean section despite its frequent occurrence and how it is often rationalized. Although there is a decrease in symptoms at three months after the birth with an 8/9 cut-off (it was not possible to comment on the results with a 12/13 cut-off due to the limited number of subjects), it does not reach the levels from before birth. In the planned CS group there is a progressive increase in depressive symptoms at the three month mark, and despite the sample of these subjects is limited, it is still possible to conjecture about the psychological experience of the birth which has not been elaborated. The NB women show an increase in depressive symptoms in the third trimester and postpartum, periods normally characterized by intensified depressive and persecutory anxiety, whereas three months after birth there are lower levels present compared to the 20–24 week stage unless the data is analyzed using a 12/13 cut-off which indicate serious depressive symptoms which obviously lasts longer.

Regarding latent, manifest, and global anxiety, which nevertheless do not reach pathological levels, they are present more in the NB women compared to the CS women at the second meeting, signaling a greater expression of emotions triggered by the proximity of the birth and the confrontation between imagined parent-child and real parent-child.

The compiled lists of adjectives providing indications on personal functioning and interpersonal and parental style were analyzed according to the type of birth and the gender of the parent. Irrespective of the variability, both groups represent the baby in more positive terms than themselves or their partners and think of themselves as more affectionate, available, etc. parents than their own parents. This can be considered an idealization process which functions like a scaffold compared to the imagined identity in construction, the newborn and the new parent, which, if not stabilized becomes disturbing. The "preciousness" of the planning and birth needs support from the environmental network because the idealization process is protective and defensive compared to fantasies of inadequacy which, if not tolerated, risk damaging construction occurs.

The CS group emerges more satisfied and affectionate, but also more anxious. CS women present themselves, the baby, and the partner more positively than the NB group apart from where they rate the baby more "messy" and their own mothers as more "anxious". It is possible to associate this minimal expression of anxious feelings with a more idealized representation of themselves which seems to protect the image of a baby "born out of a mess". Understanding parental representations involves rethinking, observing, listening, and favoring the development of the sense of intimacy and inwardness, taking into account that these are emotions that give meaning to experiences in that they are "sources of information on the person's own identity and own personal needs and the necessary actions to satisfy such needs" (Dafter, 1996).

The complexity of "work" of the psychological maternity and its impact on the health of the individual and society requires a collective responsibility, making a conscious effort in taking care by means of an equally complex "work" of the après coup.

"The keyword of the environment is reliability,
human reliability and not mechanic...
a hospital whose organisation does not inform the
woman who is to be her doctor and nurse,
is not a good hospital even if it is the nation's
best equipped, most sterilised and nickel-plated."
Donald Woods Winnicott

Conclusions

The delivery and birth of a child are fundamental moments of development constituting a "turning point" in the development of female identity and a couple's life (Ammaniti, 1992). Hospital institutions have the duty of taking care of the biological and emotional aspects of such events which are the basis, on an intrapyschic level, of the redistribution of the libidinal and narcissistic investments and, on an interpsychic level, of co-construction of affective bonds.

Along with the idealization of pregnancy and birth, there is a lack (sometimes complete) of psychological support for the woman, during pregnancy and postpartum. In the western world, hospital departments allow a very brief stay. The possibility of having an obstetrician, who like the midwife of past days, accompanies the mother postpartum is, in actual fact, very rare today. In addition, family support becomes difficult due to the distance between the woman and her family or the disintegration of the family. The lack of a network which can look after the psychological elements of the maternity experience exposes the risk of defective parenting. "Until recently, maternity was nearly always a collective experience. The mother was part of a network which included not only the family but also the context and environment. These days, maternity tends to be an individual, if not a solitary, experience. There is nothing to indicate that this is normal. First of all, it is important that the baby has a mother who is a mediator for the human context; secondly, the requirements of maternity can be excessive for the shoulders of only one person, and finally, compounding the conditions of maternity in this way contributes to the amount of maternal disfunctionality, even though many of these cases go unreported due to because of an even growing access to the pediatrician." (Delassus, 1995)

Supporting parenthood by giving more space and time to the emotional quality of relationships, favors the individual's resources and social context, trying to lessen the great difference between technological abilities advancing all the time and abilities to live and regulate the emotional experience, which are only deteriorating. It is therefore important to aid the maternity process in the sense of the inwardness, of intimacy, understanding maternal and paternal representations in order to rethink and observe and listen to the maternal narrations "the accounts do not wear out, they retain the energy in themselves like the long-lasting grain of corn in the pyramids maintained the ability to germinate intact" (Benjamin, 1991). It is about listening not only to the physical reality of pregnancy, already monitored medically but also giving space to the psychological reality of pregnancy which is often ignored or silenced: "Becoming a parent has the particular value of joining the subject to the succession of generations and giving the power to transmit life" (Houzel, 2005).

Observing the most significant exchanges before and immediately after the birth means the discovery of the most intimate bonds, in the ontogenetic, biologic and social senses of communication, exchanges which take place by means of the body's unconditional language and which develop in the most delicate weave of mutual understanding. The adult finds her/himself bare of the semantic power faced with the complexity of procreation and birth where the delicate transition from the workings of biological relationships to the coordinated and harmonic combination of social relationships probably comes into play. "We begin as simple rhythmic structures and receivers of other rhythms, becoming capable of rhythmic productions in a continuous process which makes use of previous predispositions transforming themselves thanks to new internal and external meetings and creating new harmonies in renewed interactions" (Giovanelli, 1997).

The current viewpoint is a multidisciplinary approach in which the complexity of prenatal and perinatal development is considered in the interaction of somatic, psychological, relational, and emotional aspects. It is this unity that allows the recognition of the importance of these phases, from the point of view of development of the organism as well as the inborn individual personality made up of its hereditary, individual, and socio-environmental aspects. This is confirmed in the assumption of the fundamental psychobiological unity of the human being with the decisive overcoming of dual Cartesian which still often makes the communication between medical disciplines of body and mind very difficult. Perhaps today in relation to a culture which should be more tolerant and pluralistic, there will be a context that will enable the baby to be held closer as child and as our own infantile self: "So close that we can even see him from afar, so close that we can hear him inside us, in our memories of the past but even more in the resonance of our internal experience". (Manfredi, Imbasciati, 1995).

References

Ammaniti M: (a cura di) La gravidanza tra fantasia e realtà. Il Pensiero Scientifico, Roma 1992

Ammaniti M, C Candelori, M Pola, R Tambelli: Maternità e Gravidanza. Studio delle rappresentazioni materne. Cortina, Milano 1995

Barrett G, J Peacock, C Victor, I Manyonda: Cesarean Section and Postnatal Sexual Health. Birth 32 (4) (2005) 306–311

Benjamin W: Ecrits Français. Gallimard, Paris 1991

Brazelton TB: La nascita di una famiglia. Unicopli, Milano 1987

Bydlowski M: Sognare un figlio. L'esperienza interiore della maternità. Pendragon, Bologna 2004

Clement S: Psychological aspects of Cesarean section. Harcourt, London 2001

Cramer B: Cosa diventeranno i nostri bambini. Cortina, Milano 2000

Dafter RE: Why "negative" emotions can sometimes be positive: the spectrum model of emotions and their role in mind-body healing. Advances 12 (1996) 6–19

Devitt ND: Cesarean Delivery and Native American Women. Birth 33 (1) (2006) 86–87

Edwards DRL, SAM Porter, GS Stein: A pilot study of postnatal depression following cesarean section using two retrospective self-rating instruments. Journal of Psychosomatic Research 38 (1994) 111–117

Fisher JWR, RO Stanley, GD Burrows: Psychological adjustment to Cesarean delivery: a review of the evidence. Journal of Psychosomatic Obstetrics and Gynaecology II (1990) 91–106

Fornari F: Il codice vivente: femminilità e maternità nei sogni delle madri in gravidanza. Boringhieri, Torino 1981

Francome C, W Savane, H Churchill, H Lewinson: Cesarean birth in Britain. Middlesex University Press, Middlesex 1993

Ghetti C, B Chan, JM Guise: Physicians' Responses to Patient-Requested Cesarean Delivery. Birth 31 (4) (2004) 280–284

Giovanelli G: Prenascere, Nascere e Rinascere. Lo sviluppo neuropsicologico nei primi mesi di vita. La Nuova Italia Scientifica, Roma 1997

Goer H: Patient Choice Cesarean and Informed Consent. Birth 33 (1) (2006) 87–88

Henderson E, EJ Love: Incidence of hospital-acquired infections associated with Cesarean section. Journal of Hospital Infection 29 (1995) 245–255

Hillan EM: Research and audit: women's view of Cesarean section. In: Roberts H (ed): Women's Health Matters. Routledge, London 1992

Houzel D: Le dimensioni della genitorialità. Interazioni 1 (2005) 11–26

Kaes R, H Faimberg, J Enriquez, J Baranes: Trasmissione della vita psichica tra generazioni. Borla, Roma 1995

Kendell RE, JC Chalmers, C Platz: Epidemiology of puerperal psychoses. British Journal of Psychiatry 150 (1987) 662–673

Klein MC: Quick Fix Culture: The Cesarean-Section-on Demand Debate. Birth 31 (3) (2004) 161–164

Klein MC: Epidural Analgesia: Does It or Doesn't It. Birth 33 (1) (2006) 74–76

Lebovici S: Il neonato, la madre e lo psicoanalista. Borla, Roma 1988

Lydon-Rochelle MT, VL Holt, DP Martin, TR Easterling: Association between method of delivery and maternal rehospitalization. JAMA 283 (2000) 2411–2416

Lydon-Rochelle MT, C Gardella, V Càrdenas, TR Easterling; Repeat Cesarean Delivery: What Indications are Recorded in the Medical Chart. Birth 33 (1) (2006) 4–11

Madar J, S Richmond, E Hey: Hyaline membrane disease after elective delivery 'at term'. Acta Paediatrica 8 (1999) 1244–1284

Manfredi P, A Imbasciati: Il bambino allontanato e il bambino ... da lontano. Attualità in Psicologia 4 (1995) 315–326

Maternity Center Association:. What Every Pregnant Woman Needs to Know About Cesarean Section. MCA, New York 2004

Mercer RT, MC Stainton, S Ferketich: Perceptions of the birth experience: a cross cultural comparison. Health Care for Women International 5 (1984) 29

Monti F, F Agostini, B Divizia, R Chattat, R Fava: Modalità di parto a confronto: impatto psicologico del parto spontaneo e del parto cesareo. Psychofenia VIII 12 (2005) 79–95

Prezza M, D Di Mauro, MG Giudici, C Violani, S Vaccari, F Faustini: Studio longitudinale sulla disforia post parto. In: Montemagno U, L Zichella: (a cura di), Psicosomatica ginecologica ed ostetrica. Monduzzi, Bologna 1984

Racamier PC, S Taccani: Il lavoro incerto. La psicodinamica del processo di crisi. Del Cerro, Tirrenia 1986

Raphael-Leff J: Split Milk perinatal loss and breakdown. Institute of Psychoanalysis, London 2000

Reichert A, M Baron, J Fawcett: Changes in attitudes towards Cesarean birth. A longitudinal study. Gynaecologic and Neonatal Nursing 22 (1993) 159–167

Riley D: Perinatal Mental Health: a Sourcebook for Health Professionals. Radcliffe Medical Press, Oxford 1995

Sabbadini LL: Gravidanza e parto: una nuova coscienza femminile, un nuovo protagonismo maschile. ISTAT, Roma 2001

Salvini A: Personalità femminile e riproduzione umana. Lombardo Editore, Roma 1993

Signorelli C, MS Cattaruzza, JF Osborn: Risk factors for Cesarean section in Italy: results of a multicentre study. Public Health 109 (1995) 191–199

Solano L: Psicoanalisi e ricerca empirica nell'ambito della salute. Rivista di Psicoanalisi LI (3) (2005) 695–718

Soulè M: La vita del feto: studio per comprendere la psicopatologia perinatale e gli inizi della psicosomatica. In: Righetti PL, L Sette: Non c'è due senza tre. Le emozioni dell'attesa dalla genitorialità alla prenatalità. Boringhieri, Torino 2000

Stern D: Motherhood costellation. A unified view of parent-infant psychotherapy. Basic Books, New York 1995

Tang CH, MP Wu, HC Lin, CC Hsu: Delayed parenthood and the Risk of Cesarean Section – Is Paternal Age an Indipendent Risk Factor? Birth 33 (1) (2006) 18–26

Vegetti Finzi S: Il bambino della notte. Divenire donna. Divenire madre. Mondatori, Milano 1990

Winnicott DW: Sviluppo affettivo e ambiente. Armando, Roma 1970

Walker R, D Turnbull, C Wilkinson: Increasing Cesarean Section Rates: Exploring the Role of Culture in a Australian Community. Birth 31 (2) (2004) 117–124

World Health Organization: Appropriate technology for birth. Lancet 2 (1985) 436–437

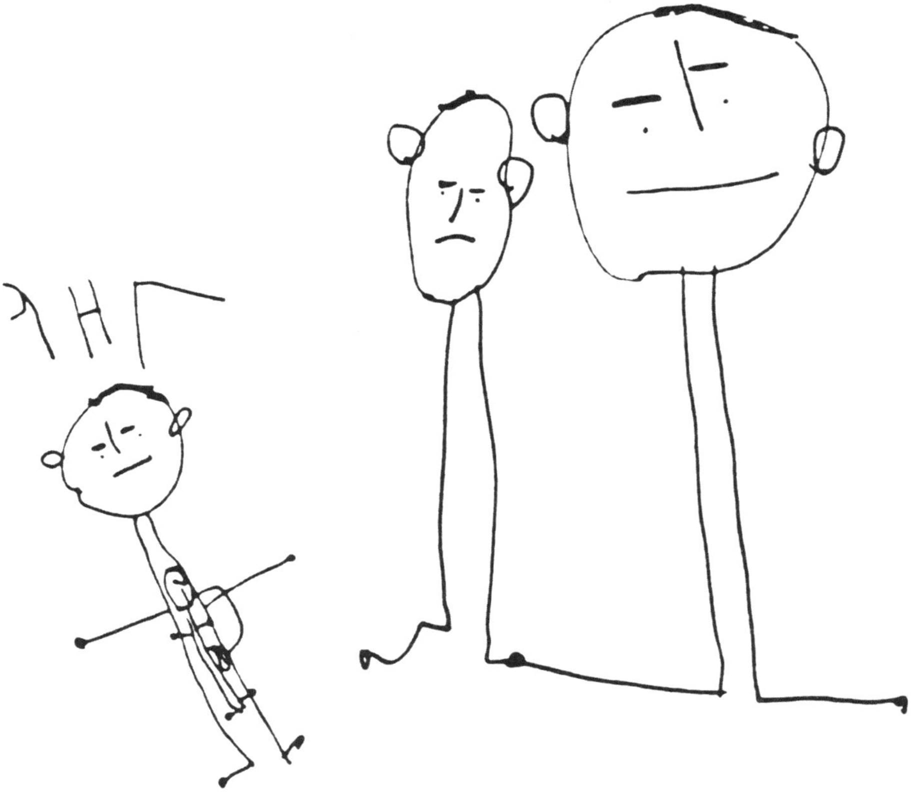

(Chloé, 4 yrs. 2 mos.)
Now I'm growing and growing and growing.

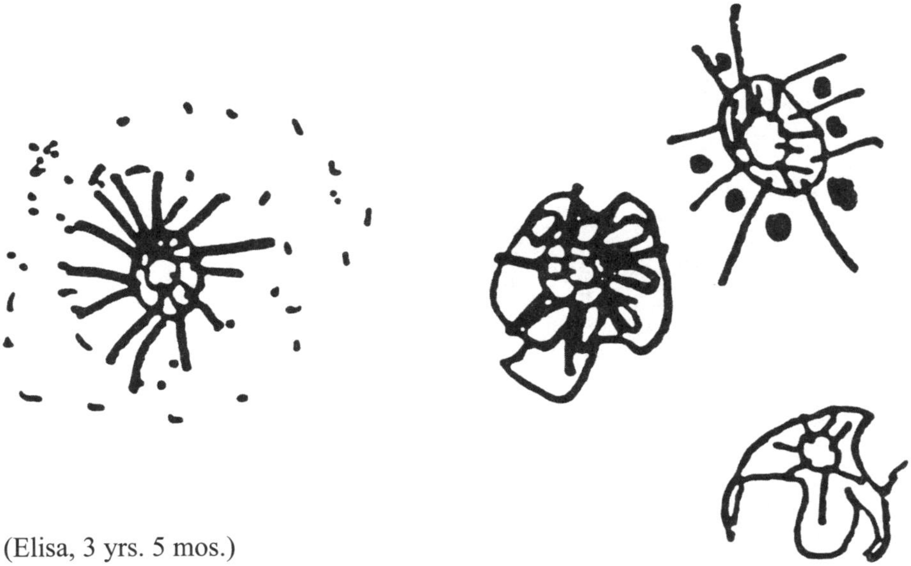

(Elisa, 3 yrs. 5 mos.)
Stars get born from their mommies, too, with all the little points.

21. From foster care to parent training – The emergence of a socio-educative approach to 'parentality'

Paul Durning; Department of Educational Science,
University of Paris X-Nanterre, France

This chapter proposes an analysis of the evolution in progress in socio-educative interventions aimed at helping parents in the education of their children by showing them an increasingly significant emergence of socio-educative perspectives. This research, centred on the educational processes within the family, which has been developed in our language (French) in the course of the last twenty years, enriched the long limited approaches to the mere consideration of affective and relational dimensions between parents and children. Taking these educational dimensions into adequate consideration leads us to examine the changes in progress in intervention strategies, instead of taking up again the question of parent training which constituted a taboo for many years. The evolution seen towards earlier and less stigmatizing actions however, does not preclude a tension, sometimes exacerbated, between approaches privileging aid to the parents and more repressive perspectives which commend more rapid placements and sanctions of "maltreating" or "weak" parents.

Family education is classically defined at the same time as a field of social practices, as training discipline, and as a university research object. This considers the parental activity of education which constitutes its central hub but embraces the multiple social interventions put into practice to prepare, sustain, aid, and observe the parents substituted in the task of educating their children (Pourtois, Desmet, 1998; Pourtois, 1989; Durning, 1998, 1995 a, 2006; Boutin, Durning, 1994, 1999).

Research activity has developed since the mid-1970s in the United States, notably in relation to the start of pre-school programs called Head-Start compensation (Westinghouse, 1969; Zigler, Valentine, 1979) and Follow Through (Weiss, Jacobs, 1988) which have given researchers in education, social work, psychology, sociology etc. the opportunity to come to observe family educational processes *in situ* (Bronfenbrenner, 1974; Shonkoff, Meisels, 1990). Ten or so years later, we may note a rapid development of this field in the French language in Belgium (Pourtois, 1979, 1989a; Desmet, Pourtois, 1993, 2000), Quebec (Terrisse, Boutin, 1994), then in France (Durning, 1988, 1995 to 2006) and in Switzerland (Kellerhals, Montandon, 1991). Just as on the other side of the Atlantic, this was the achievement of researchers studying different subjects. The majority were trying to understand early deficiency in the scholarly success of children entering school (Pourtois, Terrisse), others were specialists in the education of handicapped children (Bouchard, Lambert), and still others had studied primarily the education of children in nursery school (Tremblay, Hellinckz, Durning, Fablet, Corbillon).

The development of Francophone works, starting from the mid-1980s, is reflected by the introduction of family education study programs in Belgium and then in France, the multiplication of interviews and publications widely incited by the creation in 1986 of AIFREF – *l'Association Internationale pour la Formation et la Recherche en Education Familiale* [the International Association for Training and Research into Family Education] and finally, more recently, by the publication of the journal "*La revue internationale de l'éducation familiale*" since 1997. Thus, in the course of the last decade, family education, after training the adults, has appeared a legitimate domain of research in the educational sciences even if the school quite obviously remains its principal object.

We discuss here the analysis of actions conducted in the direction of parents by professional educators, child welfare workers, and social service assistants by sketching a chronological approach to the evolution of socio-educative interventions, specialized interventions under mandate and so-called 'early' or preventive interventions. Last but not least, we briefly touch on the ideological context covering the strong opposition between the standpoints of aid and repression.

Evolution of socio-economic and familial contexts

Current development has to be rewritten within an economic context, marked by nearly thirty years of economic crisis which has led to a real pauperization of certain social groups. In a similar perspective, it is worth taking into account the great changes in family life since the mid-1960s.

Changes in the socio-economic situation

The crisis, sometimes called "that of 1974", whose effects were not visible until some years later, largely fashioned the social situation in Western countries as a whole. Even if the signs of a recovery in Western economies are multiplying, the socio-historic contexts, in which interventions regarding families are taking place, are inconsistently marked by the economic crisis which started in 1974.

The scale and duration of unemployment explains, in a major way, the pauperization and difficulties in the cities. Western societies remain faced with an elevated number of long-term unemployed who accumulate familial, accommodation and positioning difficulties which make their return to the job market problematic. Moreover, unemployment has particularly touched the young coming out of the school system without any real qualifications, creating a divide between the initial training and their entry into the world of work which often happens via the repetition of precarious "temp" work.

These problems are correlated to those found in the school field: massive gaps, illiteracy, depravation, violence and rackets, notably in certain institutions in the suburbs, as much in France as in the USA and Canada. We could add to this list the difficulties met by the youth "resulting from immigration".

However, the significance of poverty is the subject of current debate. The fact that this is not a sufficient cause to make it the object of socio-educative interventions leads intercessors to minimize its importance and to emphasize the psycho-pathological dimensions which the families themselves underline to explain their voluntary or forced recourse to such interventions. A report by ODAS (*Decentralized Observatory of Social Action*), analyzing the "principal familial problematic danger factors" as the origin of signs of maltreatment in 55 French regions, shows the minor importance accorded to socio-economic factors.

While educational deficiencies, in our view are a modality of maltreatment and not "a reason for maltreatment", they would be the first factor with 73% of the alerts, followed by divorces and separations (10%) and psychiatric problems (9%), and substance (alcoholism and drug) abuse (4%). The other factors appear as marginal factors; financial difficulties (0%), unemployment/unstable work (2%), habitat (2%) and sickness and handicap (0%). These results are biased because of the methodology of the investigation which relates only to stress that is supposed to be the principal cause, but later, it was possible to underline three items. (ODAS, 2000) The author of the study thus stresses "the significance of relational problems and the restricted influence of problems of an economic character" (ODAS, 2000). The fact that the intercessors only point, in another study, to the economic factors in order to interpret 11% of the alerts, does not mean that 11% of the families are poor, but perhaps relies on the fact that the information on their economic situation features are very rarely found in files, even at the time of educational measures by AEMO.

Velpry et al. (2000), analyzing the files of children leaving the charge of ASE in 1980, emphasize that 63% do not mention the profession of the father and that in 1990, 57% are without information on the same point. In the study conducted by Corbillon et al (1999), information on the professional and economic situation is not found in the many family files which were the object of open-field educative action.

When these facts are known, they confirm that many families are poor. Velpry et al. (2000) underline an absence of problems or delay in advising the problems punctually only for 20% of the families benefiting from an AEMO; in 38% of the cases, they note debts or unstable work, 3% greatly being precarious. Finally, 5% of parents are absent or deceased.

The General Inspectors Naves and Cathala (2000) having been charged with verifying the statements of ATD Quart Mond, according to whom numerous placement decisions are taken for socio-economic reasons, have specially enrolled a cohort of 114 families where a child had been placed. Despite 43 of these having three or more children, none had resources greater than 10,000 Francs per month: "Most often these households lived only with various payments; family allowance, RMI". Two thirds of the cases known thus disclose social problems. The families with economic difficulty constitute the essence of the families receiving such interventions, but, quite obviously, many families (even poorer) are not the object of alerts and specialized care.

The question is, therefore, related to a profound link between the socio-economic situation and the psycho-pathological problems in the family groups, particularly in situations of great poverty. These results confirm that the psychological and relational difficulties keep pace with health, accommodation and income difficulties in accounting for the educational deficiencies at the origin of the alerts. This debate is in part comparable to concerns about the link between the threats of maltreatment and certain family forms.

Transformations in family life and the place of the child

Thoroughly planned births; "a child if I want, when I want"

The decrease in the number of children is a characteristic of all Western countries. In fact, the global birth rate has passed in France from 2.9 children per woman in 1965 to 1.7 with some limited variations over a decade or so. Altogether, Western countries show birth rates of less than two children per woman. Even if the nadir in birth rates preceded the generalization of oral contraception, the most fundamental change in family life is surely the control of birth through the development and universal use of contraception techniques, and in numerous Western countries by the liberalization of the interruption of pregnancy. During the last thirty years, unwanted births have much decreased and relate, above all, to women from disadvantaged social milieus, or those encountering psycho-social problems.

The control over procreation conditions by avoiding unwanted births is accompanied at the same time by a development in expectations and aggressive techniques against sterility or hypo-fecundity. The development, since the 1980s, of artificial insemination with donor sperm, then with 'in vitro' fertility techniques, has permitted numerous couples to procreate despite the impossible difficulties. The psychological and high financial cost of medically assisted procreation is an indication of the price parents and societies are ready to pay for a child.

A de-institutionalization of conjugal relations

Beyond the strict control of fecundity, it is indisputable that familial ways of life are following an evolution which began in the mid 1960s. Certain manifestations of which are evident. Parents are less often married and, much more often than previously, they divorce and separate, only to reform a new conjugal couple. In France, the birth rate out of wedlock has increased from 6% to 45.2% between 1965 and 2003. At the same time, the rate of marriages which have terminated in divorce has tripled, from 10 to 30%. We must underline, however, that the great majority of children are still raised by their two parents (this is the case in France for nearly 85% of minors).

These figures do not translate into a rejection of family life but rather a questioning of social institutions and especially that of marriage. The ways of familial organization are becoming in some manner private choices and inter-individual contracts, to be re-negotiated at any time. Louis Roussel (1989) maliciously evokes the family "club" which lasts just as long as the benefits drawn by each of its members appears satisfying as regards to the consented investment. The diversity in the forms of familial life is reflected especially in the multiplication of those familial forms other than strictly two-parent: the massive growth in the number of one-parent families, consisting of one adult (9 out of 10 mothers), the growth of familial re-compositions, but also homosexual families or even couples who do not live together. The obvious fragility of the familial cell therefore seems evident, even as far as the children are concerned: the experience of their peers and the mass media confirm their risks and upsets less from death in families as was in the past, than from the conflicts and separations of the parental couple.

These transformations are incontestable and well-known; they pose for numerous families difficult questions related to maintaining the parental roles after the dissolution of the conjugal couple. However, the majority of these so-called new families, one-parent, re-composed or homosexual, do not request interventions from the social services. It is known that the great majority of the children living in a one-parent family, or within one or two re-composed families, seem to behave as well as their peers that are raised within traditional two-parent contexts. In contrast, the situation is very different if we consider the families in difficulty who constitute "the clientèle" of social work. These are, if not among the "new breed", at least rarely a stable two-parent couple, but more often one-parent or a re-composed family. Furthermore re-compositions are often transitory, as the Quebec expression states "unstable couples". Studies even show that two-parent families rarely see their children in care and are scantly followed by the AEMO (Durning).

We are going to successively examine traditional socio-educative interventions before describing the emergence of publications and interventions centred on "parenthood" about which we would underline that these call for important transformations in the practices of social intervention. Finally we must recall that the development of these approaches does not exclude certain appeals for explicitly repressive interventions.

The development of specialized open field interventions

Our discussion develops the experience gained in a work carried out with my Quebec colleague Gérald Boutin (Boutin, Durning, 1994, 1999, 2006). Both of us were shocked by French or Quebec professionals, during work placement or training in another country, and we share the difficulty of putting into perspective the work of North American or North European origins concerning parent interventions with the experience and work of the French. We have therefore taken on the task of describing and analyzing the different modes of parent intervention put into practice in the principal Western countries, leaning heavily on our knowledge of French and North American realities.

Place to repair

Historically, the first educational parental intervention mode was the removal of the child and its placement in a specialized establishment, hospice, and then nursery. The re-placement in these institutions was most often justified by a separation from an ordinary environment considered incompetent or dangerous. In certain cases, particularly serious physical handicap, it is the need to benefit from specific substantial and costly awards which justifies the transfer to a nursery.

This policy was progressively questioned after the 1970s because of its cost but also because of the difficulties the young children had to re-enter society after being raised in these institutions (Fablet, 1993, 2005). The educational authority of children placed in "situations of familial substitution" (Durning, 1985) has been the object of research work since the end of World War II (Redl, 1973). In France, since the mid-1970s, researchers have given emphasis to the study of the relations between educators and children (Durning, 1985, 1992), between professionals (Fablet, 1998), and between parents and professionals (Mackiewicz, 1998). Other research has focused on the efficacy of placements (Tremblay, 1980) and the study of what becomes of the young after the placement (Corbillon-Assailly-Duyme, 1987, 1990). Lastly, we highlight a development of the research centred on maltreatment in institutions (Durning, 1982, 1997; Tomkiewicz, Vivet, 1991) which leads to the consideration that placement does not automatically constitute a measure of protection for a child maltreated in his family.

Specialized interventions in the ordinary environment

The reduction in the number of placements (effective from the beginning of the 1980s) was preceded and accompanied by a development in specialized interventions with a preventive aim (or alternatives (Fablet, 1993) to a placement carried out in the normal environment, most often, inside the family (AEMO, SESSAD, etc.) or in institutions of normal care (Corbillon, 1993; Miron, 1998).

In France, three principal interventions are distinguished.

- The interventions by the PMI [*Maternal and Infant Protection*], i.e., visits called "post-natal" by a child welfare officer constitute a very early intervention, most often the first, which is able to help the parents in their educational tasks (Durning, Mackiewicz, 1994).
- The actions for parents after the birth of a handicapped child have developed considerably to allow keeping of the child in a normal familial and then school environment. These have led to re-deployment of those actions previously carried out in open-field institutions called SESSAD (Treminitin, 1998; SESSAD, 1992).
- Finally, the educative actions carried out in everyday environments for parents encountering difficulties with their children. Here, we must distinguish between the actions justified by a crime against a young child, to those justified by the danger incurred by the same. The measures can be "voluntary" or ordered by a magistrate. (Corbillon et al., 1999). A summary of the last five years is being elaborated, listing many hundreds of articles in professional journals but only some tens of research works, leading to a corpus of knowledge of some importance (Breugnot, Durning to appear in June, 2007).

The research specially conducted by our team shows that child welfare workers identify (most often on the first visit) those families in difficulty well (PMI 1&2). It is true that these families have often accumulated many problems: insufficient income and accommodation lacking or precarious (Corbillon, 1993). These difficulties induced by unemployment are often associated with health problems and, above all, a social isolation of the mother. It would be easy to admit that such conditions favour familial conflict and the development of psycho-pathologic problems. The real difficulty is therefore not to shift the responsibility but to propose and put into practice an action capable of improving the situation (Durning et al., 1993; Durning, 1998; Olds, Henderson, 1989).

The research centred on the intervention practices themselves is recent, still not abundant and only partial. In fact, professionals often emphasize situations linked to sexuality such as the revelation of incest and the inter-generational transmission of a secret. These choices founded on psychoanalysis-inspired theorizing, accentuate the relationship dimensions at stake, emotions and, above all, counter-transfer of the intercessor. At the same time, they are less concerned with banal educational difficulties, frequent but with heavy consequences: a parent badly controls or then again gravely neglects their child – a youth does not know how to interact with his/her peers except with violence. From such situations other models are recalled, other theoretical references, and other knowledge in practice.

The situations of negligence are, however, extremely numerous (Gabel, Manciaux, 1998) and their consequences for the development of the child are the most serious and irremediable. But, above all, these situations are those in which well-constructed socio-educative procedures have demonstrated their efficacy. (Palacio-Quintin et al., 1995; Durning, 1998).

Finally, evaluations give a mitigated image of the efficacy of certain interventions. The studies by ODAS have shown that among the situations due to maltreatment, a significant proportion had already been the object of a previous alert, or even an intervention. The systematic assistance of the young leaving a placement, albeit rare in France, gives only partial and sometimes contradictory results. (Weiss, Jacob, 1988; Olds, Henderson, 1989; Cebula, Horel, 1994; Velpry et al., 2000). These evaluations, associated with the development of an incivility and under-age delinquency ever younger and more and more violent, has led to a more repressive treatment of the young themselves, but also led to questioning the responsibility of their parents, by envisaging earlier and sometimes more authoritarian interventions. In both cases, the objective is to modify parental practices without the professionals replacing them in their educative responsibilities.

Recent developments: a double centring on the parents

For the last fifteen years or so, it has been possible to notice a double movement of earlier prevention and an appeal for more than just authoritarianism; these two movements question the responsibility of the parents and lean on the recent emergence of the term "parentality" (Durning, 1999 b). At first, the parents, especially the fathers, were accused of being the cause of bad treatment of their children (towards the end of the 1980s in France). Some years later, it was the "dismissal" of the parents, again the fathers in particular, which was evoked to explain the ever earlier acts of delinquency. It became a question of sensitizing the parents to their responsibility – in effect to "re-parentalize" them.

The success of the neologism "parentality" intrigues by its rapidity and extent. Over the last three years, a huge number of publications on this theme can be found, written especially by psycho-analysts. These works underline the role of the parents (most often limiting the processes considered to solely emotional and affective dimensions) to explain the educational insufficiency of their children, but also more recently the violent and delinquent behaviour of young adolescents in so-called "difficult" schools and neighbourhoods. It is nonetheless remarkable to realize that the properly educational dimensions of the parental role remain most often evoked by one word. If the term "parentality" comprehends the importance of parents' actions, it can also lead to relieving the professional services of their responsibility for the difficulties manifested by the children in their care. In fact, even for the children sent to school after the age of two, or taken into care in institutions for early family support (nursery schools, specialized family placements), we realize that the difficulties found are more easily charged to the family rather than to the interventions which the children have sometimes benefited from during their life. As Ulla Björnberg said (1992), the parents do not have a great deal of control over the socialization outside the family but are held responsible for these difficulties.

Repression or prevention

For many years we have been able to clearly identify the outlines of a policy of repression for those parents who do not keep hold of their pre-adolescents, a dismissal, proclaimed with firmness or even threats. Police services, the courts, or even schools propose coercive measures towards certain parents (withdrawal of family allowance, corrective measures, prison penalties, parental removal) as well as towards certain measures for the young. At the same time, those responsible for French social policies attempt to develop earlier action to support families, an action supposed to help parents before recourse to more severe and stigmatizing interventions.

There is a real tension between these two approaches: while one puts groups of parents "in the open" to fight against maltreatment, the other calls for financial sanctions, treatments which are imposed increasingly, without evaluating the consequent parental damage. Here we can find quite obviously the double offer of the carrot and the stick.

Supporting "parentality"

The actions to support "parentality" developed by the Inter-Ministerial Delegation in charge of the family have as an objective the development of preventive mechanisms, preceding more formalized actions which are the responsibility of the PMI and above all open-field educative action. The project of the earliest possible prevention leads to an interest in the practices of care and parentage of the young child and not only to the relationship of attachment even if this crosses and influences the entirety of daily practices (Beckwith, 1990). We are thus lead not only to consider the educative dimension of the parent-child interaction, and, for example, to question the knowledge thus transmitted instead of the modalities of transmission, but also to consider the educative dimension of the interaction between parents and professionals.

While the AEMO has proposed or imposed on those families identified as in difficulty that the intervention be individualized, family by family, these initiatives consist of reuniting groups of families initially voluntarily, but who, in reality, are often largely oriented by the PMI. The introduction of this mechanism reflects a political will to improve the conditions of life of children and their families borne by the Inter-Ministerial Delegation.

Current studies should permit us to discover which are the parents who effectively participate in these groups, persons already in great difficulty, parents "without a problem", or perhaps those feeling themselves "passed by" in their role and who would be the first interested in the mechanism. Currently, these few groups, of whom certain refer to the "Maison Vertes" inspired by Fr. Dolto, often bring together parents of young children. Experience abroad would suggest attempting to unite heterogeneous groups on the one hand, so that the parents can come to help each other (the main aim of these meetings); on the other hand, however, this same heterogeneity (very difficult to encounter) would be the best protection against risks of stigmatization.

Evolution in debates in France (March 2006)

Taking into account recent analyses of the French child protection system (ONED 2005), a law is currently being prepared. Among other important decisions, we highlight here the creation of diversified measures allowing us to overcome the conflict between placement (in kindergarten or foster family) and educational action within the family. The law should create mixed measures associating, according to diverse modalities, these two forms of aid to parents and children in difficulties, thus allowing actions which are more varied and adapted to the specificity of each situation.

The conditions for a renewal of interventions

Without casting doubt on the ensemble of professional acquisitions elaborated over the last fifty years, the choice of developing interventions of a preventive nature and less specialized actions which diminish costs and reduce the risks of stigmatizing the persons followed, calls for certain rather important modulations of socio-educative action. These lie especially in a wider analysis of the situation not limited to an evaluation of the problems, but integrating the resources of the family group, instead of those of their social environment, and ultimately taking into account the educative dimensions of the process at stake.

Consideration of family resources

This reorientation leads to considering the conditions favouring a "good" education of children in the diagnosis of situations, as in putting an intervention strategy into practice. The insistence on the positive dimensions of situations and not only on the problems and parental insufficiencies, helps to favour an "appropriation of the parents' situation". Such an approach enters the more and more widespread theme of resilience (Werner, 1992; Manciaux, 1996; Vinay et al., 2000) and can contribute to those parents benefiting from socio-educative interventions being considered as partners, co-responsible along with the intercessor for the actions introduced. This change in the way of relating to the parents being helped would lead to confiding in the strong points of the family workings, without limiting the action to an awareness of the parents' difficulties.

The re-insertion of the family group in their environment

On a broader scale, the innovative interventions are often founded on eco-system analyses (Brofenbrenner, 1986, 1987; Belsky, 1980, 1981, 1984, 1986; Belsky, Vondra, 1989; Pallacio-Quintin et al., 1995) in an attempt to overcome an approach limited to the family group. We can note, from some works, especially North-American, a move from the apprehension of a triangular parents-professionals-children system to the consideration of a more complex system in which the context and social environment plays a major role (Whittaker, Garbarino, 1983; Dunst, Trivette, 1990). Such a point of view can reorient the action of the intercessors called to "help the helpers", rather than trying themselves to modify the family workings. Traditional analysis reveals a potentially conflicting relation of rivalry between parents and professionals, in which the child is the pawn, with the uncertainties, which we have already indicated, on whether the professional is intervening regarding the child or the parents (Durning, 1999 a). The introduction of a fourth plural player leads to a radical transformation of the system, since, particularly when the professional is supporting the natural helpers, he disengages from a position of direct rivalry with the parent, but then he needs a global analysis of the processes at stake, which largely overcomes that of the parent-child and parent-professional relationships.

Some recent works have highlighted the diversity in the practices induced by an elaborate consideration of the social environment of those families in difficulty. In a Quebec project carried out for some years on negligent families (Palacio-Quintin et al., 1995), some so-called "supportive" families are given a mandate to establish a quality relationship with the target family which should lead them to leave their isolation by bringing them to move among the different services where they can obtain some aid . At best, links with friends of the supportive family would create a re-knitting of the social fabric. In France, militant community action such as that of the ATD Quart Monde (Fourth World) also accords great importance to the network which the families in a neighbourhood or street constitute, and whose supporting role is essential.

Here, the originality would be less the discovery of the importance of the social network than the execution of concrete practices to improve the integration of a subject in his social network (Sanicola, 1994) or to animate the members of a network into aiding a family.

The re-evaluation of educational and training dimensions

Raising children presupposes the mobilization of numerous skills which evolve step by step with the growth of the children, from taking charge of the neonate to that of the adolescent (Kellerhals, Montandon, 1991; Durning, 1999b).

For a long time, the principal reference point of parents was their own education; the rapid evolution of the surrounding world, of the school system, and the requirements of employment has incontestably weakened and confused the remnants to which the parents refer to raise their children. Analyzing the situation in Scandinavian countries at the end of the 1980s, Lars Dencik (1988) underlined that it was completely new that parents as a whole be so aware of the evolution of situations that they would admit that the reference to their own education was insufficient to guide them in their parental role.

In France, however, there is a diffidence which is understandable but exacerbated, regarding the normative side of an educational or training action, according to which "parents are moulded by teaching them *the* good way of dealing with their children". Nevertheless, we can, at the same time, discuss the inverse position which considers that no knowledge can be useful and that every request for information by a parent should be dismissed as non-pertinent. We recall, for example, that professionals often maintain that what they learn through their métier is useful to them in their familial activities (Durning, 1996; Erny, Jeong, 1996).

The actions of "parentality" support postulate that it is productive to favour the exchange of experience, and to allow groups to see that "when you cannot succeed in a certain way with your child, you can try another ...". That is to say, (to be just a little normative) in agreeing to debate questions such as: what should I do if my child does not want to eat, or takes drugs ... Beyond the radical alternative between imposing on the participants a model of "good parenthood" and casting them back to their relationship difficulties, one viewpoint of support proposes the mediation of reflection shared with other parents (Pourtois, 1984).

Such a practice remains strictly reserved for professional training in our common culture. It is astonishing that we partake of an overt concept of the training of intercessors, teachers, psychologists etc., as being very different from what the training of parents could be. The first is thought of as a practice of co-construction of knowledge and interaction with others, referring directly to the consolidated knowledge, the erudition of the trainer and the experience of the participants, whereas the concept of parental training is that of indoctrination, without discussion or debate, of a reactionary familial model in students stripped of any critical sense.

Many conditions appear necessary for facilitate such evolution. We mention three:

- Re-consider the training, largely nurtured by psychological approaches elaborated during the 1970s and too rarely enriched by works on educative processes or even on social interventions. This situation is a consequence of too big a divide between the world of research and that of intervention.

- Re-consider the technical background of psycho-socio-educative intercessors (reflection about the ethical background of the intervention). Currently, the majority of training based on this background is centred both on a knowledge of public politics, and team management; it only rarely benefits from instruction centred on the actual technicality of the interventions it is charged with directing. The DESS proposed in Paris X by Michel Corbillon explicitly subscribes to this point of view.
- Develop assessment and research by partnering social intervention institutions and research laboratories.

The consideration of the multiple relational and affective dimensions, certainly, but also the cognitive dimensions of the educative process (knowledge and representations at stake) and axiological dimensions (values) opening numerous paths are able to contribute to better understanding and to intervening deep within complex educational situations. Such an approach leads to an analysis of the incidence of educative practices raised by the various familial and professional educative cases involved, without forgetting the role played by the personality and behaviour of the child himself.

References

Beckwith L: Adaptive and maladaptive parenting. Implications for intervention. In: Meisels SJ, JP Shonkoff (eds): Handbook of Early Childhood Intervention. Cambridge University Press, New York 1990

Belsky J: A family analysis of parental influence on infant exploratory competence. In: Pedersen F (ed): The Father-infant Relationship: Observational Studies in a Family Context. Praeger Special Studies, New York 1980

Belsky J: Early Human Experience: A Family Perspective. Developmental Psychology 17 (1) (1981) 3–23

Belsky J: The determinants of parenting: a process model. Child Development 55 (1984) 83–96

Belsky J: A tale of two variances: Between and within. Child Development 57 (1986) 1301–1305

Belsky J, J Vondra: Lessons from child abuse: the determinants of parenting. In: Cicchetti D, V Carlson (eds): Child Maltreatment. Theory and research on the causes and consequences of child abuse and neglect. Cambridge University Press, New York 1989

Björnberg U: La fonction parentale en Europe, tendances évolutives. In: Du politique et du social dans l'avenir de la famille. La Documentation française, Paris 1992

Boutin G, P Durning: Les interventions auprès des parents. Bilan et analyse des pratiques socio-éducatives. Privat, Paris 1994

Boutin G, P Durning: "préface à la deuxième édition". In: Les interventions auprès des parents. Bilan et analyse des pratiques socio-éducatives. Dunod, Paris 1999

Bronfenbrenner U: Is early intervention effective? Teachers College Record 76 (2) (1974) 279–303

Bronfenbrenner U: Ecology of the Family as a Context for Human Development: Research Perspectives. Developmental Psychology 22 (6) (1986) 733–742

Bronfenbrenner U: Foreword-Family support: The Quiet Revolution. In: Kagan SL et al.: America's Family Support Programs. Yale University Press, New Haven 1987

Cébula JC, C Horel (dir): Le placement familial de l'aide sociale à l'enfance. Étude Nationale mai 92 à septembre 93. Comité de pilotage de l'étude 1994

Corbillon M (coord): Enfant Présent, une crèche familiale entre accueil et prévention. Évaluation d'un mode d'accueil innovant, rapport de recherche GERIS. 1983

Corbillon M, JP Assailly, M Duyme: Le placement à l'aide sociale à l'enfance: la reproduction inter-générationnelle. Les Cahiers du CTNERHI 37 (1987) 1–33

Corbillon M, JP Assailly, M Duyme: L'enfant placé. De l'assistance publique à l'aide sociale à l'enfance. La Documentation française, Paris 1990

Corbillon M, P Rousseau, P Durning: AEMO administrative et judiciaire en Seine-Saint-Denis, analyse des moments-clés de l'intervention. Ronéo, ERISFER 1990

Dencik, L: Grandir aujourd'hui. Étude des contextes et modalités de socialisation du point de vue du jeune enfant. In: Durning P (dir): Éducation familiale. Un panorama des recherches internationales. Matrice, Paris 1988

Desmet H, JP Pourtois: Prédire, comprendre la trajectoire scolaire. PUF, Paris 1993

Dunst CJ, CM Trivette: Assessment of social support in early intervention programs. In: Meisels SJ, JP Shonkoff: Handbook of Early Childhood Intervention. Cambridge University Press, New York 1990

Durning P: Éducation et suppléance familiale en internat. C.T.N.E.R.H.I., Paris 1986

Durning P: Éducation familiale. Panorama des recherches internationales. Matrice, Paris 1988

Durning, P: L'enfant, enjeu des interactions entre familles naturelles, milieux de suppléance familiale et travailleurs sociaux. Communautés éducatives 80 (1992) 51–60

Durning P: Éducation familiale, acteurs processus et enjeux. PUF, Paris 1995a

Durning P: Exploring parenting roles. In: Colton M, W Hellinckx, P Ghesquière, M Williams (eds): The Art and Science of Child Care. Arena, Aldershot 1995b

Durning P: Faut-il éduquer les parents? Sciences Humaines 64 (1996) 10–15

Durning P. Maltraitance familiale, maltraitance institutionnelle, similitudes et spécificités. Les Cahiers de l'Actif 248–249 (1997) 37–44

Durning P: Pour une approche socio-éducative des familles maltraitantes. Le Groupe Familial 158 (1998) 88–99

Durning P: Le partage de l'action éducative entre parents et professionnels. Relevé des travaux en langue française et propositions de recherches à développer, Rapport de recherche effectuée avec la collaboration de S. Pascal, Ministère de la Justice. Instruments et méthodes 1 (1) (1999a)

Durning P: Répression, soutien ou formation des parents. Informations Sociales 73/74 (1999b) 192–199

Durning P: Nouvelles familles ou nouvelles approches des familles en détresse? In: Actualités Sociales hebdomadaires. L'avenir du social à l'aube du XXI ème siècle 2148 (7 Janvier 2000) 26

Durning P, D Fablet, MP Machiewicz: Les processus de décision et les pratiques professionnelles en œuvre lors des visites à domicile effectuées par les puéricultrices de la PMI du

département des Hauts-de-Seine, recherche conduite en convention avec le Conseil Général des Hauts-de-Seine/D.V.S. 1993
Durning P, MP Machiewicz: De la visite à domicile à la consultation de PMI. Suivi d'une cohorte de 190 enfants durant 18 mois. Ronéo, Rapport de recherche GREF 1994
Erny P, MR Jeong: Expériences de formation parentale et familiale: France, Allemagne, Belgique, Amérique du Nord, Corée du Sud. L'Harmattan, Paris 1996.
Fablet D: Dispositifs innovant de suppléance familiale et prévention de l'exclusion. Connexions 62 (1993) 91–106
Fablet D: Les modalités de coopération entre professionnels et parents d'enfants placés dans les pouponnières à caractère social. Tome 1: Les pratiques des professionnels des pouponnières en direction des familles d'enfants placés – Approche institutionnelle. Rapport MIRE/DEP 1996
Fablet D: Les modalités de coopération entre les équipes de PMI et leurs partenaires. Rapport DVS/GREF 1998
Fablet D: Suppléance familiale et interventions socio-éducatives analyser les pratiques des professionnels. L'Harmattan, Paris 2005
Gabel M, M Manciaux et al.: Enfances en danger. Fleurus, Paris 1998
Kellerhals J, C Montandon et al.: Les stratégies éducatives des familles. Delachaux, Niestlé, Lausanne 1991
Lavenu D: Des anamnèses de cas de réussite scolaire. La réussite à l'école. Contribution à la recherche de facteurs de compréhension. Thèse Université de Caen, Caen 1993
Mackiewicz MP: Suppléance précoce et parentalité: une étude de la coopération entre parents et professionnels dans les pouponnières à caractère social. Thèse de doctorat dirigée par P. Durning. Paris 1998
Manciaux M: La résilience: mythe ou réalité? In: Gabel M, S Lebovici, Ph Mazet (eds) : Maltraitance psychologique. Fleurus, Paris 1996
Miron JM: Les services de garde comme lieu de formation et de soutien pour les parents. In: Éthier LS, J Alary (dir): Comprendre la famille. Presses de l'Université du Québec, Sainte-Foy 1998
ODAS: L'observation de l'enfance en danger: Guide méthodologique. ODAS, Paris 1994
ODAS: Quinze ans de décentralisation: de l'action sociale au développement social. ODAS, Paris 2000
Olds DL, CR Henderson: The prevention of maltreatment. In: Cicchetti D, V Carlson (eds): Child Maltreatment. Theory and Research on the Causes and Consequences of Child Abuse and Neglect Cambridge University Press, New York 1989
ONED: Premier rapport de l'Observatoire national de l'enfance en danger ou gouvernement et au Parlement. Paris 2005
Palacio-Quintin E, G Couture, J Paquet et al.: Projet d'intervention auprès des familles négligentes présentant ou non des comportements violents, Rapport de recherche GREDEF 1995
Pourtois JP: Comment les mères enseignent à leur enfant (5–6 ans). PUF, Paris 1979
Pourtois JP: Éduquer les parents ou comment stimuler la compétence en éducation. Ed. Labor, Bruxelles 1984
Pourtois JP (ed) Les thématiques en Éducation familiale. De Boeck, Bruxelles 1989a
Pourtois JP: L'éducation familiale, note de synthèse. Revue Française de Pédagogie, 86 (1989b)
Pourtois JP, H Desmet: Tendances actuelles de la recherche en éducation familiale. In: Durning P (dir): Éducation familiale. Un panorama des recherches internationales. Matrice, Paris 1988

Redl F, D Wineman: L'enfant agressif, tome 1. Le moi désorganisé. Fleurus, Paris 1973 a
Redl F, D Wineman: L'enfant agressif, tome 2. Méthodes de rééducation. Fleurus, Paris 1973b
Roussel, L: La famille incertaine. Éditions Odile Jacob, Paris 1989
Sanicola L: L'intervention de réseaux. Bayard, Paris 1994
SESSAD: Les Services d'éducation spécialisée et de soins à domicile. Mouv'Ance 8 (1992)
Shonkoff JP, SJ Meisels: Early childhood intervention: The evolution of a concept. In: Meisels SJ, JP Shonkoff (eds): Handbook of Early Childhood Intervention. Cambridge University Press, New York 1989
Terrisse B, G Boutin (dir): La famille et l'éducation de l'enfant de la naissance à six ans. Les Éditions Logiques, Montréal 1994
Tomkiewicz S, P Vivet: Aimer mal, châtier bien. Enquêtes sur les violences dans des institutions pour enfants et adolescents. Seuil, Paris 1991
Tremblay RE: Les caractéristiques des internats de rééducation susceptibles d'avoir un impact positif sur les mineurs en difficulté avec la loi: étude critique des résultats de recherche. Université de Montréal, Montréal 1980
Tremintin J: Les SESSAD misent tout sur la famille. Lien social 465 (1998) 4–6
Vinay A, S Esparbes-Pistre, P Tap: Comportements d'attachement et de coping chez l'individu résilient. Revue internationale de l'éducation familiale 1 (2000) (à paraître)
Velpry L et al.: Analyse des dossiers d'enfants sortis en 1980 et 1990 de l'Aide Sociale de l'Enfance de Seine-Saint-Denis. (Rapport multigraphié provisoire recherché en cours) 2000
Weiss HB, FH Jacobs: Evaluating Family Programs. Aldine de Gruyter, New York 1988.
Werner EE: Protectives Factors and individual resilience. In: Meisels SJ, JP Shonkoff (eds): Handbook of Early Childhood Intervention. Cambridge University Press, Cambridge 1992
Westinghouse Learning Corporation: The impact of Head Start: An evaluation of the effects of Head Start on children's cognitive and affective development. Ohio University, Athens 1969
Whittaker J, J Garbarino: Social support networks. Aldine Publishing, Hawthorne 1983
Zigler E, J Valentine (eds): Project Head Stard: A legacy of the War on Poverty. Free Press, New York 1979

22. Migration, a risk for identity?

Tajeb Ferradji; Centre of Ethnopsychiatry, University Hospital of Avicenne, Bobigny, France

If, in psycho-pathology, we consider that the capacity to resolve intra-psychic and inter-personal conflicts depends on the stability of identity and racial questions, in the clinical setting, identity goes back equally well to the view of its genesis and its trouble within the perspective of understanding the world, oneself and others. If the Oedipus complex knew the success that it has since its description by Freud, it is not only because of its universality but also because it refers to a fundamental question for all men: that of their affiliation.

In fact, a name is not a simple graphic imprint on some identity papers, it is an adventure of being, a destiny. It is history with or without the history of its affiliation. Ever since *The Book of the Dead* of the ancient Egypt with its "your name is your destiny" to the Talmud, passing through the father's name of the Christians and the amber rosary of the ninety-nine names of Allah of the Muslims, we all recall that we are the creatures of that affiliation, whether it is hereditary or arbitrary and, that it is not without effect on our life.

With immigration, maternal depression in its relations with affiliation constitutes a paradigm of the puzzle of identity. The consideration of the socio-cultural context and, especially, the radical and rapid changes which affect those populations on all planes and particularly in the psycho-sociological field, an unconfined frame of the beginning of maternal depression in good measure or for a great number of patients, the etiology, the psycho-pathological expression, and taking control of the problems equal the reference to the terms sick, woman, spouse, mother, citizen, worker etc. This is in an environment of a transitional world marked by the wake of a rapid, massive, and radical integration. In this context, the puzzle of the place of the child is essential in relation to its number, just as the socio-cultural life-experience of the familial group counts on the weight of the school or religious figure.

Desire for maternity, desire for a child, to have children, make children, all are series of expressions which in the life-experience of the group and in the subconscious of the mother are crucial in the plan of certain depressive decompensations. If the depression, loss of the vital élan and loss of positive expectations, is characterized by a pathological sadness and pessimism, one cannot underline that it is going to represent a depressive pathology to be resolved when the child is born, and while, as B. Betelheim underlines, precisely being a mother and being a father questions the sense he must give to his existence. Because the child emerges in a privileged manner, one should exclusively see the ethic of the group, through the place that he and other children occupy in the projects of every man and every woman, and in the life of every couple, in the models of procreation and education of every group.

The transformation from a traditional society to a modern world is going to affect, among other things, the status and the place of the woman through the question of affiliation and identity, and this in a context of a cultural conflict that is much more exacerbated when the changes are rapid and weigh heavily on the 'historic' women. In this context, maternity appears as the privileged expression of the affirmation of belonging to the group through the proclivity of the affiliation structuring. Birth, life, and death are lived and accepted in a dimension where belonging to the group "collective 'I'" is the basic datum. The dyad mother-baby constitutes a sort of micro-cosmos of the milieu and the ambient culture. It is in this field that anticipatory illusion must come into play, whose organizational and structuring role in the interaction of the child with the fantasy of the mother, as Diatkine underlines. Sex, age, lineage, all condition social status, and the structure of the group is based on the concordance between biological procreation and familial genealogy. The status of the adult man, and even more so, the woman, is linked to the authority of the group.

The woman does not comply with a certain authority until the marriage of her children and especially her sons; that is to say, when she enters the status of mother-in-law. These facts are 'classical' in the patriarchal structures of the Mediterranean world. Marriage has procreation as its first aim and the status of the woman is a function of her fecundity. The pregnant woman benefits from a certain status which makes her significant. The secondary benefits are numerous, and the traditional practices which surround pregnancy and birth, are on the preventive mental health level and not inconsequential. Multiple maternity was a blessing; nonetheless premature birth, repeated deliveries, and pregnancies close to one another bring a physiological weakening with qualitative and quantitative deficits as well as untimely aging of the mother. This process is accelerated by the impact of the domestic and external work which the woman is often obliged to do. Hence, the increased risk of tiredness, asthenia, anemia, spontaneous abortion, and fragility in the lastborn – facts which have an important impact on the psychological equilibrium of the mother.

Being fertile, and remaining fertile, adds to the anxiety of being endured as an inadequate marriage. It is equally significant that in certain regions the menopause should be designated not by the correct Arabic word "retreat", but by the expression "age of despair". The customary and religious proceedings facilitating divorce and polygamy on the simple decision of the husband (should he be the sterile partner) reinforce this anxiety. "Anxiety of empty casts, terror of false parturition, obsession with repeated female births, the misfortune of infant mortality: such is the quadruple fixation of the woman" (Boudhiba, 1973). This acknowledgement, that is still valid in the Arab-Berbère and Mediterranean rural environments, often agrees with the reality of traditional culture.

Still today, we can find a practice of prolonged breast-feeding for two or even three years which is important for its impact physically and mentally for the child as well as of the mother. This tradition has an implication for the spectre of incest which hovers over the conjugal relationship as long as the woman is in the situation of breast-feeding. In fact, in the Coranic tradition, the simple fact of tasting the milk of a woman initiates a relationship of a dependent link to her. This shows the complex affective climate in which the couple and the baby mature during that long period of maternal narcissistic joy and megalomaniac power of the baby.

In 1968, in the "*Enfants d'hier et d'aujourd'hui*" [*Children of Yesterday and Today*], Zerdoumi describes the intimate relationship of investment of the Magreb mother with her child, underlining how much her future depends on her status as mother of a boy; "The woman makes herself a slave of her child, who uses her as her sovereign master. The mother belongs totally to her child. At night he sleeps in her lap, his flesh against hers, while the father is relegated, alone in another bed. The baby, for the mother, comes before everything. He allows her to realize herself one day, to find her place in society and when married, he offers her the chance to reign in his house. She does everything to satisfy this child, bearer of her deliverance and of her extirpation from nothing, to find her Self, in a society which only makes her a woman once she is a mother".

Multiparity, pregnancy, and prolonged breast-feeding form an uninterrupted rhythm, in which women may be often confronted by the loss of a child at a young age. When multiparity is the case, the preeminence of the collective "I" means that, paradoxically, the mourning was done rapidly, apparently excluding all blame. All the same, the late cessation of breast-feeding which is described as being generally brutal, motivates a new pregnancy, attenuating the modalities and the affective repercussions which cannot be as marked as they are presented by the authors who have approached this question regarding the black African child. Storck (1988) highlights in *Enfances indiennes* [*Indian Childhoods*] that methodological prudence is necessary, as Ainsworth observed during his study in Uganda on the reaction of babies separated from their mothers.

In this context, the problem of the mother (especially young) is inseparable from the radical evolutionary movement of the gigantic social puzzle. The resistance to change is going to grow and make the woman as target. She, the guarantor of values and traditions, and at the same time an agent of restricted alliances, is abruptly projected on the fires of the ramp. She decides more and more to remain there, even if for a time she eventually chooses the veil, which we too often forget does not mark precisely the return to cultural tradition, but the divide from parental culture and often a breakthrough into the external social space.

Desire – prohibition – blame, key terms of Oedipal positioning, are at the centre of this individual movement which is accelerating, growing within the group level. Meanwhile, aggressive reactions become increasingly important, so that every day possible developments and particularly teras between generations emerge.

How to mourn in a traditional way is the key question. To eliminate the ancestor without betraying him is the question for today's young parents. It is obvious that the young mother is not often prepared to bear that situation, hence the great vulnerability of some women. Besides, increasingly more, socio-demographic realities (such as the increase in life-expectancy) and the novel aspirations that the coming generations bring the individual face to face with social dynamics where inter-generational problems are growing, and where, above all, the young couple on the triple sociological, psychological and metaphysical level, are confronted by their own desire and especially by their desire for a child.

In fact, one of the fundamental questions which increasingly more mothers and fathers face is that of the control of their fecundity, and through this to assume their sexuality by surmounting traditional taboos. These taboos are, paradoxically, contrary to the advanced ideas and are not those of Islam. In fact, in Islam, there is no view of sins of the flesh, and the concept of the irremediable importance of the original sin linked to Adam and Eve does not exist. From this point, increasingly more often the dynamic of the traditional-modern confrontation, with all its cleavages and all the nuances which this type of dialectic presupposes in an evolutionary socio-cultural context, is expressing itself in a perspective identical to that sketched by ethno-psychiatry regarding the children of immigrants. The universality of human psychological functioning does not exclude particularities such as socio-cultural importance. The bio-somatic realities, such as the place of affection, remain however the fundamental structuring elements; organizers of an ever present individuality.

Cases of depression of minor intensity often remain unrecognized, being capable of spontaneous healing, sometimes at the expense of traces whose evidence only appears later in the emotional, affective or cognitive equilibrium of the child, but show frequent psychosomatic pathologies in the mother and in the infant. The rate of these pathologies seems to be growing; sometimes including new pathologies, even if not identified as such at the time.

Among the clinical tableaux quite particular in a traditional context, some seem to be prominent:

1) The association "state of depressive-delirious persecution" is, in fact, one of the principal clinical forms in the traditional milieu. Beyond the psychotic aspect, the depressive dynamic must be perceived, recognized and assumed by the group or by the psychiatrist not known for example in Europe. As Migarel underlines, the psychological problems hark back by the originality of their expression to the inherent productions of the individual's cultural tradition. The discussions and the attitudes of the state of suffering refer to the feeling of persecution concerning practice of sorcery. The subject uses the primordial categories of these cultural props in clinging to the beliefs

from which the subject branches. In the same way, certain kinds of depression affect a representation of bouts of delirium. Here we can find points raised by, among others, Collomb in Dakar, of which Ortigues, Show, and Ammar have underlined the link to the level of clinical expression with the educational and cultural that played a role in the organization and development of the personality.

2) Varied somatic symptoms are frequent, being able to include the affected in a diagnosis of hypochondria. These express the importance of the body in traditional culture, and the fact that it often remains the refuge and the privileged means of expression of psychological suffering, whereas the models of communication have known radical modifications. A certain decelerating psycho-motor manifestation is often discovered, and is clearer when it triggered the affected individual to take control.
   Similarly, certain clinical expressions bring to mind the picture, well summarized by Féline, under the name of hostile depression, associating the triad: Pain-Depression-Aggressiveness. This syndrome was described by Cidro-Franck and Gordon in a study dedicated to women suffering from pelvic pain in situations of marital frustration and who develop sentiments of impotent rage towards their husbands and their children with a tendency to anxiety and depression.
   The fragility affecting the woman in labor is classic, with depression being its principal form of expression, and with the weight of maternity-related conflicts and problems that it raises in the current transitional world and, particularly, because of the choices it imposes: stopping work not only for material reasons such as the lack of daycare, but above all, and primarily because of conflicts with the husband, and mother-in-law, among others.
3) The depressive states of the multipara: beyond socio-economic reasons, multiparity is a severe risk factor, as shown by the great vulnerability of the last-born of these great fraternities. In fraternities with great numbers, the infant at high risk is often conceived after a spontaneous abortion.
   The problem of those with constitutional vulnerability (Anthony, 1980) is to be restricted with reference to the bio-somatic state of the mother especially during pregnancy. Moreover, it is upon this scheme that the first relations are marked by "softening" of the potentialities and capacities of maternity of the multipara (Boucebci, 1977, 1985). In certain cases the bio-somatic woman has even a more unfavorable role than the ecological conditions that aggravate the bio-somatic state and depression.
   The dis-endowment of the multipara which is exhausted on the physical and affective levels, provokes an anticipated culpability which interferes by accentuating the difficulties of elaborating a mother-child link, precisely there where the child would have needed more significant attention and more intensive care, considering maternal vulnerability, the fragile suckling, and sometimes growth resticted and premature infant.

The evolution of sociology accentuates this risk since it would support the potential disappearance of multiparas, a group modality which efficiently, partially, or totally compensates by influencing a psycho-motor stimulation, or even by other members of the clan involved in weaning.

4) Since often a woman is roughly confronted by solitude and left alone with her anxiety and feelings of culpability, socio-cultural changes expose the mother increasingly often to situations which are highly enfeebling due to the affective problems they induce. Lebovici underlines how normal it is that the situation of psychological transparency observed during that exceptional period allows action at low cost on the psycho-therapeutic level, as in adolescence. The shared functioning of the traditional group probably had here a major therapeutic action which was extremely beneficial on a preventive as well as on a curative level. This leads to underscoring of the double mourning of the imaginary child and the required medical control at birth. However, when control stops, the situation is complicated in an inextricable fashion in the case of the young mother living in an underdeveloped socio-sanitary environment and in the context of a transitional world, whose remains are mad and inconsistent on all levels, all being introductory indicators for a high-risk situation for the health of the mother and the baby.
Certain cases show the sum of all risks. In the traditional context, the high mortality rate affected, in a significant way, the highly vulnerable neonates, who are fragile or even malformed or handicapped. Certainly, in the same line of thinking, twins are also, in various ways, objects of refusal and rejection. In today's transitional world, the woman can find herself facing these situations and sometimes in a situation of isolation which triggers-off a depressive functioning, which might be temporary but sometimes chronic, as the following observation illustrates: the case of Mrs. N. shows the role of the mother-to-be in the field of desire and the socio-cultural facts of the imaginary child. Mrs. N. was examined for a stupor depressive state gradually increasing over the last ten days. Psychiatric antecedents were absent. She had been married for two years and is pregnant. A threatened abortion led to the consultation. The ultrasound carried out was medically reassuring, but on that occasion, she learned brutally that she is probably expecting a daughter. The iatrogenic phrase created an incident at the family level, her spouse having many times advanced his intention to divorce after the long "sterility", and the incapacity of his wife to assure him a male descendent.
This brutal confrontation in an anonymous context of an unforeseen moment is a major event in a socio-cultural context where tradition and absence of clan references, the pregnancy always in progress does not allow a functioning without the group, take control and the removal of blame in a perspective where the prevalence of the collective "I" is essential. This conduct is reflected in a de-compensation. The anxious expectancy in limbo, the anes-

thetic and the maximal psycho-motor inhibition, express a depressive anticipation as witness of a time without future.

But yesterday's reality elsewhere, is present here today, and underlines the irreversible socio-cultural evolution which, with its positive and negative effects accompanies the entrance into modernity. On the whole, caricaturing the remark by Freud that there is no increase in the number of neuroses but an increase of their de-compensations, we can say that in reference to the qualitative and quantitative changes which affect the Magreb socio-culturally, politically, and economically, the entry into democracy shows at the same time an increase in the number of citizens, but also the increase in those who, here as elsewhere, know psychological suffering linked, deriving from, or concomitant to their status as a mother. This reality rests (once we have turned the page of the return to the Golden Age, in which traditional cultures would have been) on the fundamental question of Huxley and the reply of Diatkine:

Give me a better world, and I would make better mothers
Give me better mothers, and I would make a better world.

Is it necessary because of this to include women in the prevalence or the exclusivity of their role as mother? In her privileged affective intra-uterine dialogue with her baby in the first months and the first years, the mother induces and transmits an emotion, reflected by a consequential part in the stakes and the anxieties of which she is the object and the pawn. It is then, in a privileged way with her daughter, wife-to-be, that she will be tempted to transmit a message of liberation but also of defense, a reflection of her depression in our civilization.

Bibliography

Ammar S, S Douki, M Boucebci: Aspects cliniques et psychopathologiques de la dépression au Maghreb. Psychopathologie africaine XVII 1/2/3 (1981) 16–26

Anthony EJ, C Chiland, C Koupernic: L'enfant dans sa famille, l'enfant à haut risque psychiatrique. PUF, Paris 1980

Bendahman, H. Personnalité maghrébine et fonction paternelle au Maghreb (œdipe maghrébin). La Pensée Universelle, Paris 1984

Bettelheim B: Les blessures symboliques. Gallimard, Paris 1971

Boucebci M, A Yaker: Psychopathologie infanto-juvénile dans les pays en développement. In: Diatkine R, S Lebovici, M Soule: Traité de psychiatrie de l'enfant et de l'adolescent. PUF, Paris 1985

Boudhiba AA: La sexualité en Islam. PUF, Paris 1975

Collomb H: Les aspects culturels de la dépression. Revue du Praticien 28 (1978) 3025–3042

Ortigues MC: Œdipe africain. L'Harmattan, Paris 1984

Sowi I: Psychiatrie dynamique africaine. Payot, Paris 1977

Storck H: Enfances indiennes. PUF, Paris 1986

Zerdoumi N: Enfants d'hier et d'aujourd'hui. Maspero, Paris 1968

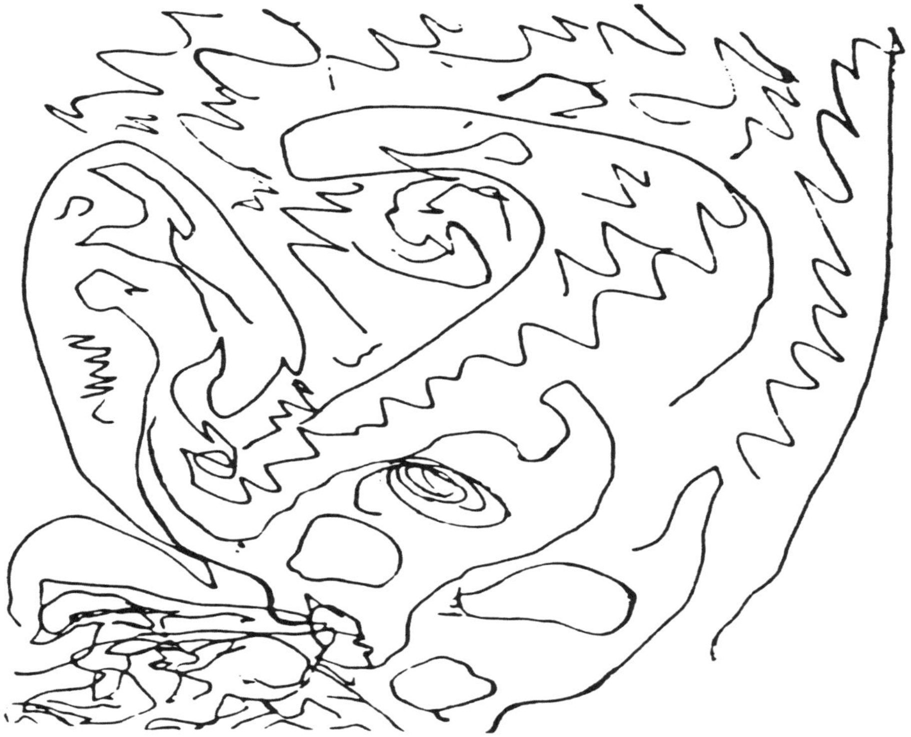

(Valeria, 3 yrs. 8 mos.)
The sea is born from the mother wave.
Time is born from the tempest.
The wind is born from the air and has the right shape to bang things.
Time is born from the years.

23. Scenarios of pregnancy and birth in immigrant families

Angela Maria Di Vita; Faculty of Educational Sciences, University of Palermo, Italy
Manuela Errante; Tourist Marketing, University of Palermo, Italy
Maria Vinciguerra; Intercultural Pedagogy and Didactics University of Palermo, Italy

For my mind-of-man
Now seeks the nature of the vast Beyond
There on the other side, that boundless sum,
Which lies without the ramparts of the world,
Toward which the spirit longs to peer afar
(Lucretius, *De Rerum Natura*, II, verses 1044–1047)

The bond with the land, places, and space in which we live has a particular meaning for all of us, in relation to the emotions they arouse, the memories connoting them and past events. They are part of our background, even though we may not always be aware of them. This is an emotional reality which cannot be disregarded. Therefore, leaving one's environment, even only for a short holiday, may be destabilizing for some and a source of anguish for others.

During an individual's lifetime, made up of a personal life-story and archetypal elements, the cultural unconsciousness is structured and interwoven with smells, flavours, colours, myths, emotional bonds of daily life, "through education and staying in a specific social and cultural group, with its language, traditions and territory of residence, and also with the events that the group experiences" (Liotta, 2005 p. 32). Leaving one's place of origin, therefore, causes a critical situation of crisis, due to the interruption of the sense of continuity that space and time guaranteed in the country of origin, leading to a sense of extraneousness with regard to the new environment. This may have a positive solution, if the subject is able to maintain internal continuity and a sense of belonging, while adapting to a new environment. Otherwise, the land will take on a connotation of conflict, representing a place of rigid and exclusive identification.

The immigration experience can be configured, on the one hand, as the guarantee of acquiring greater affluence, and on the other, as a process of being cut off from one's belonging and distance from one's loved ones. As Losi observes, "Separation from the context of origin must find a meaning in the context of arrival. And vice versa, the context of arrival, the new one, must find a meaning in that of origin. Probably it is this that allows making projects and defining a sense of the self and a tolerable future" (Losi, 2000 p. 304).

In this sense, the immigration process can be seen as a critical event, or critical transition, with consequent tasks of development. Regarding inter-family relations, members of immigrant families must coordinate their personal experiences of immigration; they may refer to times of nostalgia for their country, as well as to factors of stress, solitude, emotional closure. With respect to the social context, the members of immigrant families must face up to the difficult task of managing elements of continuity and change, as takes place in general in the dynamics of all family relationships (Monacelli, Mancini, 2005).

It is sufficient to think of the extent to which the social and family role of women changes in the migratory experience; they necessarily have to redefine the boundaries of their identity, in a process of emancipation that very often cannot be concluded in their country of origin. It is not always easy to change one's life and take on different ways of being and of imagining oneself, abandoning prior roles and spaces. The migratory experience of women is characterized by abandoning the elements of femininity of the homeland, made up of communication, practices, knowledge and exchange, memories and traditions, in which each woman had her own status. Women, needless to say, have always been the custodians of family bonds and traditions, and therefore, strong feelings of abandonment and loss in those they leave may be aroused with their departure, but also serious internal conflicts. As Cattaneo and dal Verme observe (2005), the aspiration for a different state, greater autonomy and freedom, could cause ambivalent feelings towards one's own culture. The stories which the women presently tell of depression and difficulties that do not derive so much from having embarked on a life in a country other than their own, but from the conflicts relative to the difficult and contradictory representations that they have of themselves as women.

This state of suffering may be more evident at particular times, such as when expecting a baby: having a child and bringing it up elsewhere is one of the challenges that immigrant women often have to cope with, sometimes almost immediately on their arrival in the country of emigration, both for those who immigrate on their own, and for those joining their husband. The event of maternity takes on different meanings depending on the life-stories of the women and what immigration means to them, but for all of them, this "challenge brings with it the experience of separation from their origins and the loss of the affective and cultural objects of reference" (Balsamo et al., 2002 p. 12). Each woman has her own subjectivity and her immigration path is unique.

With respect to the event of maternity, all women make choices in relation to their social conditions, their experiences, their representations, and aspirations. There are desired pregnancies, as well as unexpected and unaccepted ones. For the majority of women from developing countries, being a woman fundamentally means being a mother: "the essence of femininity coincides with that of maternity...The meaning of maternity becomes perhaps more important and more intrinsic with her biology, almost to become taken for granted to a certain extent, because procreation is an obligatory and continuous fact... The decisive stage in the life of the woman is the birth of her first child which gives her the possibility of accessing a higher level in the hierarchy of female power" (Parolari, Sacchetti, 2001). This important time in a woman's life makes her particularly vulnerable and it is in this sense that Moro (2005) speaks not only of psychological transparency but also of *cultural transparency*. Being far away from home brings out cultural representations, linked with traditions and beliefs. Furthermore, Missonnier (2005) underlines how psychological transparency, a source of anguish and fantasy, is linked with the concept of creative anticipation innate in the mental representations of the future mother: "Anticipation is an underlying theme that allows understanding the normal and pathological variations of the development of parenthood and of the child" (Missonnier, 2005 p. 60).

The study

The study is part of a series of analyses on collective imagination in pregnancy which has taken into consideration male and female aspects in both difficult and normal situations, as well as a first comparison of the representations in pregnancy of Italian first-time mothers and first-time immigrant mothers (Di Vita et al., 2005). During the analysis, the need to readapt the instruments adopted, due to the objectives and hypotheses of the research became clear.

The study we present is part of a trans-cultural perspective, assuming that cultural belonging represents an essential factor in the study of individual differences. This work is a continuation of a pilot study on the psychodynamics of birth, the initial results of which (Di Vita et al., 2004) encouraged us to continue the work; in particular, we envisage studying in greater depth our knowledge of both the present and the original family context of immigrant women expecting their first child, making a comparison between different cultures, looking at relations between generations, reflecting specifically on the repercussions that the immigration project has on the functions and experience of parenthood in a foreign country. Through the analysis of the instruments, the specificity of coming into the world in immigrant families is also looked at in depth, in order to identify how the birth of a child in a foreign country can determine a time of further disruption or, vice versa, of greater integration in relation to the culture of birth, indicating any weak points and strong points that may be useful to promote this process.

In short, the hypothesis guiding this study is that the different articulations of the stories and mental representations of future immigrant mothers are an index of the complexity of coming into the world in different cultures and can therefore become valuable indications in the organization and management of the increasingly numerous services for health and social care for immigrants.

To study the experiences of expectant immigrant women, two clinical instruments have been used: "IRMAG (Interview for Maternal Representations in Pregnancy) (Ammaniti et al., 1995) which studies the contents and narrative structure of the woman's experience in relation to herself, her child, her partner, and her own mother; and the SDFLS (Symbolic Drawing of the Family Life Space) (Gilli et al., 1990), to assess the representations with respect to the changes in the family organization. We have sized this opportunity, as in the wide range of studies on pregnancy (Di Vita, Giannone, 2002), to compare what is "said" during the interview and what is graphically "represented" in the drawing.

The **IRMAG** is a semi-structured interview that is given in about the seventh month of pregnancy.

The 41 questions of the IRMAG have been numerically reduced and readapted for immigrant women with the aim of gaining in-depth information in the following areas: **1**) the desire for maternity in the woman's personal history and in that of the couple; **2**) personal emotions, emotions of the couple and of the family on the news of the pregnancy; **3**) the emotions and changes during pregnancy in the personal life, in the life of the couple and in the relationship with the woman's own mother; the prospect of the birth; **4**) the perceptions, the emotions and the fantasies related to the unborn child; **5**) the future expectations regarding the characteristics of the woman as a mother and of the child (we want to know, in a temporal perspective, how the woman prefigures her style as a mother); **6**) the historic perspective of the mother, concerning her present and past role as a daughter.

Thanks to the system of codification proposed by Ammaniti et al. (1995), after giving a score to the seven dimensions that make up the two representational models (one in relation to the self as mother and one relative to the child) it is possible to assign one of the following three representational categories:

1) **Integrated/Balanced** maternal representations: these are women who give a rich and coherent picture of their experience in pregnancy, considered as the full conclusion and integration of their female identity;
2) **Narrow/Disinvested** maternal representations: these are women who face their pregnancy as a necessary stage in their lives, maintaining strong control over themselves and giving a fairly poor story, with few references to their psychological experience and corporal transformations;
3) **Non-Integrated/Ambivalent** maternal representations: this is characteristic of women who appear contradictory in relating their pregnancy, showing the coexistence of different attitudes towards maternity and the future child and giving a poorly integrated picture that may become confused.

Further sub-categories can be distinguished in these three categories.

The **SDFLS** is an instrument with a projective nature, produced by Mostwin at the end of the 1970s for easy access to complex family dynamics. In the test, the family life space is represented by a circle on a sheet of white paper. As an expression of completeness and unity, it marks out the borderline between the real family and the environment, represented by the external part of the circle.

The projective nature of the test means that this space is interpreted and used in a highly personal way; the basic theoretical methodological presupposition is the concept of "spatial representability of psychological reality" (Gozzoli, Tamanza, 1998 p. 24).

In the first place, the subject has to place herself and all the most significant people for her on the paper. Secondly, the subject is asked to indicate particularly significant events which have marked her history. Subsequently, the subject is asked to represent the quality of the bonds between the members. The dotted, unbroken or hatched lines do not only indicate the quality of the relationship (good, conflicting or poor) but also show, at a symbolic level, what creates uniting, binding, and trapping relations.

There is an evaluation of the Symbolic Drawing of the Family Life Space (SDFLS) which is developed on two levels: global and elementistic. With the former, the aim is to analyze the place in space of the bio-psycho-social significations, whereas with the latter the relations, the family structure, the interpersonal dynamics and the intra-personal dynamic are defined, as well as the socio-cultural dynamic. The quantity and place of the elements shown, the presence and the nature of the lines/bonds marked out and the overall configuration of the drawing is taken into consideration. The centrifugal and centripetal tensions emerge from the overall configuration, indicating the direction of the elements and how they are placed (far from or near the subject); the presence of tension or "static-ness"; the occupation of space in a diffused or coarctated manner, which indicates the capacity of enriching the SDFLS in such a way that each element has its own "place" or of suffocating the elements by excessively bringing them together in order not to occupy all the space in the circle.

The study is configured as *almost experimental*, as it was conducted in the field, i.e. in natural environments, such as the waiting rooms of gynecological centres in Palermo. Therefore, the *independent variable* is given by the culture, the *dependent* one by the experience of the woman in relation to herself, her child, her partner and her own mother.

Analysis and interpretation of the data

Of the 74 women met, 21% came from Bangladesh and Sri Lanka, 20% from eastern Europe (Romania, Poland), 15% from Mauritius, 14% from Guinea (Ivory Coast, Ghana, Nigeria), 12% from China, 5% from the Maghreb, another 5% from the Balkans, 4% from Latin America (Ecuador, Dominican Republic and Peru) and the remaining 4% from other countries.

Of all the women, 58% show maternal representations belonging to the restricted/disinvested categories with a prevalence of the accentuated sub-category, 26% have limited integrated/balanced maternal representations and the remaining 16% show non-integrated/ambivalent maternal representations; for the majority, the sub-category is confused.

Women from Bangladesh and Sri Lanka

The role of women in Bengalese society remains very difficult, although considerable progress has been made in the past ten years: the majority of the female population live in complete submission without any kind of education or health-care and in fear of domestic and social violence. The important steps forward recorded in the field of female schooling have triggered-off a violent and paradoxical reaction in some men, who, in the face of this revolution of the traditional system, have adopted a negative attitude that has degenerated, in many cases, into episodes of vendetta, a sort of jealousy of women who in a few years since their access to schooling, have succeeded in reaching graduate level and in actively taking part in social life.

With respect to marriage, many girls in these countries are married immediately after puberty, partly to free their parents from an economic burden and partly to protect the sexual purity of the girl. When a girl comes from a very poor family or has lost her parents, she may be married to a man much older than herself, as his third or fourth wife, and take on the role of sexual slave or servant. In relation to the first tool, examining the material at our disposal, the analysis of the data has allowed us to observe how the **integrated/balanced** representations, characterized by a coherent narration of the experience and by a wealth of perceptions relative to maternity and the child, appear infrequently (12%). The answers that can be included in this category provided by the women do not refer to a life experience particularly rich in perceptions and fantasies, although as a whole they are sufficiently balanced. Therefore, they were put into one of the three sub-categories distinguished by the authors, and specifically into the *"limited"* one: *"Yes, when I wasn't well I was afraid and I would cry sometimes ... – I dream a lot, when I sleep, he moves and I dream about him ... my husband is pleased that I'm pregnant but he is afraid too, because it is our first child ... that's normal! I was happy ... it was lovely! – When the baby moves, I tell my husband and take his hands to feel the baby moving ... and when he doesn't move I am sad. – In the fifth month I felt him moving. Now he doesn't move very much ... in the day he doesn't move much, more at night, I think he's hungry and he moves more"*.

The majority of the first-time mothers belong to the category of **restricted/disinvested** representations (81%), albeit through different sub-categories, according to the different nuances emerging from their stories and also confirmed by the analysis of the drawings. This category includes the women who, in telling their stories, show a certain rigidity, abstraction, resistance, and generic-ness: during the interviews, they show a particular emotional distance, as if the experience of pregnancy was not theirs. In particular, we have identified some cases as referable to the *accentuated* sub-category, where the perceptions and fantasies appear particularly poor. For example, a woman from Sri Lanka, when asked about moments of particular emotion during her pregnancy, replied: *"Yes, I was very frightened because feeling unwell, being sick ...very frightened! – No, never dreamed of baby .... I spoke to my husband and my friend .... – Husband happy for baby girl but he's afraid too"*. Other women were included in the *self-oriented* sub-category, showing greater attention to themselves and their maternity, rather than towards the baby; a woman from Bangladesh told us "*When I noticed the first changes I didn't feel well then with my tummy growing I was ... ashamed – My husband is more worried*".

Lastly, a small number of first-time mothers show **non-integrated/ambivalent representations** (6%), referable to the *confused* sub-category. Images which are not very elaborated and stories difficult to understand emerge, in a picture showing little openness towards change and contradictions : *"I am pleased .... my life hasn't changed ... I don't work, I stayed at home ... No, the same ... we get on well together ... like before, he is more careful ... he is worried when I don't feel well ... it's normal."*

In relation to the second tool used, it appears from the global evaluation of the drawings, how prevalently these have been carried out implementing a method from the diffused type of representation; the majority of women do not represent themselves as the graphic-geometric centre of the drawing and many of them are neither the psychological centre, nor do they represent the focal point, the catalyst of the family dynamics.

Women from Eastern Europe (Romania, Poland)

These lands of extraordinary beauty are in the heart of Europe: lands that have been conquered over the centuries and coveted by invaders and Medieval heroes as a stage for battling factions.

Moldavia is today a region of Romania which together with Poland has returned to the heart of Europe, after having being dominated by Russia and Communism, and regained its traditional culture with hints of Byzantine influence, where pastoral traditions remain alive and respected.

The majority of the population lives in the countryside, their lives regulated by a calendar of traditional rites which have remained extraordinarily impermeable to external influence. This may explain the words of a woman who said that the child to be born must get used to following sleep-waking rhythms but if it is not happy with those imposed by the mother, it will find its well-being on its own: *"There have to be times, but if it isn't happy with something I tell him to do I won't do it any more. Only his well-being."* It is as if an area of autonomy were left to the natural inclinations of the child.

In addition, when a child is born, before being officially presented to the orthodox community, it is looked after by all the women in the new mother's family. The strong bond along the female axis can be seen in the words of an interviewed women, who says that she would like to be: *"good like my mother because I have always been close to her and she has always been close to me and when I needed her she was always at my side ... Maybe my mother will help me, I don't know about my sister yet, I don't know if I want to have the baby in Romania, I haven't decided yet."*

In particular, in relation to the categories of interview of Romanian and Polish women, the majority (53%) present *accentuated* **restricted/disinvested** representations: the sensations expressed, the investment and fantasies are very poor, the slice of life that emerges is not supported by concrete experiences, the child is seen more in the future than in the present. For example, one woman tells us: *"I don't want to imagine it, I don't know, happy, I'm waiting because I don't know what a first baby can be like ... I don't have dreams about the baby, for the moment ... I saw it in the scan but you can't see anything, I didn't understand very well, I saw its head and the doctors told me it is fine, everything is fine now we'll see what they tell me"*. Only one of these women belongs to the self-oriented sub-category; in this case maternity is experienced as an obligatory stage for her self-realization. The remaining 26% of these women have *confused* **non-integrated/ambivalent** maternal representations and in these cases again, there emerge partial fantasies and a story that is not very well organized; on the basis of our observations, this confusion in parental identification could be attributed to the difficulty of adapting to a new culture and environment, but also to the absence of the female network of reference of their family (an issue which almost always emerges in the interviews). For example, a Romanian woman tells us: *"My mother is still in Romania .... My father is dead ... my mother-in-law is here in Sicily ... – In this period, we speak every week, every Saturday or Sunday. My mother is pleased that I'm pregnant but is more worried because she is not close to me .... My mother was 20 when she had her first baby, I am not young to have a child but I am far away and that's why she is more worried!"*

Lastly, in the interviews of the remaining 21% of this group of women there emerges a very rich and coherent picture of the experience; maternal representations belong to the *child-oriented* **integrated/balanced** category; there is a strong emotional investment in the baby that seems to give meaning to the sense of sacrifice of migration and thanks to this, the women are able to plan their lives in "another" place. One woman and her husband see the hope for something new in the child: *"No, I don't think that my relationship with my husband has changed, it's the same, our habits have changed, in that now we talk about the baby, that's new! – When he comes home from work, before saying hello to me, he says hello to the child, there is an extra presence between us... Yes, a little! A little fear and hope again"*.

The majority of the women who show **restricted/disinvested** or **non integrated/ambivalent** representations in the interviews, place themselves in a peripheral position inside the circle in the SDFLS and, although they show different significant figures of their own family, they are almost always shown far from themselves even when relations are good, as if to indicate the physical distance of important people but who, at this time, cannot offer them concrete support with their presence. Otherwise the future mothers with **integrated/balanced** representations show themselves at the centre of the circle with all the figures of their family around them, as if the physical absence of these people does not prevent them from feeling that they are close.

Women from Mauritius

The archipelago in the Indian Ocean considered "Paradise on earth" for its natural beauties is a multiethnic patchwork where religious and cultural differences coexist in a climate of general respect and great harmony. This great wealth of collective ways of celebration and encounter together with their peaceful coexistence fully express the cultural climate of Mauritius: a great respect for different faiths and traditions and an extraordinary capacity to live in peace and harmony.

From an analysis of the interviews, **integrated/balanced** representations appear a high number of times (60%). There are present elements relating to the representation of the self as a mother and of the future child, although the stories are not particularly rich in perceptions and in imagination: therefore they were all put into the *limited* sub-category. When asked to tell us how her life had changed during her pregnancy one woman told us: *"Yes, I don't work any more, I stay at home, practically everything has changed for me, even the way of thinking, everything, before, how can I put it, it was easier in everything, maybe I would spend money more easily, now, since I've been pregnant I've become more careful because I think that I don't want to buy useless things to show people, no, maybe when the baby is born …"*.

Other stories (20%), however, belong to the **restricted/disinvested category**, characterized by impersonality, rigidity as well as by reduced points of view of the interviewees, who mainly refer to aspects that are not very personal and concrete, but more abstract: *"My belly and my bust are bigger and I don't know what else …. I'm afraid of problems for the baby's health…in the scan I saw its hands, I saw everything"*. We therefore put them into the *accentuated* sub-category.

Lastly, other first-time mothers (20%) present **non integrated/ambivalent** representations, characterized by a confused and contradictory picture, where both involvement with the baby and the conflict against it coexist. In particular, as they are prevalently focused on themselves and on their own unsolved conflicts, they belong to the *self-absorbed* sub-category. Here are the words of one woman: *"My life has changed, there was some sadness but I've got over it, at* *the moment I am spending too much money, I do nothing but spend money, but my life has not changed, it is still the same and I am happy… My mother was upset, for the time being we do not live together, she feels a bit out of it, she has not rejected me but she has not accepted my pregnancy."*

From the drawings it can be observed how the partner is seen by all the women as near, although he is not always the first to be distinguished: very often it is the woman's mother who is shown immediately after the self, as if the women still considered their own families as more important or rather as if the most significant person considered as an element of support continues to be the mother, despite the formation of a new family bond. The maternal figure is present in almost all the graphic productions.

Women from Guinea (Ivory Coast, Ghana, Nigeria)

We are in the presence of a system that lives in deep symbiosis and harmony with the surrounding world, guaranteeing, in this way, the existence of the social system and of society, in a continuous representation and re-actualization of the past in the present, for the purpose of maintaining group identity, its benefit and thus guaranteeing cohesion, defence, and the reinforcement of traditional society.

For many of these women, life in Palermo appears an upheaval; the pace changes, habits change, traditions change.

The answers that can belong to the **integrated/balanced** category supplied by the women (30%) appear sufficiently balanced, although they do not refer to an experience particularly rich in perceptions and fantasies. Therefore they were included in the *"limited"* sub-category. *"My friends realized but I didn't realize; after they told me then I realized because I am a very strong woman, I don't feel pain immediately; after they told me maybe because I was worried, I began to feel sore in my bust, with a headache and feel tired. I could no longer do the housework because I was too tired."*

Fifty per cent of the interviewees belong to the **restricted/disinvested** category; in telling their stories the women show a certain rigidity and generic-ness. During the interviews, they show a particular emotional distance, as if the experience of pregnancy was not theirs: we therefore included them in the *accentuated* sub-category *"No ... not yet ... no name chosen ... new name ... for child choose name we like ... with husband."*

Lastly, 20% of the maternal representations belong to the **non integrated/ambivalent** category, which can be referred to the *confused* sub-category. The images are not very elaborate and the stories are difficult to understand, in a picture of little openness towards change and contradictions. *"It came so suddenly ... I was a bit afraid because I still did not have a good job, so to do what you want, the child, I don't know, if tomorrow you want something how do you manage, because I don't like to go and see someone and say give me this to buy* *something for my baby ... No because my husband is always with me so ... I'm not afraid; (dreams?) yes, that I had a baby (she laughs), because when I dreamt this I forgot it all morning".*

From the overall analysis of the drawings, the women do not represent themselves in the centre of the life space, but place themselves in a more decentralized position together with their husband. These drawings often represent emblematically the affective restriction and the condition of physical (psychological) isolation experienced in this period of time. Significant family members are not present, the future child is not present and groups or services such as the preliminary reception centre and the hospital, where the women go, are not present either.

Women from China

Taoism, Confucianism, and Buddhism are the three doctrines that have moulded Chinese culture, establishing the family models that traditionally see women as an object, an instrument to give birth to a son destined to inherit the family wealth. Although equality of sexes is legally recognized today, this has not eliminated the situation of inferiority of Chinese women, especially in the less developed regions (Slepoj, 2002). Chinese traditions of filial devotion and patriarchal authority mean that "the parents take on the economic and emotional costs connected with the birth and the education of the children, then the children are obliged to pay back their debt helping their elderly parents. Sa-dai-tone-tang (cohabitation of three generations) is considered the ideal solution for the elderly and for the children, the way to express their filial devotion. The eldest married son is obliged to live with his elderly parents and to provide for their needs. In practice, however, this function of caring for the elderly parents is performed mostly by the wife" (Ehrenreich, Hochschild, 2004 p. 173–174). As a consequence, the woman is subjugated to the power of her mother-in-law; a woman tells us how, on the death of her father-in-law, her husband, who is the eldest son, asked his mother to join them in Italy: *"Mother-in-law plus little brother and sister too, he is the eldest (referring to her husband) because his father is already dead. Said: we together bigger, come ... there is joy".* The authority of the parents-in-law in the family structure also appears confirmed by the drawings where the women almost always place themselves in a peripheral position and represent their parents-in-law in the centre, as if out of a sense of respect, although in actual fact the parents-in-law very often stay in China and do not follow their children to another country. This allows the new family to have a greater space of autonomy as they are not obliged to live with their parents. Despite this apparent freedom, the absence of the support of the family at the time of the birth of a child is something that all the women we met miss, and they feel they do not have adequate support at this time in their lives.

In addition, the perceptions, the emotional investment and the fantasies of Chinese women are very limited, especially for cultural reasons. The shame of talking about subjects related to the private sphere, typical of Chinese culture, does not allow the women we met to deal openly with the aspects of pregnancy related to their body, showing little wealth of perception of pregnancy in its various aspects. Therefore, the majority of these women (78%) show maternal representations that belong to the *accentuated* **restricted/disinvested** category. *"Yes, yes, it moves ... – It doesn't move very much, mmm ... more in the evening or early morning. – I don't know why! (she laughs)"*. The remaining 22% are equally distributed between *confused* **non integrated/ambivalent** representations *("Pregnancy is the same here .... I have found a family that is really good with me. I try to respect their habits.... They celebrate Christmas, whilst in China when a baby is born, there is a huge celebration... Here I do the celebrations as in China, like the Chinese New Year, I cook Chinese food and my husband's family eat at my house and they are happy, they wish us a Happy New Year. The Chinese New Year is different from here! We follow a lunar calendar and sometimes it is in January, other times in February! I celebrate my Chinese traditions and the Italian ones as well")* and *limited* **integrated/balanced** representations *("Not frightened, worried a little...now calm. When I go to bed, I dream about the baby playing (she smiles). I have spoken to my husband, he is always touching my tummy... yes yes he is happy.")*.

Women from the Maghreb

Women from the Maghreb come to Italy mainly under family reuniting programmes to join their husbands, many years after they have moved here: *"with my husband, family reuniting (did you speak Italian?). No I learnt it here"*.

The traditional model of the family in these countries is the result of an articulation and a combination of two elements: the pre-Islamic tribal structure and that laid down by Islam. The foundation of the Muslim family model lies in patri-linearity and in endogamic marriage. The legislation on family law sees an overlapping between the traditional-religious sphere and the juridical-social sphere; the head of the family is the man who is acknowledged as the only interlocutor of the institutions, the guarantor of all the members of the family.

Women belonging to this culture are still greatly submitted to family authority, which legitimizes them in their female identity only in their capacity to have children. A woman will remain united in her name and her affections to her own family, even if she goes to live with her husband's family after marriage (patrilocal system). But her entrance into the family will take place only indirectly through her children: she will always remain the outsider with her husband having the power, through the institution of repudiation, to send her back to her own family.

Not having children means a break between the world of the living and that of the dead, in that there will no longer be, when you are dead, someone alive who will think of you as their ancestor. This is in close relation to the cyclical representation of life that exists in these countries; a child comes from the world of the ancestors. As a newborn, the baby is not yet human, but suspended between two worlds; following processes and rites of humanization, it will become a human being as it grows up. It will become an adult and then die and in this way become an ancestor once again. The world of the ancestors will once again give life to children, in the form of reincarnation. This system of representation of life is cyclical, and death and life in this sense are united.

Hence the importance attributed to procreation and from the interviews there emerged the central theme of the continuity of the generations through expecting a child. A woman from Tunisia told us: *"I wait 10 years from God ... Yes (she laughs) happy, pleased because I wait so long*". Another theme that the two women from the Maghreb have in common is fear. Monia's first answer appears emblematic: "*yes, there is something different. The first baby (dead after birth) from Tunisia different. I had injections, what are they called ... eh you have vaccination from pregnancy, eight months there is vaccination. Normal hospi-*

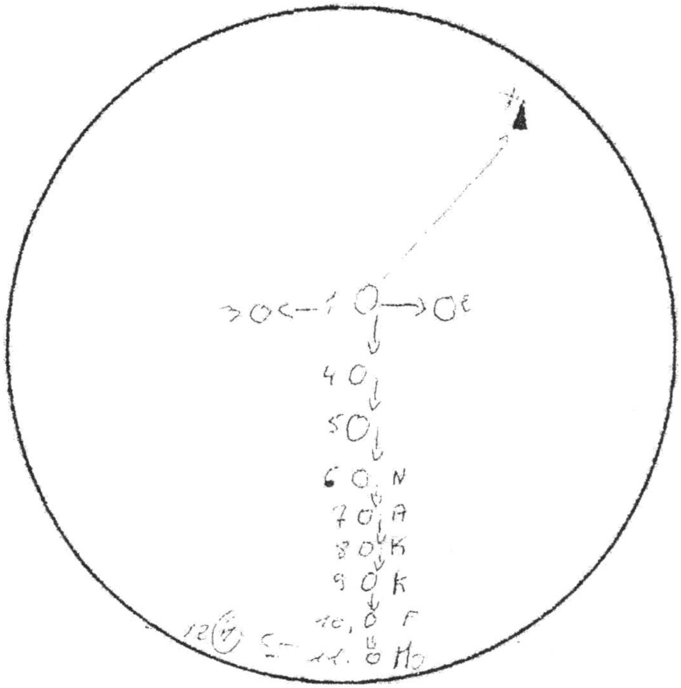

Figure 1

tal ... No no only three brothers here, one dead like all mothers ... No baby before dead". Fears and dreams about both personal physical discomfort and any illness or loss of the child clearly emerge in almost all the women, many of whom have had negative experiences of miscarriages or losing their first child after birth. These analogies in the contents of the interviews are confirmed by the evaluation according to the coding system of the representational categories: they all belong to the *restricted/disinvested with fear category.*

Once again anguish and the fear of solitude are evident in the graphic representations where the women put themselves in a central position inside the circle, placing the significant people outside or crowding all the most important people inside, including children lost previously, with a coarctate graphical representation (see Fig. 1).

Women from the Balkans area

In these lands, the population is mainly rural and lives in extended families, whilst the urban population tends towards a certain degree of emancipation; the family has a central role in the social structure, and relations are important. The extended patriarchal structure includes the parents, their sons and their wives and children, as well as any unmarried daughters. A typical rural family (and the families of rural-urban immigrants) is made up of fifteen members but families of thirty or more people, who contribute to a common economy and who eat and work together, are not infrequent. Coherently with this ideal, marriage is seen as a dream and as a responsibility (Ndreko, 2002).

Legislation gives the husband the right to marry several wives only in certain cases, for example if the first is sterile and gives her consent to a second marriage. We could say that marriage has as its purpose the control of women's sexuality. One of the women interviewed expresses her concerns about the fact that she thought she could not have children: "*yes, at first I was afraid, because I thought that I could not have children ... then, after a year, when I came here the doctor told me ... that I was pregnant we were pleased ... – There have been times when I was not well, I felt sick, I vomited ... and I was worried, I would cry. Now I am more relaxed ... – No, I haven't dreamt about my pregnancy! – When I cried or felt bad, my husband helped me... – He had more love for me." She is happy now because her husband's love is protected by the baby she is about to give him".*

In this culture, a man's greatest desire is that the first child be a male, to guarantee his lineage; this also emerged from the words of this woman: *"Before I thought it was a girl, then I found out it was a boy! I hope he'll be calm .... – My husband wants a boy so he is happier. I don't know .... My husband wants him to be calm ... My husband calls him Kevin ... I've never thought about it (she laughs) ... Yes! My husband chose it, he likes the name!"*

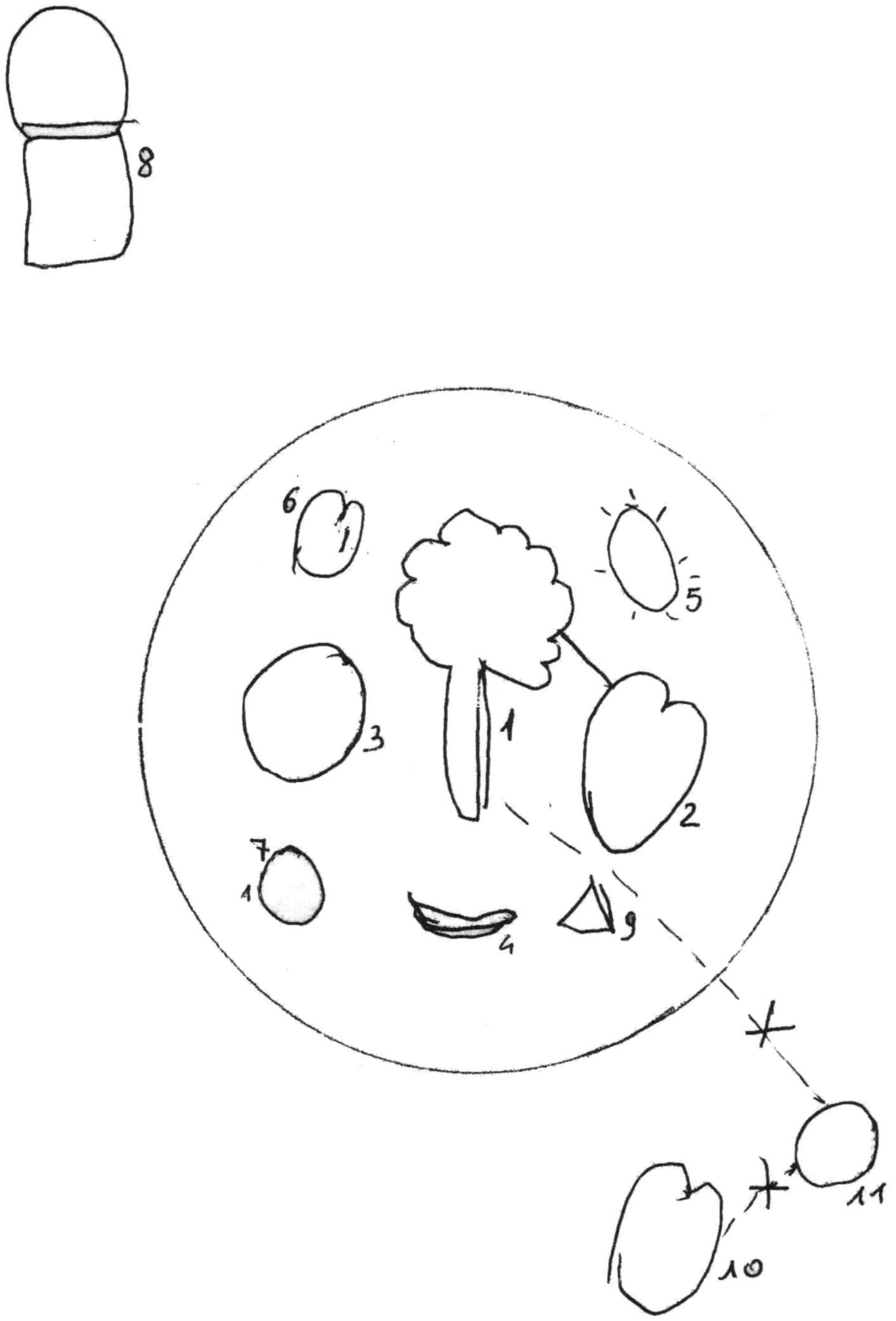

Figure 2

Many marriages are arranged by parents or relations; in some regions the engagement is agreed by the families when the children are still in their teens and in some cases they do not meet even before the evening of their wedding.

Some narrative nuclei that are in common with the women from the Maghreb emerge in the interviews with women from the Balkans; in particular, once again the presence of contents of fear and fantasies on death and illness can be noted, in the general picture of disinvestment. Fifty per cent belong to the **restricted/disinvested** category, in particular, referable to the *accentuated* sub-category, where perceptions and fantasies appear particularly impoverished.

Lastly, some 25% of the three women from the Balkans area belong to the *limited* **integrated/balanced** category and another 25% present *confused* **non-integrated/ambivalent** representations.

The importance of the family system emerges strongly from the drawings where not only the significant figures in the family nucleus are included, but also part of the extended family (grandparents, parents-in-law, etc.). The drawings have been made implementing a diffused type of representation. In addition, some of the significant figures are shown with a heart, the symbol denoting a strong bond of affection; in this sense, the importance of the family structure is understood. The women often use two different symbols to show themselves and their husband, in particular one of the women draws herself as a flower (symbol of her fertility) and her husband with a heart (see Fig. 2).

Women from Latin America (Dominican Republic, Ecuador and Peru)

The women from the Dominican Republic show a good capacity for initial adaptation and a certain initiative in encountering new situations; one woman tells us: *"I am Dominican, I come from Santo Domingo, I am here because there is my cousin here who is married and lives here, I came to work and I met my husband ... It was difficult for me when I arrived for work .... everything! – because I didn't have the papers then gradually because first I was in Rome with my sister and then I came here and I found a job as a maid, I met this family and they liked me very much from the beginning, then I got married and I am here".* The maternal representations of these women belong to the *limited* **integrated/balanced** category, the representations of maternity and of the child are quite rich and characterized by a strong emotional investment, pregnancy is planned and greatly desired. *"This baby was planned, I wanted it very much, even before actually ... we decided before getting married and then we got married. Before I knew I was pregnant, I was sad because I was hoping in the results of the tests then when I knew I was pregnant I was pleased. I spoke to my husband then everyone was happy".* The drawings are also very rich, with the presence of many figures belonging to the woman's own family and the child about to be born is always shown.

The countries formed after the wars of independence led by Simon Bolivar include, as well as Bolivia, Colombia and Venezuela, Ecuador and Peru. Ecuador is in the north-west of South America and borders on the north with Colombia, to the south-east with Peru and to the west with the Pacific Ocean. The group of women from Peru or Ecuador is characterized by a high rate of illegality, due to their very recent arrival and the presence of many single-parent nuclei. The presence of women who have come to Italy alone is very high. One Peruvian woman tells us: *"I have been in Sicily for almost five years, I came illegally. Now all my papers are in order. I'm not working any more (she points at her belly). Yes, I learnt Italian hearing it at work. (what did you do?) everything, I did cleaning, I was a carer, a babysitter, yes ... No I arrived safely, I came with a false passport, but it was OK, I got in (she laughs). No no, all the same but it's expensive because there it's not like here where everything is free, there you have to pay for everything: the examinations, the scans, the medicine. It's much harder to be pregnant there"*. This woman has already had a miscarriage and lost a baby girl, she is very rigid in speaking about her present pregnancy, her maternal representations are (like those of the other women in the same group) *accentuated* **restricted/disinvested**; in the drawing she places herself in the centre with her dead daughter next to her, whilst the child about to be born is drawn in a peripheral position and far from her. We think that her individual story of suffering and loss does not yet allow her to find any mental space for the new baby.

As far as the group of women from Ecuador is concerned, this country is made up of different social groups who are united by a common history, speak the same language, and belong to the same culture. The economic crisis has forced men to emigrate en masse and women have to play a role of primary importance because, alone in the community, they have to take care of the house, the children, the productive activity and take a more active part in community life. Women, who have always been the depositories of native culture, are compared to the "Mother goddess" and as such give life, feed and bring up the children and transmit the traditions of their people. One of the women interviewed tells us, in reference to the role that she had in Ecuador in her own family: *"my smallest brother no, because he had more love than me. Now he feels put to one side"* and also: *"I have always been a little rigid with myself to do everything well. If I could not do a thing well I got angry with myself, I like everything to be right"*. This rigidity also emerges from the *confused* **non integrated/ambivalent** maternal representations that emerge from the interviews of the women from Ecuador: it is as if the concerns inherent in other spheres of their lives provides a confused and disorganized picture of their identity as a mother. *"I know that it will be difficult when my baby is born because now I am looking for another house to change because where I live I don't like it, it's too small. I live with another family I don't like. Yes, I don't like lots of things. I'm worried about this"*. The drawings show a coarctate representation with the self placed in the centre surrounded by all the most important significant figures, the church and the people that belong to her community as if to show a need for protection and belonging.

Conclusions

Over the past few years, the births of children who are not Italian citizens, as well as the number of immigrant women admitted to hospital for maternity-related reasons, have increased considerably in Italy. The health service is unprepared and inadequate to deal with this new situation. Immigrant women are often seen, unfortunately still today, as an inconvenience that creates problems and difficulties of a medical, social, and organization order; attention for foreign women is limited therefore, in the majority of cases, to the general availability of a health operator who often does not have even the basic notions on the particularities of immigrant women.

In daily life, all this has created various problems of communication, information, relations which are all the more urgent as they are linked to a particular time of life, maternity. This often entails a situation of incomprehension and isolation and a relationship between the patient and health service where detachment and distance prevail. Due to the difficulties in communication, medical assistance that is not always strictly necessary is often given merely to be sure that there are no complications. Greater attention and understanding, including empathy, must be given to immigrant women in the health and social services as well as easier and better known access to health services.

The risks faced by immigrant women of situations of strong emotional tension are considerable and can lead to destabilization expressed with evident states of malaise, which can appear in the experience of motherhood and child care. These situations of depression can be caused by the separation from their context of life and by coming into contact with different value systems, where women are torn between maintaining the norm in an unknown place and complying with the norms that they have not yet internalized because they are inappropriate to them.

Access to parenthood is a universal and fundamental experience on which all societies place great value, surrounding it with words, ceremonies or ritual gestures. Every society accompanies this passage with different models of "becoming parents" (Giraud, Moro, 2002). In the individual life story, becoming a parent implies the need for reorganizing representations of the self and relations with others, with parents in particular, a change which is often well received but which is also highly ambivalent, as Serge Lebovici underlines. The immigration event does not fundamentally modify this process, but gives it a particular resonance due to the reorganization that is carried out in a context which is not only different from the cultural point of view but in a subjective situation of relative destabilization which is commonly called "immigration trauma". In other words, the fact of becoming a parent, experienced in one's own country, in the presence of one's own family and society, a considerable change and rich in potential, is at times endured in the immigration situation as a painful episode without any reward.

The difficulties encountered by immigrant families, and by women at this particular time, have in themselves risks and this should encourage us even more to change techniques and perspectives, adapting to new and increasingly complex clinical situations. The women we have met represent, with their life-stories, the multiple ways of coping with this important passage, which is, however, influenced only in part by the migratory state and therefore by cultural differences. For this reason, in our research on maternal representations, we have only underlined the important function of anticipation compared to the competences of parenthood (Missonnier, 2005); in particular, this protective/defensive function in the parent/baby relationship allows creating through the ritual of birth a space of transition which helps the path of parents and operators. Taking this theoretical assumption as a starting-point, the presence of the organization and management of an increasing number of specialist services for the social and healthcare for immigrants, could reduce the difficulties and obstacles related to the cultural aspects of the situation.

Acknowledgement

We thank Dr Alessandra Fontana and Caterina Lamionica for supplying and evaluating part of the tools.

References

Ammaniti M, C Candelori, M Pola, R Tambelli: Maternità e gravidanza. Studio delle rappresentazioni materne. Cortina, Milan 1995

Balsamo E, G Favaro, F Giacalone: Mille modi di crescere. Bambini immigrati e modi di cura. Angeli, Milan 2002

Bayle B: L'identité conceptionnelle. Tout se joue-t-il avant la naissance? L'Harmattan, Paris 2005

Cattaneo ML, S dal Verme: Donne e madri nella migrazione. Prospettive transculturali e di genere. Unicopli, Milan 2005

Chinosi L: Sguardi di mamme. Modalità di crescita dell'infanzia straniera. Angeli, Milan 2002

Di Vita AM, F Giannone: (a cura di). La famiglia che nasce. Angeli, Milan 2002

Di Vita AM, M Errante, A Salerno, M Vinciguerra: Simboli e significati della gravidanza e della nascita nelle famiglie immigrate. In: Salerno A, AM Di Vita AM (des): Genitorialità a rischio. Ruoli, contesti e relazioni. Angeli, Milan 2004 pp. 170–209

Di Vita AM, M Errante, M Vinciguerra: L'attesa e la nascita nelle donne migranti. Un'indagine esplorativa. Biblíon 1 (2005) 49–63

Ehrenreich B, AR Hochschild: (a cura di). Donne globali. Tate, colf e badanti. Feltrinelli, Milan 2004

Gilli O, O Greco, C Regalia, G Banzatti: Il Disegno Simbolico dello Spazio di Vita Familiare. Vita e Pensiero, Milan 1990

Giraud F, MR Moro: Parentalité et migrations. In: Solis-Ponton L: (a cura di). La parentalité. Presses Universitaires de France, Paris 2002 pp. 325–338

Gozzoli C, C Regalia: Migrazioni e famiglie. Percorsi, legami e interventi psicosociali. Il Mulino, Bologna 2005

Gozzoli C, G Tamanza: Family Life Space. L'analisi metrica del disegno. Angeli, Milan 1998

Kristof A: Ieri. Einaudi, Turin 1997

Liotta E: Su anima e terra. Il valore psichico del luogo. Edizioni Magi, Rome 2005

Losi N: Vite altrove. Migrazione e disagio psichico. Feltrinelli, Milan 2000

Missonnier S: La consultazione terapeutica perinatale. Psicologia della genitorialità, della gravidanza e della nascita. Cortina, Milan 2005

Monacelli N, T Mancini: Appartenenze culturali e dinamiche familiari. In: Fruggeri L (ed): Diverse normalità. Psicologia sociale delle relazioni familiari. Carocci, Rome 2005

Moro MR: Bambini di qui venuti da altrove. Angeli, Milan 2005

Moscardino U, G Axia: Psicologia, cultura e sviluppo umano. Carocci, Rome 2002

Ndreko M: Le donne albanesi di fronte alla transizione. www.medmedia.org, 2002

Parolari L, G Sacchetti: Donne immigrate: gravidanza e maternità. Carocci, Rome 2001

Slepoj V: Le ferite delle donne. Mondatori, Milan 2002

Tognetti Bordogna M: Le famiglie dell'immigrazioni. I ricongiungimenti familiari. Istituto Transculturale per la salute, Department for Social Affairs 2000

24. Family preparations for birth

Bernadette Tillard; Department of Educational Science, University of Paris X-Nanterre, France

Based on ethnological research into birth carried out in families living in a housing scheme in Lille, France (Tillard, 2002), this paper investigates the family preparations for birth. In preparing for the infant's arrival, the future parents progressively enter into the idea of their future roles. This preliminary stage is closely linked to the institutional mechanisms of medical assistance in pregnancy and to the technological means of medical surveillance.

Diagnosis and declaration

In France, by civil law, the declaration of birth is compulsory. However, since 1945, social rights have actively encouraged the declaration of pregnancy, its medical and social services.

Link between diagnosis and medical/social services

The ordinance of 2nd November 1945 instituting the Protection of Mothers and Infants (PMI) came into practice just before the law of 2nd August 1946 which established family support (Norvez, 1990). Thus medical services would be defined and generalized, establishing the right to financial support paid by family allowance bureaus. Medical diagnosis precedes social services, since the diagnosis of pregnancy is registered with the PMI who choose whether to provide medical/social assistance or not.

In effect, when the question of diagnosing a pregnancy arises, and the woman does not wish to have an abortion of the pregnancy, the declaration of pregnancy is made by a doctor. This declaration is made simultaneously to the family allowance bureau and the PMI. Medical and social services continue until birth and beyond, in a more or less intensive way until the age of six. At that time, the first visit by the service to promote health in pupils takes place on the occasion of the child starting primary school. The diagnosis is therefore the first stage in the acceptance by society of the promise of human life that is being carried by the mother.

Link between perceptions of the woman and the diagnosis

In order for a medical diagnosis to be carried out during the first three months, it must be preceded by the woman approaching the health services. Sometimes, however, pregnancy is perceived late by the woman because of lack of perception of physical signs.

Francine presents a general malaise at the beginning of her pregnancy (nausea, vomiting, mammary tension). These are interpreted by her partner as signs of pregnancy. Francine is not convinced by her partner's explanations, she goes for a consultation two months later. If this 20-year old woman has opted for an abortion during the previous year, an abortion will be "impossible" this time and the declaration of pregnancy will be made late, requiring special permission from the Family Allowance bureau, a procedure permitting the team of the relevant PMI to be informed of the pregnancy and leading to a special intervention on behalf of the social workers of the Family Allowance department.

As for Monique, she learns that she is in the middle of a fourth pregnancy when she goes to consult the PMI about placing an IUD... she is six and a half months pregnant.

Martine is twenty five. She stopped taking the pill a year ago. In January, she finds that her periods are particularly painful. She feels swollen like a balloon. She goes for a consultation and finds out that she is pregnant and that she will give birth in three months' time.

In a study carried out into the birth issues of young women (Tillard, 1997), the frequency of diagnoses made on the threshold of maternity, even when the young woman is in labor, has been estimated. Two young women from among the fifty met at Calais, Beuvry, Roubaix and Mauberge were typical, given that about four percent of young mothers are under 20 years of age. In these cases, the medical diagnosis of pregnancy was still not carried out, and the declaration had not been made. One went to the emergency room because of abdominal pain; she had not realized her condition. The other came for her first pre-natal visit. For a long time she had put off facing her family on the subject of pregnancy. It had been the neighbours who had come up with the hypothesis of a pregnancy, talking of it with the future grandmother. This outside opinion on the young woman had worried the mother who had taken the initiative to accompany her daughter for a consultation.

The denials of pregnancy are quite disconcerting. Social outlaws, these babies arrive with a fanfare even when nothing has announced them. They upset the expectations of the family, as well as those of the medical and social workers. The forms of these denials seem variable. It is very difficult to know for each woman where the denial is: disregarding the presence of the fetus or the fetus is perceived but the information is not communicated to her immediate circle? Certain women are aware of being pregnant, but delay as long as possible the arduous moment of revelation, foreseeing the upset that this pregnancy will bring into their family, educational, or professional circle. Sometimes a first attempt to speak about the pregnancy leads them to withdraw into solitary waiting. Hence, the woman may share her impressions with her partner, who "doesn't want to hear of any pregnancy", a wish which will be followed right up to the day of giving birth. Other women seem not to perceive the changes in their body. This ignorance, or lack of awareness, has its effects on their surroundings and blinds their immediate circle. To "surprise" (a term often used to speak of *accidental* conception), we should add astonishment at an advanced pregnancy in the moment of its revelation, but at least the announcement should have been honest. There will not be pressure from her immediate circle to motivate the woman to have an abortion, no "showing her the door" or marital arguments. And finally, there is the newborn who announces his arrival!

The difficulty of listening to one's self, to one's body in particular, is not attributable to negligence. Certainly, the body of those women who do not notice that they are pregnant sometimes bears the stigmata of evident disease indicating an insecure life (dental pathology, obesity, dermatological pathology, etc.), but this is not always the case. The coquetry of these two young women, aged 28 or 30, expecting their fifth child but who pay particular attention to their appearance cannot pass unnoticed. Denial affects also those women who care for their appearance, but, in the case of unrecognized pregnancies, the perception of the body in question is not a visual impression and a surface aesthetic. It concerns the indulgence that the person is capable of settling herself in a way that she feels a thrill (Duden, 1996). Even in the popular or urban milieu where the body is often at the service of the machine and has been dignified by the accession of industry, one learns *not to listen,* and it is in this self-disdain that a part of the pride resides, which one accords oneself and which others show one.

However, these situations of denying pregnancy are "the tree which hides the forest". A good number of pregnancies are precious, sometimes planned and followed by the declarations of birth and maternity as much for the facilities as for the allowance instalments. On the other hand, certain young women live, from the moment of declaring the pregnancy, with the feeling of a social usefulness. *"Getting the paperwork"* at the same time as the fetus is growing is thus lived as a prelude to maternity.

Sometimes this task is presented as a female duty. It is true that mothers see in the family allowance payments a sort of maternal salary (Selim, 1984), particularly when they live alone with their child(ren). The difficulties encountered in administrative applications and the time passed completing dossiers and justifying their situation enhances the feeling of a remuneration acquired after a job.

The declaration of pregnancy

As has been discussed in the preceding section, the medical diagnosis of pregnancy can only take place if the woman submits herself to a medical examination. Similarly, the declaration of pregnancy by the physician or gynecologist cannot be made without a new agreement with the woman. In effect, this declaration is "obligatory" in matters of social rights. Its function is to allow medical/social assistance but it does not replace civil rights. Civil rights include the obligation to declare birth but not to declare pregnancy. Certain women who confuse medical and social assistance, and thus civil and social rights, want to keep their distance from the medical and social hierarchies after first showing the child; that is to say, their child is not tended by a doctor or the health service: no medical diagnosis, no declaration of pregnancy, no social assistance. Others, who understand the different natures of medical and social services, sometimes want to accept one and refuse the other. Different strategies are then possible. One of them consists in being followed by a private establishment not including the social service, the other is to demand the doctor not to perform the declaration of pregnancy.

Maternal sensitivity

The pregnant woman is sometimes perceived and sees herself as a being possessed. She manifests sudden and irrational envy (Arnaud, 1994; Ravolomanga, 1991; Laurent, 1989; Loux, 1990). She is unusually irritable. At certain times, this irritability is a departure point from which the partner discovers her state. This possession of the mother by the fetus, which originates from the idea of a woman besieged by the future human life was already represented by the [French] expression *"j'ai été prise" – "I was taken"*. This is sometimes expressed by the relation between the search for a first name and the intuition regarding the sex of the infant without there being any traditional symptoms attached to one or the other sex or a particular position of the child.

> "I didn't find any boys' names, only girls' names. Anyway, I told my husband that it wasn't worth looking for a boy's name at any cost. You always have the sex that you prepared the name for."
>
> "It doesn't surprise me that I had a boy, I couldn't find a girl's name anyhow, we could never agree!"
>
> "Before the ultrasound, I knew it was a boy... just like that!"

These symbiotic relationships between the bodies of the mother and the fetus have always been a point of discussion between medical workers and those giving birth. The history of this theme seems to evolve in a parallel manner with representations of the individual in our Western society. Claudia Pancino, in an article in the magazine *Ethnologie Française*, showed the evolution of the ideas regarding maternal envy. The proposals retained regarding these irrational impulses are related to the notion of the woman's power of imagination over the fetus. The author remarks that the culture of wisdom, after putting women on guard against their imagination, was then charged with explaining the unfounded character of this belief (Pancino, 1997).

The development of fetal medicine has permitted the elaboration of the physical relationships between the mother and the fetus. Conversely, the existence of commingled psychosomatic illnesses has also been recognized in adults. However, the links between maternal psychology and fetal development are not the object of research. Everything happens as if a physical link is recognized without a psychological one. The pronouncements regarding mother-fetus psychological links, whether we are dealing with an influence of the mother on the fetus or the fetus on the mother, tend to be considered as archaisms contrary to the manner in which they are considered by other civilizations (Dufour, 1998). Apart from being thought about, or forming the object of studies which do not touch medical specialists, these mother-fetus relationships are sometimes expressed as forms on the fringes of medicine, when health professionals are interested in them. Thus Maurice Titran, pediatrician at a medical social action center for premature birth, tells us his reflections: *"Nothing has been established scientifically. I would thus be modest, but I have my own little idea all the same: a woman, depressed, suffering, misunderstood during her pregnancy, will give birth to a baby who will pose us a lot of problems. If we have the chance to be able to listen, keep her company, help her while she is pregnant, we will save ourselves hours of pediatric work. We are also beginning to sense that certain kinds of psychological suffering originate in the life pre-birth ..."* (Potekov, Titran, 1996). In this passage, the idea is expressed that caring for the mother acts on the future infant, if the words, the medical assistance, and material aid to the mother (and parents) conjoin to support the mother. The thought of a mother-fetus symbiosis allows us to envisage a positive action for the child being carried. Popular expressions speak equally of these links:

> "You have the sex you prepare the name for,"
>
> "After my fall, I didn't feel any change in my sensations, so the baby is all right."

This language evokes, then, the same idea of the transparency of the maternal body or the symbiosis between mother and fetus. Thus, it seems that certain ideas being currently elaborated and ideas coming from tradition, share the same representation of the pregnant woman.

A question of vocabulary

Before anything else, the "potentiality of the person" (Fédila, 1996) and a first embarrassment that follows must be designated. How can we speak other than in medical terms that are not used by the standard family?

Medical vocabulary distinguishes the embryo from the fetus. The embryo is "the product of conception" during the first three months of pregnancy. The fetus follows the embryo, a term reserved for the second and third trimesters of pregnancy. The newborn is defined as an infant from birth to six weeks. The suckling is the child of less than two years. The terms employed are therefore relatively precise, but the limits evolve with medical practice, and have repercussions on the life of the family. Thus, the progress made in taking charge during newborn reanimation has contributed to the modification of the limit of viability of the fetus. After 1975, the limit of viability was 28 weeks of amenorrhea. In 1993, this limit was lowered by six weeks to be now 22 weeks of amenorrhea. *In case of death of this greatly premature baby, all signs of life at birth of the infant or all births beyond the limit of viability allow the consideration of the fruits of the pregnancy as an infant, providing him with a status, making him a figure in the family annals, in the civic registers and attributing him a burial.* Such a limit leads therefore to events which remain inscribed in the annals of the family and which are socially recognized as such.

Medical terms exist thus to designate 'he you are expecting'. The importance of biological criteria in defining these terms is highlighted. By comparison, the vocabulary currently used by families is extremely scarce. More often than not, the future parents, the brothers and sisters, and the immediate circle want to speak of the "baby". This underlines how much confusion exists between 'he you are expecting' and 'he who is born' since only one term allows you to speak of him. This designation by anticipation has particularly developed by the use of ultrasound. Before envisaging the repercussions of this exam before and during birth, we must remember that the parents and their immediate circle have always envisaged the future infant. Hence, in this lie the preparation of names and the hypotheses regarding the sex of the infant.

The sex of the fetus

Popular knowledge regarding external signs feeds the predictions concerning the sex of the infant. These signs most often make reference to the shape of the mother's abdomen which results from a particular position of the fetus in the uterus. The women in the popular quarter where I did my survey knew these external signs. *"Carrying forward"* means you are going to have a boy. *"Carrying on the right"* imposes the same prediction. Of course, by the opposite token, the abdomen a little prominent with back pain or more generous forms or a more significant perception on the left with lead to the birth of a girl. In every culture, one side is attributed to the female, while the other is attributed to the male. In the article *Le sang des guerriers et le sang des femmes (The blood of warriors and the blood of women)*, Françoise Héritier indicates that *these discourses are built on a system of binary categories, of dualistic pairs, which oppose face to face series such as Sun and Moon, high and low, right and left, light and dark, brilliant and dull, light and heavy, front and back, hot and cold, dry and wet, male and female, superior and inferior* (Héritier, 1996). This discussion is one of the vectors of the sexual division of the qualities and marks attributed to men and women. But, as Margaret Mead underlines, *one or other of these qualities is to be found sometimes attributed to one, sometimes to the other.* (Mead, 1948)

We should add that, often, the dualistic opposition of the terms carries for certain pairs a more positive side for one than for the other. As it is for 'right' in relation to 'left'.

The predictions of women from the immediate circle have always existed. These vaguely attract the attention of pregnant women who refer to them, indicating the importance of such and such a person to their family or one of their neighbours who has said that... they do not say so to believe it but to make regular references to it. This form of popular knowledge is a bearer of representations which, by definition, are empirical elements which do not rest on scientific experience or do not always need to be verified in order to find themselves upheld.

In contrast to the preparation for the pregnancy which is often associated with the worry of attracting bad luck for the infant, it should be noticed that the speculations regarding the sex of the infant are not concerned by the same taboo. Tradition authorizes the proclamation on the subject of the sex of the infant who will be born. This has constituted a particular fertilizer for the growth of the ultrasound scan.

Ultrasound

The ultrasound scan developed very rapidly during the eighties. It has become the object of an acclamation just as much among families as among practitioners. This exam has made *"ne plus se voir"* – *"no more to be see"* (an expression used by women to describe the stop of their periods) correspond to *"voir le bébé"* – *"look at the baby"* thanks to the ultrasound apparatus. The appearance of the fetus and its movements are consequently translated into two dimensions on the surface of the screen and offer the family *"the first image"* of the child according to the expression of Michèle Fellous, an image sometimes inserted in the photo album.

The realism of the ultrasound image is refused by those parents who do not care to know the sex before birth and to continue to imagine the child to be. The confident expectation of the realization of the birth is very clear on the ultrasound scan. "Look at the baby" they say and not "Look at the embryo or the fetus". Moreover, this episode of visualizing the embryo via ultrasound has been presented by some women wondering whether to continue their pregnancy as a deciding factor when choosing not to abort the pregnancy.

A mother hesitates while employing the term *baby* and the expression *"something living inside us"*. Sometimes, the woman puts her perception of some movements on the secret side of pregnancy *"I feel it"*, a perception which is hers and which belongs to no one but her, while the ultrasound image belongs to the objective awareness *"everything is seen"* which passes beyond the limits of the human body's interior and exterior, and which, at the same time, permits others to witness what she perceives. Faced with this technology, the parents are forced to take a position. The majority of them wish to know the sex of the child, but once the secret of the sex has been revealed, what do the parents do with the information? New norms of healthy behavior are establishing themselves little by little. Sometimes, the parents are not in agreement: one wants to know, the other prefers not. In certain circumstances, one or the other learns that he or she would have wished to remain ignorant. Everything happens as if, once the medical forecast has been expressed, the parents consider themselves the revealers of an embarrassing secret or of a piece of information which, in anticipation, they communicate to all or part of their immediate circle. Following the manner in which the parents of the unborn child voluntarily or involuntarily circulate the information, the immediate circle is going to be able to hear or must be discreet. The consensus on this occurrence seems to be that the wish of the parents to know or not to know must be respected, and then to share or respect this information. The majority of parents take into account the knowledge of the sex to prepare only one first name or to buy clothes which considers the announcement of a boy or a girl. Some begin from this point on to speak of the child using the chosen first name.

If ultrasound is an instrument of medical surveillance of pregnancy used by doctors to know the state of the fetus and detect malformations, it is similarly expected by the families to reply to their own questions such as the size of the fetus and its sex. This concern is a subject on which no taboo exists because it has always been the object of speculation during pregnancy.

Undoubtedly, the acceptance of the ultrasound scan by families is reinforced. In passing beyond medical objectives and launching into "predicting" the sex of the fetus, doctors have, in a certain manner, allowed the growth of an ultrasound culture, a manifestation of the medical culture which thus integrates itself into the ensemble of cultural variations present in France. This integration of the ultrasound scan in the preparations for birth has consequences in the development of preparations for birth as for the preparation of naming the infant at the moment of birth.

References

Arnaud V: La Naissance chez les Botel Tobago. In: Koubi J, J Massard-Vincent: Enfants et sociétés d'Asie du Sud-Est. L'Harmattan, Paris 1994

Duden B: L'Invention du fœtus. Descartes, Paris 1996

Dufour R: Femme et enfantement, sagesse dans la culture Inuit. Papyrus, Québec 1988

Fédila P, D Lecourt, JF Mattéi, C Thibault, D Thouvenin, C Sureau: L'embryon humain est-il humain? PUF, Paris 1996

Fellous M: La première image. Nathan, Paris 1991

Héritier F: Masculin/féminin. La pensée de la différence. Odile Jacob, Paris 1996

Laurent S: Naître au moyen âge de la conception à la naissance: la grossesse et l'accouchement (XIIe–XVe siècle), Édition Le léopard d'or, Paris 1989

Le Grand-Sébille C, MF Morel, C Zonabend: Le foetus, le nourrisson, la mort. L'Harmattan, Paris 1998

Loux F: Traditions et soins d'aujourd'hui. Inter Editions, Paris 1990
Mead M: L'un et l'autre sexe. Denoël/Gonthier, Paris 1948
Norvez A: De la naissance à l'école. Santé, modes de garde et préscolarité dans la France contemporaine. INED, Paris 1990
Pancino C: Les "envies" de la femme enceinte: une croyance entre culture savante et populaire. Ethnologie française XXVII (2) (1997) 154–162
Potekov T, M Titran: Vies de familles, un autre regard sur l'exclusion. Gallimard, Paris 1996
Ravololomanga B: Pour la santé et la beauté de l'enfant à naitre (Tanala, Madagascar). In: Lallemand S, O Journet, E Ewombe-Moundo, B Ravololomanga, A Dupuis, M Cros, D Jonckers: Grossesse et petite enfance en Afrique noire et à Madagascar. L'Harmattan, Paris 1991
Sélim M: Travail, distance sociale, résidence. Terrain 3 (1984) 5–19
Tillard B: Maternité chez les femmes de moins de vingt ans. Nord-Pas-de-Calais, Lille 1997
Tillard B: Des Familles face à la naissance. L'Harmattan, Paris 2002

25. Physiological pain, pathological pain, iatrogenic pain: The quality of pain and women's experience

Giovanna Bestetti; Faculty of Medicine, University of Milan and Milan-Bicocca, Italy
Anita Regalia; Gynaecology and Obstetrics Clinic, S. Gerardo; Hospital, University of Milan-Bicocca, Italy

During the late 1970s, the most important industrialized countries of the world witnessed not only the social and cultural debate on the equality of the sexes take root, but also the propagation of the necessity of eliminating the pain of childbirth. Childbirth pain is identified as an independent and negative variable of the experience of childbirth that relegated women to a subaltern role and subjugates them to nature, preventing them from taking control of their own body. It is during these years that the use of epidural analgesia became widespread in every hospital and is posited as one of the emancipator rights won by women. During the same years, various groups of operators (midwifes in particular), who demonstrated great awareness in relation to the de-medicalization of childbirth, focussed on the problem of pain during childbirth, in attempt to identify non-pharmacological methods capable of eliminating this component from the experience of childbirth (the first of these methods can obviously be identified with the antenatal classes that expectant mothers attend in preparation for childbirth, Simkin, 1989). During the late 1990s, open-minded operators tried to draw up lists of options where all the advantages and disadvantages of every alternative offered to women were discussed and organized on the basis of a scale which went from less invasive alternatives to epidural analgesia (in some cases/examples, the most invasive scale is represented by cesarean section, Department of Health, 1993; NHMRC, 1996). This way, women, in their effort to alleviate/eliminate the pain of childbirth, could exercise their right to an 'informed choice'. If we carry out a critical analysis of culture that currently characterizes obstetrics, we summarized that the debate on the pain of childbirth is essentially underpinned by two principles, which are interpreted differently according to whether the person accepts or rejects the idea of medicalization. In spite of this, these principles are basically very similar:

1) Pain during childbirth is defined in biological terms as a reaction to tissue damage; the subjective variation of the perception of pain is acknowledged as a complex phenomenon, and is essentially correlated to the woman's psychological state and her history, irrespective of the conditions of the delivery and the context of assistance;

2) The main goal of the various obstetric alternatives is always the elimination of pain. What differentiates the various options is the degree of medicalization involved by the recommended method.

Contrary to this view, we think it might be useful not to approach pain of childbirth as a uniquely biological entity, the perception of which essentially varies according to women's subjectivity. We think it is important to face the problem also from the perspective of the assistance offered to women, and distinguish pain of a physiologically spontaneous labor from that of a pathological one. At the same time, we think it is necessary to acknowledge the iatrogenic components of pain so that we can, if not eliminate them completely, at least contain them. As a consequence, it becomes fundamental to emphasize the variables of assistance, which very often are not mentioned or are kept in the background.

During a physiological labor, pain is a component which participates in the construction/definition of the normality of childbirth and characterizes it as an intense psycho-affective experience (McCrea et al., 2000). If the woman is in good health and is effectively assisted and if the fetus is in the correct position and its dimensions are proportionate to the birth canal, there is no point in trying to eliminate the pain of childbirth. In fact, this pain assumes a form that enables women to draw directly from their internal resources in order to endure it, but it also becomes functional to the eutocia itself, as it activates a harmonic neurohormonal fall, which determines a good contractile activity and a normal descent of the fetus in the birth canal.

On the other hand, in some pathological deliveries, pain can work as an obstacle against the eutocia of birth, activating an anomalous incretion of adrenaline and prostaglandin. In these cases, it might be useful to alleviate or eliminate it. On the basis of our experience and the scholarly works published on the subject, we have drawn up a list distinguishing between maternal conditions and conditions connected to labor (Epidural guidelines Monza, 2005).

Maternal pathology:
- Pregnancy induced Hypertension – preeclampsia
- Respiratory pathology (asthma)
- Cardiac pathology (valvulopathology, primary pulmonary hypertension)
- Endocrine pathology (pre-gestational diabetes with low compensation)
- Psychiatric pathology (psychosis responding to medical treatment)
- Vaginismus

Pathology of labour (*it is essential to explain to women that the conditions below could be a symptom of a mechanical dystocia and as a consequence, recourse to epidural analgesia cannot exclude the necessity of a cesarean section)*
Latent phase
- Prolonged latent phase (>24 hours)

Active phase

- Spontaneous hyperkinesis, which cannot be corrected by resorting to relaxation procedures (i.e., water) in the absence of a strong suspicion of feto-pelvic disproportion (FPD) or of a clear absence of fetal engagement.
- Diskinetic labor, which cannot be corrected by resorting to relaxation procedures in the absence of a strong suspicion of FPD or of a clear absence of fetal engagement.
- Hyperkinetic response to low dosage of oxytocin in the absence of a strong suspicion of FPD.
- Necessity of prolonging the use of oxytocin because of marked slowing of labor progression in situations where the prognosis for a vaginal delivery seems positive.
- Presence of unfavorable cervical conditions such as consistency and dilatation, which can be summarized with the expression "cervical dystocia" and which could lead to a cesarean section.
- Labor during which the woman appears intolerant and completely withdrawn, rejecting all forms of support. This might lead operators to question her psychological wellbeing, eventually leading to a cesarean section.

Finally, iatrogenic pain refers to the fact that, as demonstrated by our practical experience in the delivery room and various formal researches on the subject, some obstetric procedures clearly increase the pain felt by women. Their use must therefore be attentively evaluated, as it has important consequences for the mother and the infant, and determines a disharmony in the fall of neurohormons such as adrenaline, oxytocin and prostaglandin, increasing the probability of a cesarean section.

Which are these procedures, and how do women talk about them in relation to their experience of pain? (The quotes of the women are taken from a large sample which includes approximately 1000 interviews, collected over five years by Dr. Bestetti and her team in order to investigate how childbirth is experienced and remembered, in particular in relation to pain, expectations, clinical course and assistance modalities, deduced, whenever possible, from case sheets and medical records). These include the induction of labor, its augmentation through the use of oxytocin, limitation of movement, multiple examinations often performed by more than one operator, manual dilatation, Kristeller's maneuver and episiotomy. Delivery rooms where the stated goal is the safety of the mother and her child cannot avoid taking into serious consideration the fact that obstetric procedures, albeit useful, substantially differ in reality. For example, it was demonstrated that labor is usefully induced in approximately 10% of cases, while in most Italian hospitals it is induced in 20–25% of cases; oxytocin, which is useful to augment labor, should not be used in more than 15% of labors, but, on average, it is used in 30% of cases.

In their accounts, women describe in detail how, when *"induction begins"* or *"they are put on a drip"*, pain very quickly assumes an unbearable connotation, which is often worsened by the restraint of movement that follows because of the application of cardiotocography: *"contractions were not very strong and they induced labor another time; then contractions began to become more frequent and stronger ... I was breathless, because it really ... was exhausting ... really, one after the other, without a break! And I was there with the monitor, I had to stay still, otherwise they would lose the heartbeat, it was impossible..."*

"They gave me oxytocin ... and all the things I learned during antenatal classes I ... didn't do any of them! Neither the breathing, nor the concentration, nothing ... because when you are there, as I said, they inject this substance into your veins and this terrible pain begins ... and then, one contraction immediately follows the next ... I just said "stop! I want a cesarean section!" ... it was madness ..."

Every woman should be free to move as she wants during labor, while in 65% of Italian delivery rooms (ISS data, 2002) they are not allowed to choose their position, despite the fact that it is precisely this forced position which makes it much harder to bear the pain and concentrate on the expulsive effort of delivery: *"Lying down made me feel a lot of pain, ... I could not lie down because I was writhing like mad. For me the only bearable position was standing up, rocking back and forth, as the midwife of the previous shift had let me do ...."*

"I could not stand it any more, at the end, when I was on the bed... I couldn't stand it anymore ... I would say: "that's enough, pull her out!" The only way I could feel a bit better was to scream. During our classes they had told us we could assume the position we wanted ... the best position that could help us bear the pain. So I ... was there, leaning with by forearms onto the bed, like that, on my feet, with my forearms resting on the bed in order to push. But then an midwife entered the room and told me: 'No! you can't stay like this. That position doesn't lead to anything, lie down!'".

Another aspect worth considering is that, during labor, often more than one operator visits the patient approximately every 1–2 hours in the active phase. This is in contrast to the guidelines given by the WHO indicating four hours as an acceptable intervention time at this stage. Vaginal explorations are described by women as very unpleasant moments, which add "further" pain: *"I don't believe those people who say that it is the most beautiful day of their lives ... it is a painful, unpleasant, uncomfortable, embarrassing moment ... sometimes a hundred people visit you, you lose all sense of privacy, you feel as if you are an object, there for everybody to examine"*

"One of the craziest moments were the examinations... they were always there, rummaging ... it seemed endless".

Manual dilatation too, which should happen only in emergency cases when dilatation is almost complete in a multipara, is practised in 5–6% of cases in some hospitals: *"Every time he examined me he would say, 'now I'll help you a little bit'; yes, he helped ... but it was a terrible pain, I felt as if someone was slaughtering me ...."*

When its use is accepted, even Kristeller's manoeuvre (which in any case should be practiced in no more than 3–4% of expulsive periods), becomes standard procedure in many delivery rooms. This too, as other painful procedures, is often presented as a form of "help" to the woman who, despite the pain, accepts it as a necessary procedure to give birth to her child and, often enough, as a sign of her inadequacy in pushing: *"he would press me with God knows what kind of strength ... high up on my stomach, a terrible pain ... I felt I was dying, as if I was being slaughtered, without breath, but it was helpful, because I couldn't do it on my own, I was pushing the wrong way. Without him he would have never been delivered ... "* and when Kristeller's maneuver is associated with the use of a vacuum extractor, the pain is said to be particularly intense, even when, as in this case, the woman has had an epidural:

"One was pressing and the other, with the vacuum extractor, tried to pull him out ... an amazing pain...his little head was always there, halfway, half inside, half outside ... That is the unhappiest memory ... without doubt it's the unbearable pain I felt."

Episiotomy rate should not be greater than 10–15%, whereas in Italy "the little cut" is practiced in 60–70% of cases. Even this procedure, whose entity and pain is minimized by operators, is nonetheless defined as painful both during antenatal classes and in specialized magazines for expectant mothers. Yet, it is perceived as "necessary" and unavoidable: *"In order not to make you tear and bring about a prolapse they have to cut, and so they cut me ... you know, they do that without anesthesia, because they say that when everything is tense you can't feel a thing ... but I felt scissors cutting something thick ... I felt 'snap', as if they were using poultry shears, and I went "ouch!" ... They cut me, and I felt pain, but perhaps I was just nervous and couldn't stand it any longer".* Episiorrhaphy, too, is a procedure which most women describe as particularly painful, most of the time because of inadequate analgesia. Yet, most operators do not think the pain of episiorrhaphy is worth considering; on the contrary, they ascribe it to a "natural" intolerance of women to be "touched there" after hours of labor. If, according to the operators, the "pain of the stitches" is irrelevant, to the patients this is really a "pain without any reason".

"During labor pain has a reason, but the stitches? No ... it seems just a further pain. Why do you have to feel pain? Why do you have to feel hurt? But stitches ... when the (woman) gynecologist arrived and gave me stitches, I said "Help!", because they used a sort analgesic spray, but I have no idea, it did not have an immediate effect, in any case I don't know whether they gave me enough, but the first stitches ... I felt everything, I mean, I felt the needle going in and coming out ... Everything, a terrible pain, and in fact I said: "but I feel everything" and she went: "no, it's impossible". Actually, during our antenatal

classes they told us that after delivery you can't really stand anything any more. So, although they give you an anesthetic, you think you still feel pain, even if it is not true".

The fact that operators often suggest that the contact with the baby could work as an analgesic (clearly thinking that women could "be distracted" from pain), is clear evidence of their lack of consideration for the reality of pain during suture:

"... they had to give me loads of stitches ..., I had a lateral cut and I asked how many I needed ... they told me they didn't know, that there were too many, and that they had lost count ... and then they told my husband to put the baby on my belly, in order to distract me from pain, but I felt a terrible pain, so I said: "I don't want Francesco now", and my gynecologist "come on, relax, be a good mum", but I didn't want Francesco to feel my tension, I was rigid and I didn't want him there, I didn't even want Sergio to see this because I felt I was making him watch something at the butcher's ...."

Finally, after birth, prolonged contact with the newborn is not always allowed, which contradicts the psychological interpretation of pain often invoked in other contexts, as a form of pain caused by the separation from the newborn.

"As soon as he was delivered, they let me see him, then they took him away, they washed him, measured him, and then left him a little while on my side for me to look at. I wanted to take him in my arms, but they took him away because they said it was better to make sure he was warm enough. I felt very sad, afterwards, I did not expect this, I was there, all alone, on a stretcher, waiting for a bed ... I felt empty and in pain ..."

"... they immediately put him on my tummy, when I didn't even realize he was born, I touched him to make sure he was real, but they immediately told me "he is still dirty, we're going to wash him and then you can cuddle him!', they brought him back half an hour later because there had been lots of deliveries and they were very busy. Then a nurse came in and said "here he is, all nice and clean!'."

Furthermore, we can consider "iatrogenic" factors even the organization of tasks which, in the delivery room, does not ensure a constant support by a member of the hospital staff (a midwife in particular), in a one-on-one relationship with the patient. An appraisal of 50 studies of the Cochrane Library, carried out in 2003 by Hodnett, emphasizes that the constant presence of operators and the support they provide, reduce the request/necessity of medical intervention for pain. In addition, the operators' constant presence reduces the number of operative deliveries, cesarean sections, and women who describe childbirth as a negative experience, while increasing the Apgar score at 5 minutes.

Many women actually suggest that one of the most difficult aspects of coping with the pain of labor was the fact they were left alone: *"it was the most wearing experience of my life, precisely because I didn't know what to do, and nobody would stay there with me ..."*

"in the end, the shift changed, and Federica [the midwife] arrived ... she stayed there with me ... finally I wasn't alone anymore, there was someone I could trust"

When dealing with childbirth, then, it is important to distinguish 'physiological pain' from pathological and iatrogenic pain. When describing their experience of childbirth, women, obviously do not refer to these categories, but if the description of their experience is seen in the light of the clinical course of their labor and the procedures they had to endure, one can identify in their reports a precise relationship between the "type of pain" and the subjective evaluation of the quality of the experience. Women who, during their physiological labor and delivery did not have to endure any invasive procedure, were adequately supported by an midwife, and were allowed to spend some time with their baby from the very first hours after childbirth, very rarely describe the experience of pain in destructive terms and do not wish for any form of analgesia, should they have to go through the same thing again. On the other hand, it is more likely that women who were subjected to painful and invasive procedures, or women whose labor and delivery took a pathological course, experienced pain in a negative and de-structured way.

But how do women talk about the pain of childbirth? When you ask them to define and describe it, the beginning is often uncertain, *"well ... it's difficult."*, but then their description turns into a short narrative of an experience characterized by its uniqueness: pain is not described in itself, but in relation to the way women experience it. Very few women (approximately 10%) define pain in childbirth by comparing it to other kinds of pain, with the exception of menstrual pain or, for those who have experienced it, renal colic. From our reports, the pain of childbirth stands out as different from any other form of pain, it cannot be compared to other kinds of pain and even its localization (which, after all, should be easily defined), is only rarely invented.

The pain of childbirth is described as:

- An indescribable pain, *"You can't really describe it, you can only feel it" "it's too strong, and so personal that you can't describe it, you have to experience it" inexpressible, without equal.*
- A pain *"with a purpose"*, *"which has a meaning"*, not only because it leads to the birth of a baby – you can have this even without pain – but mainly because it shows that during childbirth, pain works as a signal and a guide *"it makes you feel what is going on, the stage you have reached"*, but it does not act as a "warning", pointing to a pathological condition of danger.
- It is a pain which belongs *"It's a pain that is born inside you but that you can't control; at times you go along with it, at times you resist it; sometimes you think you can take it, at other times you are overwhelmed by it. The conclusion is a real miracle"*.
- An extremely strong pain *"it's an extremely strong pain that leaves you breathless, but that afterwards makes you feel you have accomplished an impossible task"*.

- A pain which leads to knowledge and awareness, because it encourages the emergence of aspects of the subject that the subject herself did not know before *"it all seemed impossible, but at the same time it made me realize I had incredible resources. It's an experience which brings out totally unexpected and uncontrollable instincts." "it's easy, really, but it's worth it, and afterwards you feel brilliant, stronger". "It really makes you perceive your real limits; when you say 'I can't take this any longer', you are actually telling the truth, you don't just say those words for the sake of saying something...but then you carry on and you make it, which of course astonishes and surprises you".*
- A pain that brings together opposites: *"… with every contraction, you say 'I can't take it anymore', and, at the same time, 'I've made it, this one has gone as well" "... It makes you feel lost and strong at the same time" "you feel strong and powerful, precisely when you are at the highest of your impotency, and you feel that, in order to be there ... you can't do anything else but surrender and let yourself be carried away ... and then you realize that this incredibly strong wave which seems to come from the outside and that seems to sweep you away, in reality comes from the inside and carries you away." "It's indescribable and cannot be compared to any other pain, because the joy and the satisfaction it brings turns it into a non-pain".*
- It is a pain that takes the patient to ecstasy and joy *"it's a pain that is born from deep inside, occasionally unbearable ... that makes you reach a state of utter grace and great joy" "It brings you closer to a state of joy never experienced before" "it's a gratifying pain, too immense to explain".*
- It is a pain which can be compared to natural forces: *"An uncontrollable tornado which arrives, strikes, and disappears" "it's an eruption of great exertion, with a final flow of joy and peace". "An extremely high wave that arrives, you see it coming, slowly, and you hear it, until it gets you and you have to ride it, otherwise it gets you down and panic kicks in. And then the very last wave arrives, the highest, when you lack both breath and strength, it seems impossible to overcome it. But then she/he is born...that's it, there's a calm sea and a blue sky. And on the waves which now rock you, almost as a miracle, there are two of you resting, close to each other."*

But pain is also defined as:
- *"destructive"," inhuman", "tearing", "excruciating",*
- *"violent", "intolerable", "terrible"," exhausting",*
- *"unfair" "unacceptable in year 2000",*
- *"horrible", "meaningless", "atrocious",*
- *"that makes you experience negatively what should be the most beautiful moment of your life",*
- *"that fortunately you forget",*
- *"that can make you hate your child"*

How can we explain this difference? Is it the woman's history? Is it her psychological "strength" and "stability"? Does it depend on the mode of assistance? And to what extent does it depend on one thing or another? Those women who have experienced physiological labor and delivery, and who have been well assisted throughout the process (just like some women who, despite a non-physiological condition, have felt supported and assisted, and were therefore able to experience childbirth with great awareness, actively participating in it – for example, situations in which the midwife has been careful to position the cardiotocograph in such a way as to allow the analgesic postures), describe the experience of pain in positive terms, as an intrinsic component to the process of childbirth, which has its own meaning. Conversely, women who without any real indication in this sense, during labor and delivery, have been subjected to painful and/or invasive procedures, and who were neither supported nor encouraged, often report an unbearable, destructive and useless pain.

It is interesting to observe that women who have experienced childbirth within the boundaries of physiology (or who have in any case been supported while facing occasional difficulties), use narrative modalities that express their perception of themselves as competent subjects, as "mothers who know how to give birth" when describing their experience. For example, they use active verbs and describe pain in an articulate way, with modalities that indicate not only its intensity but also its dimension of "usefulness" and "meaningfulness". As such, pain is perceived as a guide in the search for analgesic positions, as a signal which indicates the proximity of labor and childbirth, as a bearable dimension, even in its seemingly "unbearable-ness", and as an experience that leads to a higher awareness of the Self. Conversely, women who feel they have been 'subjected', without sufficient reason, to modalities and procedures which, in spite of being considered unavoidable and necessary but lead to the impression they were unable to give birth, express themselves very differently. The narrative modalities these women use are characterized by an almost all-pervasive use of the passive form, by ascribing of the positive outcome of the delivery to the operators' intervention and, on the other hand, by the attribution of the moments of difficulty (as if they coincided with an actual fault) to themselves: *"as I wouldn't dilate, they put me on a drip" "they helped my child come into the world, thank God ... I couldn't push, so they cut me and they pushed ... so that my son was born!"*

It is, however, worth mentioning that in relation to the experience of pain in childbirth, the divide is not between purely physiological situations and situations where some intervention is necessary in order to 'correct' possible disharmonies. Indeed, the distinction is between clinical attitudes and forms of behavior which define "in advance" the necessity of "correcting" the spontaneous course of labor and childbirth, and clinical conduct which justifies intervention only in situations of documented deviation from physiology.

In fact, if the value of physiology is acknowledged, even if during labor there is a need for more intensive monitoring or for augmentation, every effort is made to support the woman in every way, helping her to perceive herself as an active subject and not as an object from which a child can be extracted: *"At a certain point, he began to give signals that he wanted to come out more quickly, his heartbeat was slowing down ... so the midwife and the (woman) doctor explained to me they had to put me on a drip in order to accelerate labor and monitor me closely to check everything was ok. The pain was much more intense, but the midwife tried to make me walk anyway ...she hung the drip to a thing with wheels, so that I could move. During delivery, he couldn't take it any longer, so the midwife called the doctor who told me 'now we push together, so that we help him come into the world more quickly!' So we pushed together and after a couple of minutes he was born! It was really good team work...yes, a terrible pain, but in the end, I was happy we'd managed it!"*

Another aspect worth mentioning relates to those communicative modalities and styles that operators assume and that can work against a positive perception of childbirth. In the first instance, operators might disconfirm the sensations that women report, something which can be very disorienting and which can determine, irrespective of the intensity of pain, a lived experience of fear and solitude:

"I was in terrible pain, and she [the midwife], kept saying 'it's impossible! I saw you half an hour ago, you are at the beginning, you can't feel pain. Sleep now! And so, I curled up under the blanket and wept in silence. That was the worst. I felt alone, and I felt really scared ..."

Even the operators' judgments which refer to stereotypes and prejudices related to modalities of expression of pain, can hurt and render this experience negative:

"With me she was nice, of course, professional, but cold, she didn't really talk to me. Then I heard her saying 'that one is a real pain ... she is a teacher!'"

The midwife kept saying "Stop making all this fuss! Where do you think you are? Stop screaming, you're just wasting your energy! This is not right. You are not getting anywhere! – and I felt more and more useless, then she would try to be nice 'Come on dear, push, come on ...', but, immediately afterwards – 'oh, come on, you can't call that a push!"

"During antenatal classes they told us we could bring our mat, so that we could stay on the floor, if we wanted, because they were not equipped for that, so I took it with me. As soon as I stepped into the delivery room, an midwife, who I discovered later was the head of the delivery room, shouted at me: 'Where do you think you're going with that thing, we're not at a camping site, you know!' I suddenly felt an idiot, I felt ridiculous ..."

But even interpretations and impositions can throw a shadow on the experience of childbirth: *"the pain was excruciating, and I was scared of pushing, and she said: 'why can't you let your baby girl go? Why don't you want to let her come out? That's enough! Shut your mouth and push underneath, holding your breath' But really, it's not that I didn't want to; I was in pain, and I couldn't do it. Afterwards I've given all this a lot of thought, and I still wonder what froze me, besides the pain ... I don't know ... when I think about it, it's a gloomy thought ...*"

Even the fear women feel to express pain: *"I wanted to scream, but I didn't give in, I kept everything inside, because I didn't want to embarrass myself, either with doctors, or with my husband, it was very hard, but I managed it and afterwards they complimented me on that. It wasn't easy with that woman screaming right next to me ..."*

Besides the differences in assistance practice, which certainly have a fundamental bearing on the way childbirth is experienced, what other variables determine women's expectations in relation to the pain of childbirth, the way it can be faced and their orientation towards epidural analgesia? It seems important to consider both the way the pain of childbirth is discussed through the media, in magazines for expectant mothers, and during antenatal classes, and what women can tell each other about this experience. This appears to contradict the fact that, in most cases, childbirth takes place in a context where pain is generally experienced negatively, a context which is characterized by a very high rate of medicalization, thus suggesting that childbirth is, in fact, no 'normal' event.

One of the variables which can influence the way a woman approaches the experience of labor, is therefore the way she has heard others talk about the pain of childbirth. Thus, in a period when "pro-epidural campaigns" are all pervasive (in newspapers, on TV, occasionally even during antenatal classes), the pain of childbirth is increasingly compared to other, often very severe, forms of pain. Women have rarely experienced these forms of pain personally, but they certainly imagine them as unbearable and intolerable. It therefore makes sense that the pain of childbirth should be quantified on the basis of "evaluation scales" which place it very close to these other forms of pain.

While seeming a neutral operation, the reduction of an extremely complex experience such as pain by childbirth to a number entails a definition and a representation of the pain of childbirth which does not do justice to its peculiarity. It is precisely this aspect that emerges from the descriptions offered by women who have given birth and who have turned pain into a positive experience. The pain of childbirth, which is established on the basis of quantitative parameters that "neutralize" its peculiarity and underline its intensity, is thus defined as "severe" and compared to other examples of pain, either to terrible and fearsome forms of pain (understood as signs of serious traumatic pathological conditions), or to the better known and prosaic toothache.

In this process, there is perhaps an unconscious manipulative effect that leads to consider analgesia as "normal" and necessary: in fact, this operation cannot but bring about reactions of refusal and fear in women, and therefore little faith in their ability to bear this pain, thereby rendering as "obvious" the necessity of having an effective analgesia such as the epidural. Who could in fact even imagine bearing the simple extraction of a tooth without some form of anesthesia?

We could wonder now why it should not be possible to talk about the pain of childbirth by referring to the words of the women who have experienced it. In addition, we ought to be courageous enough to acknowledge how much the conditions of the environment and the forms of assistance provided determine its definition. After all, even the descriptions of the pain of childbirth as one whose perception depends largely on the woman's attitude, her threshold of pain, her history, her use of accompanying practices (whatever they might be), which seem to promise they will work as some sort of analgesia, may convey a dangerous message which does not help women approach the experience of childbirth in a positive way.

Ascribing the perception of pain solely to the woman (to her preparation and her disposition to perceiving pain) means to assign her a responsibility (fundamentally, a form of guilt) that is out of her competence and that results very little in relation to assistance. In this sense, it might be useful to remember that psycho-prophylaxis has posited too much emphasis on the psychological condition of the woman, to the detriment of the assistance provided, resulting in the negation of the reality of pain. Even today, this attitude is not completely extinguished, and this is dangerous, precisely because it distracts attention from the context and, more fundamentally, because it does not give women the possibility to develop and grow through a positive experience of childbirth.

We cannot actually forget that, as attentive and sensitive operators know very well, many women who appeared "frail" and "in difficulty" during pregnancy, or who actually reported "difficult" psychological stories, thanks to attentive and "majestical" assistance during pregnancy, labor and delivery, were able to reactivate and mobilize unexpected resources at the moment of childbirth.

During pregnancy and childbirth, a physiological process of "regression" takes place, and leads women to experience their own childhood history again, for example, by becoming small again in order to be on the same wavelength with the future baby. When this regression is acknowledged and well assisted, it enables women to heal wounds and fill empty/blank spaces, thus becoming "therapeutic".

The "psychological indications" for the epidural should take these aspects into serious consideration, reflecting on how the choice of the epidural "for psychological fragility", could result in a missed opportunity. (Bergeret–Amselek, 2005; Langer, 1951; Gaskin, 2003; Revault D'Alonnes, 1976; Soifer, 1977; Schmid, 2005) As to the preparation to childbirth, which today is increasingly defined in positive terms as "assistance in childbirth", we must underline the uselessness of offering women any kind of practice (even the "natural", "non-pharmacological" and soft ones), with the promise that, if correctly applied, they will have an analgesic effect. Any kind of practice which is offered with this promise, and that has to be learnt through specific training and repetitive exercises, creates in women the idea that labor and delivery coincide with a sort of "examination" during which the reduction of pain a person might or might not obtain, assumes the meaning of a "mark" that confirms the woman's psychological health, or her being a good "student/adept" to the method proposed. Throughout the years, the conclusion was reached that the various corporal practices used during the preparation for childbirth have a positive effect, as far as they help women achieve a higher awareness of their own body and, in a cultural and historical context, characterized by a great insensitivity towards, and ignorance of, the body, enable them to familiarize with it. Yet, these practices are rather negative when they are offered as analgesic procedures, both because they are not analgesic and because they convey the message that the pain of childbirth is actually unbearable (Leap, 2005).

Another fundamental idea for the articulation of a discourse that takes into account the irreducible complexity typical of the pain of childbirth, concerns its definition, its tolerability and its possible treatment. According to the philosopher Salvatore Natoli "it is technique that largely determines the conditions in which human beings can experience pain" and "in contemporary society, science, and technique have the power to change the threshold of pain, thus determining the levels of its perception" (Natoli, 1986). As far as the experience of pain during childbirth is concerned, we cannot but acknowledge that pain is real, which occurred in the field of obstetrics only when a technique (epidural analgesia) has become available. We cannot forget that before that moment the pain of childbirth, as expressed by women, was not judged worth considering. Indeed, it was considered as an "abnormal reaction in comparison to the entity of the stimulus" (Piscicelli, 1977), or a simple "hysterical reaction" which had to be penalized and repressed. Actually, those health institutions such as hospitals and universities which today advocate the epidural for all "civilized" women who want to "give birth in a human way", until a few years ago were renowned for their "philosophy of assistance", characterized by repressive and restrictive attitudes in relation to those women who expressed pain. After all, even today it is still obvious that the definition of pain tolerability does not pertain to the subjectivity of the woman who experiences it, but, as the words quoted below effectively demonstrate, is yet again a prerogative of the operators:

"Anesthesia was only half effective and I felt a lot of pain. Then the doctor told me 'well, at least we got rid of half the pain'. In actual fact, I was very happy I had had an epidural, because I would have never been able to stand the pain in its entirety, it would have been completely intolerable!"

The words of this operator, uttered when it was no longer possible to proceed with analgesia, appear equally relevant:

"Come on, you have had an epidural all this time, for the last ten minutes you could try and collaborate!"

"Pain today is understood as something which can and should be dominated and faced as controllable. Controlling the threshold of pain means making decisions about the modalities one could resort to in order to let it come to the surface or repress it. When we speak of the threshold of pain, we do not refer solely to the quantification of its intensity but also to the locus of its manifestation in general experience" (Natoli, 1986). Even when talking about the pain of childbirth, it is worth considering how, for operators but also for women and their partners, it is pain in itself that is intolerable, and not its various manifestations which, in the particular case of labor and delivery, make clear the insuppressible affective, corporeal, and sensual charge inherent in the experience of childbirth.

A final consideration concerns the importance of the variable "time", which appears central to the choice of epidural analgesia, as it determines the evaluation of pain on the part of both women and operators. First of all, how does the evaluation of the experience of pain in childbirth change throughout time? It is interesting to notice that the reports of women who experience highly medicalized deliveries, characterized by their low relational assistance, tend to define pain in evasive, synthetic, unarticulated ways, focusing on the birth of their child, a moment which "made them forget everything". Conversely, those women who have experienced adequate assistance with low medicalization, talk about pain in a more articulate way, describe labor and delivery itself in detail, with a lot of particulars and the birth of the child is not described as a moment when "everything is forgotten" but rather as a moment when "everything passes".

After all, as it is well known, during labor and delivery most women, finding themselves facing pain, ask for help, and this help can be offered through analgesia or via a much more involving and demanding form of support on the part of a dedicated midwife who guarantees her a one-on-one form of assistance. We cannot forget that this lack of assistance modality does not depend on the lack of staff, but on a personal unwillingness to open oneself to involvement, an aspect which is often ascribed to personal qualities rather than to a specific and necessary professional training. Furthermore, a woman who during labor asks for analgesia actually does not always want the operators to proceed: *"In that moment I felt really bad and I would have accepted anything, even the epidural ... but now I'm happy nobody offered it to me".*

The positive elaboration of the experience of pain in childbirth takes place in time, and not in the immediacy of the moment (Bestetti, Vegetti Finzi, 1999). This is, therefore, that kind of awareness that operators should adopt when they meet a woman who asks for an epidural during either pregnancy or labor. This awareness should lead to articulation of the discourse on the choice of the epidural not in the simplistic terms of the "right to choose freely", acknowledging that this choice is not actually "free" at all, not at least until the same women are offered the possibility of choosing, equally "freely" and "knowingly", any of the procedures analyzed above, which determine in a substantial way the quality of the experience. One should not forget that "every woman discovers the meaning of childbirth always, and only, after giving birth" (Arcidiacono, 1985).

References

Arcidiacono C: Oltre il tabù del dolore: la fatica e il piacere di esistere e far nascere in AAVV Le culture del parto. Feltrinelli, Milano 1985

Bergeret-Amselek C: Il mistero delle madri. U n viaggio nel cuore della materialità. Magi, Roma 2005

Bestetti G, A Boneschi, GV Limonta Grezzi, PA Molina, AL Regalia, L Usuelli: La richiesta di analgesia in travaglio di parto da parte delle donne. In: Abrate, Comitini et al.: (a cura di) Atti del convegno Culture della nascita a confronto. Emilia, Reggio 1996

Bestetti G, S Vegetti Finzi: Riflessioni sul senso del nascere e del mettere al mondo: l'analgesia nel dolore del parto. Nascere 71 (25) (1997)

Department of Health Changing Childbirth (Cumberledge Report). Department of Health HMSO, London 1993

Gaskin IM: La gioia del parto. Bonomi, Pavia 2003

Langer M: Maternità e sesso. Loescher, Torino 1981

Leap N, T Anderson: The role of pain and the empowerment of women. In: Downe S (ed): Normal Childbirth: Evidence and Debate. Churchill Livingstone, Edinburgh 2004

Linee guida analgesia epidurale. Pubblicazione in proprio, Clinica Ostetrica Ginecologica Ospedale S.Gerardo Monza Università degli Studi di Milano Bicocca 2005

McCrea H, M Wright, M Stringer: Psychosocial factors influencing personal control in pain relief. International Journal of Nursing Studies 37 (2000) 493–503

Natoli S: L'esperienza del dolore. Le forme del patire nella cultura occidentale. Feltrinelli, Milano 1986

NHMRC Options for effective care in childbirth. Australian Government Printing Service, Canberra 1996

Piscicelli U: Training autogeno respiratorio e psicoprofilassi ostetrica. Piccin, Padova 1977

Revault D'Alonnes C: Le mal joli. Accouchements et douleur. Plon, Paris 1991

Schmid V: Venire al mondo e dare alla luce. Urra, Milano 2005

Sestetti G: Il dolore del parto: accoglierlo ed elaborarlo o cancellarlo? Nascere 76 (27) 1999

Simkin P: Non-pharmacological methods of pain relief during labour. In: Chalmers I, M Enkin, M Keirse (eds): Effective Care in Pregnancy & Childbirth. Oxford University Press, Oxford 1989

Soifer R: Psicodinamica della gravidanza, parto, puerperio. Borla, Torino 1985

26. Low risk delivery today

Fabio Facchinetti, Giulia Dante, Alba Ricchi, Annibale Volpe;
Unit of Obstetrics, Mother-Infant Department, University
of Modena and Reggio Emilia, Italy

In western societies, the culture of birth is expanding and the delivery itself, the core moment of this process, is seen increasingly more as an experience that has to be faced actively, with the mother, the couple, and the family all playing key roles. The most general categories of the individual cultures are applied to the means of delivery: birth must reflect the convictions, beliefs, and experiences of the protagonists and not limit itself to a biological event delegated to others, in the implicit demand for safety.

It is worth remembering that the outcome of delivery, for both mother and child, is historically linked to unpredictability and associated with individual tragedies that place privileged nobles and poor servants on the same level: not even queens could avoid the risk of dying during delivery. The extraordinary acceleration of medical culture has determined fundamental modifications in obstetric assistance which nowadays is criticized with a demand for a greater balance between technicality and humanization. This paper outlines the contours of the discussion and attempts to propose models of mediation.

Historical evolution of obstetric assistance

Tracing the historical evolution of obstetrics is equivalent to following the development of the scientific and clinical concepts of this branch of medicine. We must therefore discuss modifications of knowledge from the pre-Hippocratic and Hippocratic era onwards.

In the pre-Hippocratic and Hippocratic period (Corpus Ippocraticum), physicians gained their first knowledge on both fetus nutrition through the umbilical cord and the delivery mechanism, but the surgeons of the time, who were called only in cases of a difficult delivery, were barbers and were thus cultureless. The School from Alexandria (III s B.C.) with Herofilus and Herasistratus, favored the use of autopsy on humans and embryos and demonstrated that the concepts of the distocia were dependent on mother and fetus as well as the delivery methods. In ancient Rome, the history of obstetrics began with the so-called Lex Regia, attributed to Numa Pompilio (715 B.C.), who started the post-mortem Cesarean section. Pliny reported that Aurelia, mother of Scipio the African, was subjected to the uterus section (undoubtedly in post-mortem) in order to give birth to the winner of Cartagena.

With the conquest of Greece, Roman medicine benefited from the knowledge of Eastern doctors whose influence predominated until Galen (130 A.D.) who described pregnancy, abortion, and delivery. In the Middle Ages, obstetrics made little progress, mainly due to the advances of Arabic culture (Avicenna), which dominated for six centuries and introduced the forceps for the extraction of the dead fetus. The fundamentals of the Hippocratic School of Galen and Avicenna were also applied in the Salernitan School of the late Middle Ages by Vesalius, who derived his knowledge from Albertus Magnus, bishop of Ratisbona.

Obstetricians began to make progress, despite the fact that even in France until XVIth century, physicians were forbidden to attend deliveries. Nevertheless, in 1663, upon the order of Louis XVI, the French physician Clement assisted the beautiful favorite La Vallière and also Madame de Montespan.

Galileo carried out the first scientific applications and introduced the concept of experiment as the only means of proving and deducing the general law of facts. During the Renaissance, there was no place for the training midwives at University since medicine and surgery were taught only to men; obstetricians often trained from experience alone, becoming the vehicle of beliefs and rituals from one generation to the next.

Illuminism determined a relevant scientific and technological progress: in the XVIIIth century research institutes and the first scientific magazines were founded. This century also marks the implementation of medical specialization in obstetrics: chairs for pupils were created together with the "Schools of minor obstetrics" for the preparation of midwives (women only). These were the years of the heated attack on the part of obstetricians about the inadequacy of men attending pregnancies and physiologic deliveries. Midwives claimed that they had the diagnostic abilities to foresee pathological deliveries and therefore needed to send for the physician or the surgeon only in cases "against nature". However, they often delayed this call and carried out breech extractions and other interventions themselves.

Instrumental delivery (forceps) and soon afterwards the Cesarean section were not immediately accepted, in particular by obstetricians. This added fuel to the debate on "medicalization" intended as an attempt on the part of the "male medical power" to impose on autonomous female culture. From 1761 to 1789, "Schools for midwives" were instituted also in Italy, but the progressive scientific maturation of gynecologists gradually introduced males in attendance to physiologic pregnancy and delivery.

In the XIXth century, medicine became an experimental science based on experience. Moreover, gynecology gained a deeper and recognized cultural base with obstetrics becoming part of it. Gynecology made significant progress in the surgical domain and disease was intended as a "pathology of organ" and not as a "general dyscrasia". The gynecologist became the "doctor and surgeon" of feminine genitalia, while the obstetrician remained in the role of the midwife.

The XXth century is characterized by the rapid social changes for women and by the acceleration of the gynecological science. For a closer analysis of this recent period, the last 50 years can be divided into three phases: "post-war", "post-modern" and "globalization".

The post-war era (1945–1965) saw the acquisition of fundamental knowledge on the pathophysiology of pregnancy and delivery, the birth event was moved to the hospital and determined the institution of neonatal medicine units. At the same time, the gynecologist became the "caregiver" for pregnancy and delivery, hygiene and physiology. Delivery rooms followed more and more rigorous hygienic standards matching the appeal and coldness of the surgery rooms. In contrast, delivery rooms were developed with multiple beds, without any care for intimacy; there was a wide use of drugs (analgesic substances, oxytocin) and instrumental deliveries (forceps, vacuum). In these twenty years, however, perinatal mortality rates dropped to levels close to incompressibility throughout Western Europe; the reduction of maternal mortality rates was even more drastic.

In the post-modern period, together with the cultural revolution of late 60's, a focus on humanization was developed in contrast to previous medicalization, and subsequently, towards the end of the millennium, the "New Age" era encouraged the concepts of the "natural" way of delivery. In this period alternative birth centers were founded: these were the "Alternative Birth Centers" (ABC) and "Maternity Houses" (Vizzone, 1998).

At present, there is an ongoing critical rethinking in industrialized countries, on delivery management by hospital structures, in an attempt to bring back naturalness and spontaneity, allowing the parturient and her relatives to experience the joy of the event.

Models of alternative birth

Operative models

Alternative birth centers. ABCs spread throughout the United States in the 70's. The project originated from multiple needs: the possibility for the future "low risk" mother to control her delivery in an atmosphere similar to the family environment, together with the future father and other children; at the same time the possibility to adopt all the most updated diagnostic tools and the treatments for potential unforeseen complications during delivery. ABCs are located in the vicinity of Ob/Gyn units of the same hospital. The ABC represents an alternative to home delivery and permitted the return to the involvement of the whole family. The gynecologists of the centers have to impose strict selection criteria for admittance in order to accept only the low risk parturient. The guidelines and protocols for "low-risk deliveries" are considerably rigid, but this pre-selection is not always adequate to prevent all possible obstetrical risk.

Among the most positive features, there is the presence of a “perinatal nurse” who attends to the woman and her family from the moment she enters the institution until she goes home, examining her and her child within 24 hours after the delivery, giving continuous assistance also during the postpartum period. The medical assistance is warm, respectful, quick and, at the same time, not intrusive.

Among the basic criteria for ABC functionality, there must be a quick means in cases of emergency of transferring patients to a traditional unit. The active participation of the couple at an antenatal preparatory course lasting 10–12 weeks and starting around the 22nd week of pregnancy is also compulsory. Antenatal classes are held by midwives, physicians and “psychological managers”, who are part of the staff that the couple may have the chance to meet at delivery.

Delivery takes place with as little intervention as possible. Some centers forbid the use of oxytocin, amniorexis, analgesics and the continuous monitoring of fetal heart rate. This latter control is carried out for at least 10 minutes, about once an hour, and at the second stage, for at least 1 minute after each contraction, every 5 minutes. Gynecological examinations are limited, oxytocin is used only immediately post-partum and any treatment is preliminarily discussed with the patient. She can eat, drink, and meet her family; she can have a mirror to follow the delivery of her child. Among the criticisms that the ABCs received were that they artificially separated a proper familiar atmosphere from scientific safety and rigor. On the other hand, a positive criticism is that if the atmosphere for delivery is correct in the ABCs, every mother should have the right to take advantage of it, albeit at high-risk; the possibility of having a healthy baby by means of a pleasant delivery must be guaranteed to one and all.

The maternity house. This was founded in the Netherlands, as non-hospital structures for delivery, including the periods of pregnancy and postpartum. These houses are often managed only by midwives and are open to women and their families. They represent a place where it is possible to talk about a “social model of birth”, where the woman is the protagonist of the birth, a slow and rhythmical process where emotions and pain, typical feminine merits, are well accepted as the subject of knowledge.

In Italy, “Maternity Houses” were originally only created as projects and proposals, and are seldom active. It is not even known whether Italian women prefer this type of structure, since no research has ever been carried out. Nevertheless, the structure should be close to a high level delivery unit, managed by gynecological staff who are highly competent in perinatology and who are ready to assist the labor “with their hands behind their backs”.

Three main points appear to delineate the definition of a Maternity House: the autonomy of women who chose the structure; the role of the midwife and also the gynecologist who defines the guidelines; the concept of “structure equipped for physiological delivery” while not being classified as a small low-quality hospital. Such ideas have been continuously updated and were modified following the criteria of "evidence based medicine" (Forleo, Forleo, 2006).

Water delivery. In every culture, water has always represented the symbol of the Mother. It is possible that the presence of the midwife and the use of water are two aspects of the same fundamental need. It might be useful to remember that for many women the water method during labor is probably not just a fashion but rather an ancient need, since in many cultures water is associated with birth (Odent, 2000). Moreover, whereas on the one hand, up until a few years ago water birth was considered a rather weird and possibly endangering choice, nowadays water birth has become a frequent event, often privileged for its naturalness and kindness. Delivering with sweetness: a synthetic definition such as this, summarizes the advantages that future mothers are offered by this possibility.

Leboyer and Odent were pioneers of the water birth method and demonstrated the benefits of that "sweet partum" in a study they carried out in 1983. Water, with its relaxing effect on the whole body, is supposed to help the woman to better cope with contraction pains, setting her at a correct distance from them and freeing her mind (Odent, 1983). Nevertheless, a water delivery is limited to pregnancy at term, since the natural "diving reflex" matures in the last week of intrauterine life. Therefore it is necessary for this reflex to be present since it allows the baby to avoid water inhalation (Cluett et al., 2004).

Results

A large sample size is needed to be able to analyze the effectiveness of interventions in cases of extremely rare events; such a sample is often difficult to collect, even by means of multi-centre studies. Indeed, to evaluate a 20% difference in perinatal mortality between home-like and conventional institutional birth in a low-risk population, a sample size of 704,000 cases would be needed (Lilford, 1987). Therefore, the scientific data available comes from observational studies taken from articles published from the mid 1990's onwards, and which do not include any research carried out in under-developed countries, where social and economical conditions are very different from our own reality.

A meta-analysis of six controlled observational studies was conducted, and the perinatal outcomes of 24,092 selected and primarily low-risk pregnant women were analyzed to measure mortality and morbidity, including Apgar scores, maternal lacerations, and intervention rates. Perinatal mortality was not significantly different in the two groups. The main difference in the outcome was a lower frequency of low Apgar scores and severe lacerations in the home-like vs conventional birth (Olsen, 1997).

In the Netherlands a cross-sectional study was performed using Dutch national perinatal registries of the year 2000. In all age groups, the planned home birth percentage in primiparous women was lower than in multiparous women (23.5% vs. 42.8%). Dutch and non-Dutch women showed practically similar percentages of obstetrician-supervised hospital births but large differences in percentages of planned home births (36.5% vs 17.3%). Fewer home births were observed in large cities (30.5%) as compared with small towns (35.7%) and rural areas (35.8%) (Anthony et al., 2005).

In Norway, a prospective study reported the short-term outcome for mothers and newborns of all pregnancies accepted for birth in maternity houses. The study included 1275 women who started labor in the maternity houses, around 1% of all births in Norway during this period. Of those, 1217 (95.5%) also delivered there whereas 58 (4.5%) women had to be transferred to hospital. In the postpartum period there were a further 57 (4.7%) transfers of mother and baby. Nine women had undergone a vacuum extraction, one delivery with forceps, and three had had a vaginal breech. Five babies (0.4%) had an Apgar score below 7 at 5 minutes. There were two (0.2%) neonatal deaths; both babies were born with a serious group B streptococcal infection (Schmidt, Abelsen, 2002).

Thirty-four studies were included in a systematic review evaluating clinical, psychosocial, and economical outcomes of women planning to deliver in Maternity Houses in northern countries. Data mainly derived from small observational and poor quality studies, with a high probability of positive or negative bias. These limitations, making impossible any comparison between results from the different studies, also prevented determination of any benefits or risks associated with home-like delivery versus conventional assistance. The systematic review highlighted the need for new evaluation studies (Stewart et al., 2004).

Finally, there is only one systematic review including all randomized or quasi-randomized controlled trials that compared the effects of a home-like institutional birth environment to conventional hospital care. Six trials involving 8677 women are included. Between 29% and 67% of women allocated to home-like settings were transferred to standard care before or during labor.

However, no firm conclusions could be drawn regarding the effects of staffing or organizational models. When compared to conventional institutional settings, home-like environments for childbirth are associated with modest benefits, including reduced medical intervention and increased maternal satisfaction. Caregivers and clients should be vigilant for signs of complications. The main findings of the review are listed in Table 1 (Hodnett et al., 2005).

As far as water delivery is concerned, many studies have been carried out albeit involving very few subjects. In a randomized English trial, 99 low risk nulliparous women were considered. Women were divided into two groups: 49 were allocated to labor in water using the pool, and a second group of 50 were allocated to standard care. About half of the women belonging to the first group needed epidural analgesia in comparison to two thirds of the second group. Those who adopted the labor in water method needed in general less medical intervention to facilitate contractions and reported that they felt calmer and safer. The study also highlighted the fact that primiparas need less analgesia if subjected to labor in water and a reduced need for epidural analgesia. These results also show that women may receive some benefits from labor in water, without necessarily applying the delivery in water (Cluett et al., 2004).

Some researchers, however, are worried about the fact that a water birth may represent a risk for the baby. Indeed, a case of respiratory distress consequent to water delivery was reported. Although such events seem uncommon, this may also be the result of under-reporting. A full term male infant weighing 3150 g was born in the birthing pool to a 34 year old, healthy primigravida who went into spontaneous labor at term. The baby was born underwater and required no resuscitation. At one hour, he was grunting and then admitted to the neonatal intensive care unit, in need for supplementary oxygen for nine hours to maintain saturation level at ≥92. He was screened for infection and started on antibiotics. In view of his persisting respiratory distress he was designated "nil by mouth". Chest radiography soon after admission showed widespread changes consistent with aspiration of the birthing pool water. Further radiography on day 3, showed a resolution of the abnormalities. The infant made a full recovery. This study confirmed that immersion during labor is associated with significant reductions in the use of analgesia and in women's reports of pain, but highlighted the fact that both practitioners and parents need to be aware of these potential risks so that mothers can make a fully informed decision about the place of delivery (Kassim et al., 2005).

Table 1 Results of the study "Home-like vs hospital".

Item	Relative risk	95% Confidence interval
No intrapartum analgesia/anaesthesia	1.19	1.01–1.40
Spontaneous vaginal birth	1.03	1.01–1.06
Vaginal/perineal tears	1.08	1.03–1.13
Preference for the same setting the next time	1.81	1.65–1.98
Satisfaction with intrapartum care	1.14	1.07–1.21
Breastfeeding initiation	1.06	1.02–1.09
Breastfeeding continuation six to eight weeks	1.06	1.02–1.10
Perinatal mortality	1.83	0.99–3.38
Episiotomy	0.85	0.74–0.99

Conclusions

Both maternal and child mortality has drastically diminished since 1950. Such a phenomenon has been observed in all developed countries including Italy. The perinatal mortality rate in Italy fell from 46.6/1000 live born in 1955 to 10.1 in 1990. In terms of indexes, considering 100 as the value of year 1955, that of year 1990 dropped by about 80% to 21.8, (ISTAT, 1955 ff.). The data showed that for every 5 perinatal deaths recorded in 1955 there was only one case in 1990.

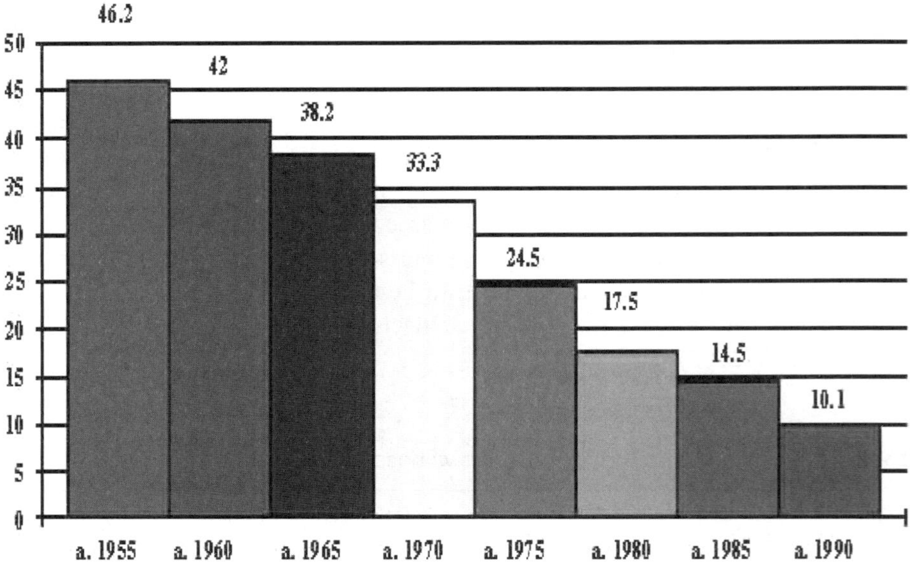

Figure 1 Perinatal mortality, 1955–1990.

At the same time, the reduction in maternal mortality was even more significant. The reasons for such a drop must be attributed primarily to the overall improvement in life conditions and also to the phenomena of *medicine socialization* and *medicine technology* (Consiglio Sanitario Nazionale, 1988). These attitudes have led to advancement in health for everyone and to the evolution from empiricism to the clinical, diagnostic, and therapeutic accuracy, respectively. It is therefore clear that the concept of risk in obstetrics, intended as anything that might happen with complications for the mother and/or the baby, has rapidly evolved, not only among the operators (Kloosterman et al., 1987).

The society of technology and information in which we are living has conditioned common thoughts and deeply changed family expectations, even with respect to a few decades ago. If health is a right (as indeed it is) and pregnancy

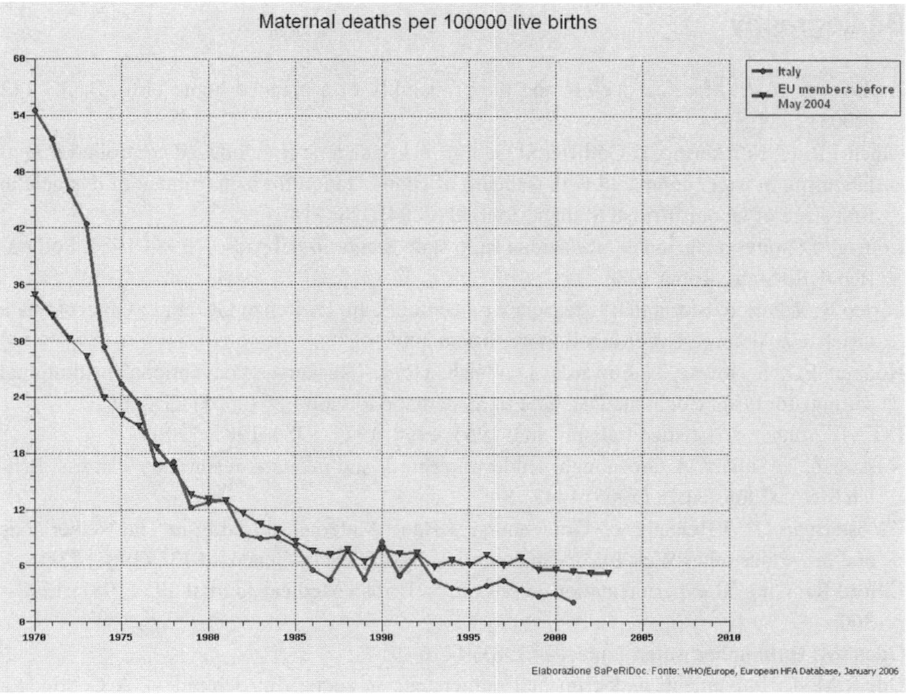

Figure 2 Maternal mortality in Italy and in Europe per 100,000 live births.

is a natural event (as indeed it is), everybody expects healthy and lovely babies to be born from complication-free deliveries. Satisfying the increased need for naturalness in the birth event and the legitimate reduction (absence) of medicalization is still a difficult challenge, considering the minimum or barely absent acceptance of complications.

Among the above mentioned alternative birth models, the home-like version with de-medicalized assistance, if active in an institutional hospital unit, seems to be associated with a good quality/safety ratio. However, every birth center has to choose its most appropriate model, depending upon organizational features on the one hand, and on the specific social and cultural conditions of the afferent population on the other. To reach this objective, it is important to stimulate the training aspect too: it is necessary (at least in the Italian situation) that midwives, the center of this kind of initiative, receive specific training both on cultural and relational aspects as well as on operative ones. This will spread the culture of institutionalized low-risk delivery and promote the activation of home-like delivery in several social contexts.

Bibliography

Anthony S et al.: Maternal factors and the probability of a planned home birth. BJOG 112 (2005) 748–53

Cluett ER, RM Pickering, K Getliffe, St George, NJ Saunders: Randomized controlled trial of labouring in water compared with standard of augmentation for management of dystocia in first stage of labour. British Medical Journal (2004) 328: 314

Consiglio Sanitario Nazionale: Relazione sullo stato Sanitario del paese – 1984/1986. Poligrafico dello Stato, Roma 1988

Forleo R, P Forleo: Storia dell'ostetricia e ginecologia. In: Di Renzo GC et al.: Ginecologia e Ostetricia, Volume 1. Verduci Editore, Roma 2006

Hodnett ED, S Downe, N Edwards, D Walsh: Home-like versus conventional institutional settings for birth. Cochrane Database of Systematic Reviews 25 (2005) CD000012

ISTAT: Annuario Statistico Italiano, anni 1955, 1960, 1975, 1980, 1985, 1990

Kassim Z, M Sellars, A Greenough: Underwater birth and neonatal respiratory distress. British Medical Journal 18 (2005) 1447–8

Kloosterman GJ, J Bennebroek Gravenhorst, J Bout: Maternal mortality in The Netherlands and in various other West European countries. Ned Tijdschr Geneeskd 131 (1987) 2380–1

Lilford RJ: Clinical experimentation in obstetrics. British Medical Journal 295 (1987) 1298–300

Odent M: Birth under water. Lancet 2 (1983) 1476–7

Odent M: I cambiamenti endocrini nell'immersione in acqua. In: Schmid V, A Contin: La casa Maternità. Atti del convegno 14-15-16 aprile 2000. Editeam s.a.s., Napoli 2000

Olsen O: Meta-analysis of the safety of home birth. Birth 24 (1997) 4–13

Schmidt N, B Abelsen, P Øian: Deliveries in maternity homes in Norway: results from a 2-year prospective study. Acta Obstetricia et Gynecologica Scandinavica 81 (2002) 731

Stewart M et al.: Birth centre review. National Perinatal Epidemiology Unit, Oxford, 2004

Vizzone A: Quando l'anomalia era segno dell'espiazione di una colpa. Artemisia News 1 (1998) 5–6